FALSE HOPE

FALSE HOPE

Bone Marrow Transplantation for Breast Cancer

Richard A. Rettig

Peter D. Jacobson

Cynthia M. Farquhar

Wade M. Aubry

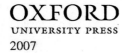
UNIVERSITY PRESS
2007

OXFORD

UNIVERSITY PRESS

Oxford University Press, Inc., publishes works that further
Oxford University's objective of excellence
in research, scholarship, and education.

Oxford New York
Auckland Cape Town Dar es Salaam Hong Kong Karachi
Kuala Lumpur Madrid Melbourne Mexico City Nairobi
New Delhi Shanghai Taipei Toronto

With offices in
Argentina Austria Brazil Chile Czech Republic France Greece
Guatemala Hungary Italy Japan Poland Portugal Singapore
South Korea Switzerland Thailand Turkey Ukraine Vietnam

Published by Oxford University Press, Inc.
198 Madison Avenue, New York, New York 10016

www.oup.com

Oxford is a registered trademark of Oxford University Press

Library of Congress Cataloging-in-Publication Data
False hope: bone marrow transplantation for breast cancer / Richard A. Rettig ... [et al.].
      p. ; cm.
   Includes bibliographical references and index.
   ISBN-13: 978-0-19-518776-2
   ISBN-10: 0-19-518776-8
   1. Breast—Cancer—Chemotherapy—United States—History. 2. Bone marrow—Transplantation—
United States—History. 3. Autotransplantation—United States—History. 4. Breast—Cancer—Chemotherapy—
Complications. 5. Bone marrow—Transplantation—Complications. 6. Autotransplantation—Complications.
   [DNLM: 1. Breast Neoplasms—history—United States. 2. Breast Neoplasms—therapy—United States.
3. Antineoplastic Combined Chemotherapy Protocols—history—United States. 4. Bone Marrow Transplantation—
history—United States. 5. Combined Modality Therapy—history—United States. 6. History, 20th Century—
United States. 7. Transplantation, Autologous—history—United States. WP 11 AA1 F197 2006]
   I. Rettig, Richard A.
   RC280.B8F353 2006
   616.99′449061—dc22

                                                                                                    2005037781

9 8 7 6 5 4 3 2 1
Printed in the United States of America
on acid-free paper

*To all women and their families faced with breast cancer
and to the continuing search for more effective treatments*

Acknowledgments

We owe an immense debt of gratitude to many individuals and regret our inability to thank them more than we do here. We thank I. Craig Henderson for help in understanding the clinical issues and for placing them in a larger context of both oncology and policy. We thank the many other clinical researchers we acknowledge as interviewees or whose papers we cite. We thank William P. Peters for a gracious interview toward the end of our research.

We thank the many women, some of whom we cite in the text, for helping us understand the women's health and breast cancer patient advocacy movements. It is difficult to know how many books remain to be written to describe and interpret these important phenomena. We especially thank Amy Langer for several extended interviews and for access to the files of the National Association of Breast Cancer Organizations. Three New York women, all breast cancer survivors, read an early draft of the final chapter. Musa Mayer, Helen Schiff, and Anne Grant challenged our lack of attention to the Food and Drug Administration and forced us to reflect on our emphasis on high-dose chemotherapy as a medical procedure not evaluated by that agency. That we differ with them does not lessen our appreciation for the help they provided. We thank Mary Ann Napoli of the Center for Medical Consumers, New York City, for providing us with the 1982 press release of the American Society of Clinical Oncology cited in chapter 2. A number of past and present board members of the National Breast Cancer Coalition provided invaluable assistance. These include Fran Visco, Kay Dickersin, Susan Love, Belle Shayer, and Betsy Lambert. Cindy Pearson of the National Women's Health Network, Sheryl Ruzek of Temple University, and Mary Lou Smith of Research Advocacy also deserve thanks for their important help. At the end of chapter 9, we feature Virginia Hetrick, Alice Philipson, Anne Grant, and Jane Sprague Zones, and thank them for their willingness to share their stories. We also feature Pam Baber and thank Ron Baber for allowing us to use his late wife's story.

Peter Jacobson thanks Stefanie A. Doebler, JD, MPH, for her outstanding and invaluable work in analyzing the litigated high-dose chemotherapy with autologous bone marrow transplantation cases in chapter 3 and in comparing the litigation results to the interview results reported in chapter 4. He also thanks Rachel Turow, JD, MPH, for her admirable assistance on the Office of Personnel Management case study in chapter 6. Finally, he thanks the interview respondents—plaintiffs' and defense lawyers who contributed to chapter 4 and those who aided in the Minnesota stage legislative case in chapter 6—for their invaluable information and insights.

Wade Aubry thanks Lawrence J. Rose for his wise counsel and research assistance in this project and in many other endeavors.

Cynthia Farquhar thanks Claudia Steiner of the Agency for Healthcare Research and Quality for her major contribution to chapter 5 in accessing that agency's Health Care Utilization Project database and in the analyses and interpretation of the data. Both she and Rettig thank Carolyn Clancy of AHRQ for encouraging this collaboration. Farquhar thanks Melodee Nugent and Mary Horowitz of the Autologous Blood and Marrow Transplant Registry, who were helpful in providing data from the registry and answering questions about how the data were collected. She also thanks Mark Jeffrey, oncologist, with the Canterbury District Health Board, New Zealand, and Belinda Scott, breast surgeon of Breast Associates, Auckland, New Zealand, each of whom read and made useful comments on a draft of her chapters. Robert Birch, of Zeryx, formerly of Response Technologies, warrants grateful appreciation for a valuable interview.

For chapter 7 especially, we thank Naomi Aronson, Dan Engel, Jerry Seidenfeld, David Tennenbaum, and Inger Sapphire-Bernstein, all of the Blue Cross Blue Shield Association, for hosting an all-day site visit for three of us. Susan Gleeson, first director of the association's Technology Evaluation Center, graciously provided an interview in her suburban Seattle home. David Eddy shared his experience in a ride from downtown Washington, D.C., to Dulles Airport. At ECRI, Jeff Lerner, Charles Turkleson, and Diane Robertson hosted a full-day site visit. William McGivney, then at the National Comprehensive Cancer Network, related his experience with high-dose chemotherapy with autologous bone marrow transplantation at Aetna. Grace Monaco and Peter Goldschmidt described the Medical Care Ombudsman in detail, for which we thank them.

We thank Andrew Dorr, Jeffrey Abrams, Edward Stadtmauer, John Glick, Russell Basser, and William Peters for interviews related to chapter 8.

Raymond Weiss provided three lengthy and detailed interviews related to the audits of the South African trials, which are described in chapter 9.

For the appendix, Cynthia Farquhar thanks Jane Marjoribanks of the University of Auckland, who assisted with the identification of the U.S. and international trials, sought additional data from many of the trialists, and helped extract the data and prepare the Cochrane reviews. She also thanks Sarah Hetrick, who assisted with the trial searches and preparation of the Cochrane reviews, and Anne Lethaby of the University of Auckland and Val Gebski of the University of Sydney, who assisted with the statistical analyses. Farquhar thanks the Cochrane Collaboration of Sydney, Australia, and especially Russell Basser, who provided valuable insight into the international trials.

Finally, thanks go to our RAND colleagues who helped in this effort. Renee Labor, an extraordinarily professional research assistant, was with us during the first year of the project. Her move from RAND Washington to RAND Santa Monica, although advancing her career, was regretted deeply by all the project team members. A special thank-you goes to Lisa Spear, project assistant, who contributed above and beyond the call of duty in preparing the final manuscript and integrating medical, legal, and social science writing styles in accordance with the preferred style of Oxford University Press. We gratefully thank her for her patience and productivity. Stephen Bloodsworth converted a crude drawing into figure 1.1. Jane Ryan, director of RAND publications, provided wise counsel and guidance throughout the publication process. We are very grateful to them. Two RAND reviewers, Jennifer Malin, an oncologist, and David Studdert, a lawyer, provided an invaluable critical reading of the manuscript. All responsibility for remaining errors rests with the authors.

This project was supported by a grant from the Robert Wood Johnson Foundation to the RAND Corporation through the Health Care Financing and Organization Program of Academy Health (grant 044128).

Contents

Introduction   3

Part I   Initial Conditions

1   Breast Cancer Patients and the Emergence of a Treatment   11
2   Jumping the Gun   35

Part II   Drivers of Clinical Use

3   Court Trials   73
4   Litigation Strategies   103
5   Entrepreneurial Oncology   129
6   Government Mandates   152

Part III   The Struggle for Evidence-Based Medicine

7   Technology Assessments   181
8   Clinical Trials   206
9   Dénouement   239

Part IV   The Significance of the Story

10   Values in Conflict   259
Appendix: Evidence-Based Reviews of Clinical Trials   287
Notes   301
References   315
Index   343

FALSE HOPE

Introduction

High-dose chemotherapy with autologous bone marrow transplantation (HDC/ABMT) emerged in the late 1980s as a promising new treatment for metastatic breast cancer, then for high-risk breast cancer. Its promise was based on high levels of complete and partial tumor response. In the 1990s, HDC/ABMT burst on the oncology scene and was catapulted into widespread use before careful evaluation. The unconfirmed promise of this procedure drove clinical practice, health insurance coverage decisions, court decisions about coverage of individual patients, and federal administrative and state legislative mandates of HDC/ABMT as a covered benefit. Entrepreneurial oncology then exploited a lucrative market.

In parallel to rapid and widespread clinical use, randomized clinical trials were begun in 1990–1991 to evaluate whether the HDC/ABMT procedure was better than, worse than, or the same as conventional treatment. But, these trials struggled to accrue patients in the face of the widespread availability of the new treatment. Estimates of the number of women receiving the procedure outside of randomized clinical trials between 1989 and 2001 range from a low of 23,000 to a possible high of 35,000–40,000. By contrast, perhaps 1000 women received the investigational treatment within a randomized clinical trial during this time. By the end of the decade, the treatment's promise had largely evaporated. In 1999, at the annual meeting of the American Society of Clinical Oncology, four clinical trials reported "no benefit" in overall survival between HDC/ABMT and conventional treatment A South African trial, the only one to claim benefit, was audited the following year and found to be fraudulent. An earlier trial by the same investigator was audited subsequently and also found to be fraudulent.

In writing this book, we have had two objectives. First, we want to tell the story of the rise and virtual demise of HDC/ABMT as a treatment for metastatic and early-stage breast cancer. Second, in telling the story, we aim to draw lessons from it for the evaluation of other medical procedures. We adopt a historical approach—partly because medical science does not systematically tell its stories, and we hope that many interested individuals will find this account more accessible than the medical literature. The story is extraordinarily complex, however, and involves not one but several intertwined histories—patient demands; conflicting roles of physicians; scientific and clinical issues; and legal, economic, and political factors. For this reason, we tell the story through a series of specific histories, successively laid one upon the other. In this way, we seek to disentangle the several stories from each other and then assemble a big picture, a mosaic as it were, from numerous small tiles.

Only a few individuals know the entire HDC/ABMT story, from its clinical science origins to its rapid decline, in great detail. Many more know it in broad outline.

But the story is neither well known nor understood by most of those in the policy community or in the general public. We have discovered during our research that many people have been involved with HDC/ABMT over time, but relatively few have been involved over all the events of two decades or more. This book brackets the procedure's emergence as a clinical treatment and the decline in its use. We emphasize the period 1988 through 1992 because these early years defined the entire decade of the 1990s but are not fully appreciated by those who encountered HDC/ABMT later in the decade. We also highlight by this emphasis the conceptual and practical importance of the *initial conditions* for the evaluation of other medical procedures.

Thomas C. Chamberlin (1843–1928), an eminent geologist and academician, wrote a paper, "The Method of Multiple Working Hypotheses," first published in *Science* (old series) in 1890 and republished in 1965 (Chamberlin 1965). He advanced his method as superior to that of the ruling theory and that of the single working hypothesis, holding that the purpose of the method of multiple working hypotheses was "to bring up into view every rational explanation of new phenomena, and to develop every tenable hypothesis respecting their cause and history" (p. 756). In this book, we attempt to describe the various drivers of the HDC/ABMT experience, which include the requirements of clinical science, patient demands, physician advice to patients, physicians' beliefs and enthusiasms, patient advocacy, litigation, economics (the cost of the procedure, insurers' resistance to pay for investigational treatment, and entrepreneurial oncology), politics, the ambivalent commitment of oncology to randomized clinical trials, and how the media reported the story.

Why a case study? Why this one? We adopted this methodological approach for several reasons. First, case studies permit examination of the many factors and multiple perspectives that shape clinical medicine but typically go unexamined in the scientific literature. Second, stories are much more accessible to interested individuals (patients, policymakers, members of Congress and congressional staff, and the general public) than are the articles published by clinical researchers in peer-reviewed scientific journals. Finally, reflection on the details of a case allows one to draw broader lessons about the future (Flyvbjerg 2001).

But, fascinating as its details are, we are not content simply to tell the HDC/ABMT story. Our second objective is to draw lessons that go beyond the immediate procedure and consider how we in the United States evaluate other medical procedures. What has been learned from this experience? We believe that the lessons we draw have relevance to thinking about the future and about how the U.S. health care system ought to respond to the introduction of new medical procedures.

There are several ways to interpret the events we describe. Prominent during the 1990s was the interpretation that the HDC/ABMT story was one of managed care denying coverage for a lifesaving treatment to desperate patients for financial reasons. A feminist overlay on that interpretation held that denials of coverage by insurers represented yet another instance of women's health needs being given short shrift. Our interpretation, benefiting from hindsight, is that the story represents a basic conflict between the demands of individual patients for access to an untested, but potentially lifesaving treatment versus the collective need of society to evaluate new medical procedures before their widespread clinical use.

Central to our access-versus-evaluation viewpoint is our characterization of HDC/ABMT as a medical procedure. Strictly speaking, it was not a procedure because it lacked a procedure code as specified in *Current Procedural Terminology, Standard Edition*, published annually by the American Medical Association. We use the term broadly to encompass the primary components of HDC/ABMT: combination drug regimens used in dosages much higher than conventional chemotherapy, narrowly defined procedures (e.g., bone marrow aspiration), and supportive care. The important distinction is that HDC/ABMT was not a therapeutic product that fell under the jurisdiction of the Food and Drug Administration (FDA). The FDA, which reviews new drugs, biologics, and medical devices for safety and effectiveness, had no role in the evaluation of HDC/ABMT or a role in the evaluation of medical procedures. This was true because the HDC regimens consisted of combinations of drugs that had been approved previously as single agents. The use of such regimens falls within the practice of medicine. Thus, as medical procedure, HDC/ABMT escaped FDA evaluation. The distinction is important because there is no regulatory oversight of medicine that requires the rigorous evaluation of medical procedures. We address this institutional deficit in the final chapter.

In part I, "Initial Conditions," we anchor the analysis in the factors surrounding the emergence of the HDC/ABMT procedure. In chapter 1, we present four vignettes of women with a diagnosis of a breast cancer. We then examine the several elements (combination chemotherapy, HDC, bone marrow transplantation, adjuvant chemotherapy, and human growth factors) that came together as the procedure of HDC/ABMT for breast cancer. The chapter also deals with the role of bone marrow transplanters and of Phase 2 studies. In chapter 2, we discuss how a procedure emerges, emphasizing how one is recognized in the awkward "conversation" involving physicians and insurers, then how procedures are evaluated, and how this differs from the evaluation of pharmaceuticals. We then examine the ambivalent commitment of both oncology and health insurers to randomized clinical trials and the decision to initiate such trials. We highlight the legitimation of the procedure as ripe for clinical use by prominent oncologists, which resulted in the fateful branching to rapid and widespread clinical use concurrent with the much slower evaluation of the procedure through randomized clinical trials. We also examine the context-setting role of the women's health movement and how newspapers and television reported the story.

In part II, "Drivers of Clinical Use," we examine the interactions among patients and physicians, insurers, and the legal system regarding health insurance coverage of HDC/ABMT. Chapter 3 analyzes the court trials in which judges and juries responded to women seeking relief from denial of coverage. Chapter 4 analyzes the litigation strategies used by the plaintiffs' lawyers on behalf of women denied treatment access by insurers. It also describes defense attorneys' strategies as they argued that exposure to this experimental and highly toxic treatment was unjustified save in a randomized clinical trial. We describe the utilization of the procedure in chapter 5 with national data and provide a case study of for-profit exploitation of the procedure. Chapter 6 analyzes two cases of government mandates—one by the federal government Office of Personnel Management and another by the Minnesota state legislature—that required coverage of the experimental procedure by all health plans under their respective jurisdiction.

Part III, "The Struggle for Evidence-based Medicine," deals with how those committed to rigorous evaluation of new medical procedures dealt with HDC/ABMT. Evaluation involves technology assessments, clinical trials, and audits of trials. It is a responsibility shared among the developers of a medical procedure, patients, practicing physicians, and third parties such as health plans and insurers. It occurs at the levels of clinical science, clinical practice, and insurance coverage decisions.

Chapter 7 examines how procedures are evaluated by technology assessments when there are no data, a challenge that faced insurers in the first half of the 1990s. Such assessments, based on systematic reviews of the scientific literature, repeatedly concluded that existing data did not support the claim that HDC/ABMT was better or even the same as conventional treatment. Yet, the absence of data on effectiveness had little if any effect on use of the procedure. Chapter 8 documents the tortuous route by which phase 3 randomized clinical trials were initiated, enrolled patients with great difficulty, and eventually reported results of no benefit in 1999. The no benefit results drained enthusiasm for the procedure from oncology. Chapter 9 recounts the audits of the only two trials claiming dramatic benefit from HDC/ABMT. These trials by a South African investigator, one trial reported in 1995 and the other in 1999, when audited, were shown to be fraudulent.

In the final part of the book, "The Significance of the Story," chapter 10 draws lessons from this account and seeks to apply them to the broader issue of the evaluation of experimental medical procedures. We conclude that initial conditions matter; that conflicting values are ubiquitous, pervade all stages of the process, and permeate the judgments of all parties to the discussion; and that an institutional deficit exists in the evaluation of procedures. Unlike the evaluation of new drugs, which occurs within a statutory framework administered by a federal agency, governed by explicit rules, and embedded in a culture and tradition, the evaluation of procedures for which there is no commercial sponsor is much less organized. We propose a public–private partnership to remedy this deficit.

Research Methodologies

We used a number of different methodologies in the preparation of this book. We made extensive use of semistructured interviews with key actors for every stage of the research and analysis. Some individuals were interviewed more than once, and we often established a continuing "conversation" with some individuals. Although some interviews were conducted over the telephone, most were face-to-face, and some involved full-day site visits.

Most interviews identify the interviewee and the date of the interview. However, the plaintiffs and defense attorneys interviewed for chapter 4 and the interviewees for the Minnesota case study (chapter 6) were granted anonymity. In the former case, 8 attorneys were interviewed: 4 plaintiffs and 4 defense attorneys. In Minnesota, 16 interviews were conducted: proponents and opponents of the state mandate, including legislators, other state officials, patient advocates, physicians, and health insurers.

One of us (Rettig) attended the 2002 and 2003 annual meetings of the American Society for Clinical Oncology simply to witness activity at this major event on the regular calendar of oncology.

We relied greatly on the published scientific literature. Typically, we would conduct a Medline search for all citations to a particular clinician-investigator. From that list, which included abstracts, we selected papers pertaining to HDC/ABMT for breast cancer and obtained and read the papers. Interviewees often identified important papers and interpreted their importance for us. In addition to the published literature, we obtained and reviewed many documents—memoranda, letters, unpublished reports—not easily categorized by Medline and that may not be readily accessible to the public. Such documents have sometimes been described as "fugitive literature." We interpreted these in the context of when, where, and why they were generated, often relying on our interviewees for help in answering these questions.

To analyze the reported court cases, Peter Jacobson and Stefanie Doebler used standard electronic legal research tools such as Westlaw and Lexis-Nexis. We also examined the law review literature and the published health services literature to learn about cases that might not have been available through an online search. To capture cases that might not have been reported, we contacted people involved in the litigation and other stakeholders. For the analysis, Doebler, a dual law and public health degree candidate at the University of Michigan, read and reread all of the cases and compiled a list of case themes and descriptive data. To corroborate the analysis, Jacobson independently read and analyzed several leading cases. Together, Jacobson and Doebler analyzed the recurring case themes and compared them to the interview results.

Cynthia Farquhar, with a research assistant, conducted the analyses of the Health Care Utilization Project database about the utilization of HDC/ABMT during 1993–2001. The database captures discharge data from 22 states from which national estimates are made. Other data were provided by the Autologous Blood and Marrow Transplant Registry, which collects approximately 50%–60% of all treatments. Farquhar, who is also involved with the Cochrane Collaboration, conducted systematic reviews of the randomized clinical trials of HDC/ABMT for metastatic and high-risk breast cancer, both in the United States and in Europe. A summary of these reviews appears as an appendix to the book.

The print and television and radio reports of the HDC/ABMT story were obtained by a Nexus-Lexus search conducted by Renée Labor. The transcripts of these accounts, which filled three large-ring binders, remain in the project files. On the basis of these reports and her own prior investigative reporting of the HDC/ABMT story, Shannon Brownlee, a freelance medical science writer, prepared an analysis of how the media covered the story; the analysis appears both in chapter 2 and in summary form in the final chapter.

Part I

Initial Conditions

1

Breast Cancer Patients and the Emergence of a Treatment

Now hope that is seen is not hope. For who hopes for what is seen? But if we hope for what we do not see, we wait for it with patience.
—St. Paul, Romans 8:24–25 (NRSV)

Hope is the elevating feeling we experience when we see—in the mind's eye—a path to a better future. Hope acknowledges the significant obstacles and deep pitfalls along that path. True hope has no room for delusion.
—Jerome Groopman, *The Anatomy of Hope*

Pamela Pirozzi, a 35-year-old mother of three, was diagnosed with breast cancer in May 1989 (Leff 1990b). After a modified mastectomy and 6 months of chemotherapy, her prognosis looked good. But, in early 1990 she learned that the cancer had returned and spread elsewhere in her body. Her physician, Stanley P. Watkins, Jr., advised her that her best chance for surviving more than a year was a new procedure involving high-dose chemotherapy (HDC) augmented by transplantation of her bone marrow. However, her insurer, Blue Cross and Blue Shield of Virginia, denied the request for coverage on the grounds that the procedure, estimated to cost at least $100,000, was experimental. Pamela and her husband, Mike Pirozzi, sued, and on April 18, 1990, a federal district court judge in Alexandria, Virginia, ruled in her favor (Howe 1990). Although the insurer had followed its policy in denying coverage, Judge T. S. Ellis III determined that the policy was flawed: "To require that the plaintiff or other plan members wait until somebody chooses to present statistical proof [about the success of a treatment] that would satisfy all the experts means that plan members would be doomed to receive medical procedures that are not state of the art" (Howe 1990, p. C1). However, after 4 months of testing and chemotherapy, the cancer had spread, and her physicians concluded that she was no longer a suitable candidate for the treatment (Leff 1990a).

Arline Betzner, 54-year-old mother of two from St. Petersburg, Florida, was also denied coverage by her insurer, Aetna Insurance Company, in April 1990 (Gentry 1990). Her husband Bill emptied their savings to make a $25,000 down payment on treatment at the H. Lee Moffitt Cancer Center in Tampa and said he would sell the family home to raise the rest of the funds if necessary. She was an ideal candidate for the experimental procedure of autologous bone marrow transplantation (ABMT), having responded with complete remission to 10 weeks of chemotherapy. A physician at Moffitt put Betzner's chances at long-term disease-free survival at 25% with the treatment but said they were slim without it. An Aetna spokeswoman, defending the coverage denial, wrote: "It is not generally accepted by the medical profession as a safe, effective and appropriate procedure for the treatment of metastatic breast cancer" (Gentry 1990, p. 1A).

Angela Davis, a St. Louis television producer and freelance writer, discovered a lump in her right breast in 1988 (Hernon 1992). She received a lumpectomy, which removed the tumor, followed by 6 weeks of radiation therapy and 6 months of chemotherapy. In mid-1991, a cough signaled that her cancer had returned. Plunging into medical textbooks, calling specialists, she learned about bone marrow transplantation (BMT) and that medical opinion was divided on its effectiveness. She decided to go ahead with a transplant, but the St. Louis University Medical Center wanted $40,000 up front. A correspondence file between Davis and her insurance company, Blue Cross and Blue Shield of Missouri, thickened between September and November. Then, on November 15 her insurer denied coverage of the experimental procedure. She filed suit in federal district court and, in early December, the court ordered her insurer to pay for treatment, which began on February 3.

Davis was treated but died shortly afterward. The newspaper chronicled her final days this way:

> The bone marrow procedure is complicated, and it can be painful. As much as a quart of bone marrow can be harvested. Davis received dozens of punctures in each hip, so that her bone marrow could be sucked out and frozen for use later. The patient then faces 3 to 5 days of intense chemotherapy. The drugs are administered intravenously, often through a catheter inserted in the chest. When it's time to transplant the bone marrow, it is taken to the bedside in frozen packages, thawed in warm water, then re-injected into the body. Within days, the danger of infection began. Davis was kept in a special dust-filtered room. She developed a 105-degree fever and was wrapped in a cooling blanket. Twice she was admitted to the intensive care unit. Her blood pressure dropped dangerously. She was given more than a dozen antibiotics. All this is normal. Two weeks after her treatment ended, her tumors had returned. Davis had spent more than 5 weeks in the hospital. Another cycle of high-dose chemotherapy that had been planned was canceled. Sent home, she entered a hospice program. (Hernon 1992, p. 1A, reprinted with permission of the *St. Louis Post Dispatch*)

In early 1996, a *Time* magazine cover featured a gagged physician, headlined by, "What Your Doctor Can't Tell You: An In-depth Look at Managed Care—And One Woman's Fight to Survive." The story by Erik Larson featured HealthNet, "one of the most aggressively cost conscious" managed care organizations in California and highlighted its opposition to investigational treatments and research (Larson 1996). The woman in question was Christine deMeurs, a HealthNet beneficiary, who had discovered a lump in her breast in August 1992. She had a radical mastectomy and radiation therapy, followed by a round of chemotherapy that ended in March 1993. A bone scan 2 months later revealed stage IV metastatic breast cancer. Her physician, an oncologist at the Rancho Canyon medical group, recommended that she consider a bone marrow transplant. A referral to a Scripps oncologist confirmed that

Christine was a transplant candidate, but that several chemotherapy cycles would be required to show the responsiveness of her tumor to the potent drugs. The encounter was unsatisfactory, partly because the procedure was not even described.

On the day of that encounter, Christine and her husband flew to Denver and she visited Dr. Roy Jones, an oncologist at the University of Colorado, on June 9 (Larson 1996, p. 48). Jones thought a transplant would still help. But, insurance coverage would become an issue as HealthNet had, on the prior day, decided to deny coverage for the procedure on the grounds of an investigational exclusion in her contract. Jones challenged this decision: "Is it reasonable," he said, "for an insurer to demand the gold standard of proof and simultaneously refuse to pay for patients to enter a trial to get that level of proof?" Unwilling to undergo months of treatment away from home, deMeurs sought referral to the University of California at Los Angeles (UCLA) from her oncologist, who refused. She requested a new oncologist, who agreed that a transplant ought to be considered and suggested she go to UCLA.

The UCLA encounter was remarkable. On June 25, Christine saw Dr. John Glaspy, described as "a fierce patient advocate" (Larson 1996, p. 50). Transplantation was an option, he thought, not one he could wholeheartedly recommend, but it "was on the rational list." Christine did not disclose that she was enrolled in HealthNet, and Glaspy did not indicate that he been a member of a HealthNet committee that earlier in 1993 had developed practice guidelines that called for denial of coverage for patients with advanced stage IV breast cancer. He had voted for coverage initially but now agreed to support the majority view against it. Christine began induction therapy. At the same time, the deMeurs retained attorney Mark Hiepler, who filed a detailed appeal seeking an injunction against HealthNet's denial of coverage.

In early September, Glaspy learned that Christine was a HealthNet subscriber (Larson 1996, p. 51). On September 9, he signed a legal declaration in support of her appeal, convinced the insurer should pay. That afternoon, he attended a meeting of HealthNet's bone marrow transplant committee. In the seesaw discussion, HealthNet wished to distribute the guidelines to all oncologists in its network, indicating what was covered and what was not. The physicians demurred, preferring a general rule that would permit exceptions on a case-by-case basis. The guidelines, which barred transplants for advanced breast cancer, remained unchanged.

HealthNet then called Dr. Dennis Slamon, the head of oncology at UCLA and Glaspy's superior, to say that it wished UCLA to support the guidelines and to ask whether they intended to perform the deMeurs transplant (Larson 1996, p. 51). Slamon had decided that UCLA, not HealthNet, should pay for the treatment, given the appeal, because the bone marrow had already been harvested, and it would be inappropriate to start the procedure and fail to complete it. He informed Glaspy after the decision. Glaspy, outraged at this interference and wishing to persuade HealthNet to pay, considered resigning but did not. However, on September 22, he did sign a second declaration, stunning to the deMeurs, opposing the injunction they sought.

But, UCLA agreed in writing to pay. Christine deMeurs began the procedure on September 23, completed it, had four disease-free months, fell ill again in the spring of 1994, and died on March 9, 1995. An arbitration panel later determined that HealthNet should have paid for the procedure, had interfered in the doctor–patient relationship, and awarded Alan deMeurs $1.02 million. A HealthNet spokesman said, "I'm sorry the panel didn't see that HealthNet was doing what was best for the patient, which was to deny the treatment as investigational, and which in the end was proven the right decision" (Larson 1996, p. 52).

The Story in Brief: A Fateful Branching

What do these cases illustrate? They indicate the intense hope and fear that drove women with a diagnosis of breast cancer to seek an experimental treatment presumed to offer better prospects than conventional therapy. They suggest the dependence of women on the advice they receive from their physicians, especially when a treatment is characterized as "the only chance for a cure." The cases show how the demands of these women were expressed forcefully to and through families, physicians, clergy, employers, and newspaper and television reporters. They demonstrate that lawyers often translated these demands into litigation against health insurers. They indicate that insurers often provoked litigation by denying coverage of the high-dose chemotherapy with autologous bone marrow transplantation (HDC/ABMT) procedure on the grounds that the procedure was experimental. An important underlying consideration was that the procedure was very expensive, significantly more than conventional therapy.

Finally, these cases reveal "the face of the patient" as reported in the daily news. A 35-five-year old mother of two small children facing premature death calls forth compassion and creates an intense desire to avoid repeating such scenarios in the future. Thus, the way the media report a story like this becomes part of the story itself.

But, the news accounts tell only part of the story. Masked at the time to both the general public and to many, if not most, women with breast cancer, the cases do not indicate the intense scientific and clinical controversy surrounding HDC/ABMT. They do not reveal the exploitation of the procedure for financial gain by both for-profit and not-for-profit oncology providers. Bone marrow transplanters were in great demand because they generated high patient volumes and revenue streams with substantial margins.

These early accounts do not display national data about the utilization of the procedure. Expanding clinical use began in 1989, rose rapidly throughout the 1990s, peaked in 1997 or 1998, and dropped precipitously from mid-1999 onward. Estimates range from a low of 23,000 to perhaps as many as 35,000–40,000 women who received HDC/ABMT for breast cancer between 1989 and 2001. But, in this period only 1000 women would receive the experimental treatment through randomized clinical trials, which were needed to provide the definitive evidence of whether it worked.

These early accounts provide no more than a hint about how events would unfold in the 1990s, which we describe in detail in this book. To orient the reader to this complex story, we present figure 1.1. It shows that HDC/ABMT emerged as an experimental procedure in the late 1980s based on developments in the 1970s and 1980s.

A fateful branching occurred, a "natural experiment," in effect, with the HDC/ABMT procedure following two parallel pathways. The clinical utilization pathway involved rapid and widespread use of HDC/ABMT, first for treating metastatic

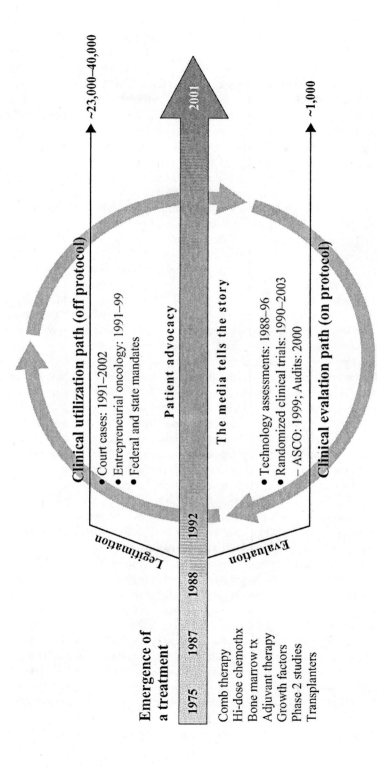

Figure 1.1. The high-dose chemotherapy with autologous bone marrow transplantation (HDC/ABMT) experience.

breast cancer, a terminal disease, but soon thereafter also for treating high-risk, poor-prognosis breast cancer that was not clearly terminal. Three of the above patient vignettes, for example, occurred in the 1988–1992 period. In these very important early years, patients began demanding access to HDC/ABMT; these demands were often encouraged by the advice of their physicians, supported by family and friends, aided by lawyers and reporters, sanctioned by the leadership of oncology, and reinforced by media reporting. The other pathway, clinical evaluation by randomized clinical trials, involved a much slower process that would show no benefit in overall survival at the end of the decade.

These parallel pathways—clinical use and clinical evaluation—began simultaneously, virtually concurrent with the emergence of the procedure, and their antagonistic relationship would define controversy about HDC/ABMT for the rest of the decade. Widespread clinical use was driven by many factors: patient demands, physician advice, and the reporting of the story in the press. Importantly, the oncology community would legitimate the early use of HDC/ABMT—jump the gun—before its thorough evaluation (chapter 2). Litigation against insurers for denials of coverage of patient care costs would make courtrooms the venue for pressing contending claims (chapters 3 and 4). Utilization of the procedure would skyrocket as both for-profit and not-for-profit oncology providers exploited it for financial gain (chapter 5). Federal government agencies, especially the Office of Personnel Management, and state legislatures would mandate insurance coverage of the procedure (chapter 6) without evidence of effectiveness.

Evaluation was much slower. The questions were these: Was the treatment as effective or more effective than standard chemotherapy? If so, what outcomes should be used to measure effectiveness? How should the procedure be evaluated? Technology assessments, basically systematic reviews of the existing literature, repeatedly concluded that the data were inadequate to support claims that HDC/ABMT was superior to conventional treatment (chapter 7). Randomized clinical trials, the gold standard of medical effectiveness, required time to organize, accrue patients, provide treatment according to protocol, collect data over an appropriate length of time, evaluate the experimental and control arms, and report results to patients, the scientific community, and the general public (chapter 8). The randomized trials encountered substantial difficulties in enrolling patients due to the widespread availability of the procedure outside such trials. But, in 1999 four trials (one in metastatic and three in high-risk patients) reported no statistically significant benefit from HDC/ABMT in terms of overall survival for patients. One South African trial in high-risk patients reported benefit, but when that trial was audited in 2000, it was discovered to be fraudulent. An audit of a prior South African trial in metastatic patients by the same investigator was then audited as well and also found to be fraudulent (chapter 9).

The HDC/ABMT experience reveals an underlying tension between two conflicting values. One value is making experimental cancer therapies readily available to patients for whom conventional therapy offers relatively little hope. The second value is the need to validate the medical effectiveness of such therapies before their widespread use and to protect patients from treatments that might be no better than or even worse than existing treatments. Commitment to this value has evolved over time, especially for breast cancer treatments, as the challenge to the Halsted radical mastectomy by randomized clinical trials of breast-conserving surgery indicates (Lerner 2001). Validation of treatment effectiveness in turn requires that the integrity of the evaluation by randomized clinical trials be protected. For these reasons, we characterize the basic conflict in the HDC/ABMT story as one of access to an experimental procedure for breast cancer outside a clinical trial versus evaluation of that procedure in a randomized trial before widespread use.

The HDC/ABMT story can be characterized in two other ways. A prevalent interpretation has been that health insurers' denials of coverage for HDC/ABMT on the grounds that the procedure was experimental typified the unwillingness of managed care organizations to pay for needed health care services for financial reasons (Anders 1996). A second view is a feminist version of the first: Managed care, health insurers, and health plans were unwilling to pay for a new breast cancer treatment that, though untested, was believed to be beneficial and even lifesaving for women, whereas insurers were willing to reimburse HDC/ABMT as a treatment for testicular cancer. In 1990, the Congressional Women's Caucus declared war on male bias in medicine. As former Rep. Patricia Schroeder explained: "I've had a theory that you fund what you fear. When you have a male-dominated group of researchers, they are more worried about prostate cancer than breast cancer" (Goodman 1990, p. 15).

We view the HDC/ABMT story as a basic conflict between demands for access to a potentially lifesaving experimental treatment by individual women with a breast cancer diagnosis versus a collective societal need to evaluate new medical treatments before their widespread use. The cost of the treatment, which was typically a multiple of the cost of standard therapy, heightened this need for evaluation. Because access versus evaluation is a theme that HDC/ABMT shares with many other new medical procedures, we draw broader policy lessons from this account in the final chapter.

In the remainder of this chapter, we review briefly breast cancer and its treatment and examine the nature and elements of the HDC/ABMT procedure: combination chemotherapy, HDC, BMT, adjuvant chemotherapy, and human growth factors. We also describe the role of the transplanters and of phase 2 clinical studies in the emergence of HDC/ABMT as a breast cancer treatment. In chapter 2, we focus on the factors that led to the fateful branching to clinical use of HDC/ABMT concurrent with its evaluation in randomized clinical trials.

Breast Cancer and Its Treatment

Breast cancer is a major killer. It is the second leading cause of cancer death among women (representing 15% of all cancer deaths), compared to 25% of cancer deaths from lung cancer (American Cancer Society [ACS] 2004). Estimated deaths from breast cancer in 2003 were 39,800 for women and 400 for men. Mortality rates for breast cancer declined significantly in recent years, mostly among young women, both white and black, falling 1.4% annually in 1989–1995 and then at a rate of 3.2% annually. Survival for women with breast cancer varies as a function of the stage of the disease at diagnosis. The ACS data show 5-year relative survival rates of 86% for all stages, 97% for local, 78% for regional, and 23% for distant (or metastasized) cancers. The ACS, relying on the SEER staging system of the National Cancer Institute, defines local-stage tumors as cancers that are confined to the breast; regional-stage tumors have spread to surrounding tissue or nearby lymph nodes; and distant-stage tumors have spread (or metastasized) to distant organs (ACS, *Breast Cancer Facts & Figures* 2005–2006, p. 1). The 5-year relative survival rates are higher for white women than for African American women.

Breast cancer is the leading type of new cancer among women. The ACS estimated that 211,300 new cases of invasive breast cancer would occur among women and 1300 among men in the United States in 2003 (ACS 2004). New cases of breast cancer represented one third of 658,800 cases for all cancers in women, greater than the 12% of new cases of lung cancer among women. The incidence of breast cancer among white women increased at about 4.5% in the 1980s but has risen more slowly in the 1990s. The cumulative probability of developing breast cancer increases as a function of age. Lifetime chances for women from birth to age 39 are 1 in 228; for those aged 40 to 59, they rise to 1 in 24, and they increase to 1 in 4 for those aged 60 to 79. All women, from birth to death, have a 1 in 8 chance of developing breast cancer (ACS 2004).

Breast cancer is treated today by surgery, radiotherapy, chemotherapy, and hormonal therapy. Primary treatment of breast cancer may involve surgical removal of the lesion, either by total mastectomy (modified radical or simple) or by lumpectomy, axillary (arm pit) lymph node dissection (less frequent today), and postoperative local radiotherapy (ACS 2004). The principal surgical procedure well into the 1980s was radical mastectomy. The century-long dominance of this procedure was challenged by randomized controlled trials comparing it with breast-conserving surgery, or lumpectomy, followed by radiation therapy (I. C. Henderson and Canellos 1980a, 1980b; Lerner 2001).

Breast cancer is classified as noninvasive or invasive according to a complex staging system developed and continuously updated by the American Joint Committee on Cancer, which includes the National Cancer Institute, American Cancer Society, American Society of Clinical Oncology, and other professional societies, as members. *Noninvasive* breast cancer includes lobular carcinoma in situ (LCIS) and ductal carcinoma in situ (DCIS). *Invasive* breast cancers are classified as stages I, II, III, or IV, which are described in table 1.1 based on the NCI Dictionary of Cancer Terms.

Stages I, IIA, and IIB differ according to tumor size (2 cm or less, greater than 2 cm but less than 5 cm, and more than 5 cm, respectively) and lymph node involvement (none, 1–3, 4 or more, respectively). Stage IIA or IIB breast cancers involve a high risk of relapse after primary treatment (more than 50% recurrence within 5 years of initial diagnosis). Consequently, in addition to primary therapy, *adjuvant* or secondary chemotherapy and hormonal therapy may be considered for both node-negative and node-positive cancers, depending on tumor size, histology, hormone receptor status and age.

Stage IIIA and IIIB breast cancers are classified as operable or inoperable, respectively, depending on the size of the tumor (for IIIA), the size of the breast, and the degree of inflammatory changes. Primary treatment for operable breast cancers smaller than 5 cm is either total mastectomy with axillary node dissection or lumpectomy, axillary dissection, and radiation therapy. For tumors greater than 5 cm in size,

Table 1.1 Breast cancer staging

Breast cancer stage	Description
I	The tumor is no larger than 2 cm and has not spread outside the breast.
II	Divided into stage IIA and stage IIB based on tumor size and whether it has spread to the axillary lymph nodes (the lymph nodes under the arm).
	In stage IIA, the cancer is either no larger than 2 cm and has spread to the axillary lymph nodes or between 2 and 5 cm but has not spread to the axillary lymph nodes.
	In stage IIB, the cancer is either between 2 and 5 cm and has spread to the axillary lymph nodes or >5 cm but has not spread to the axillary lymph nodes.
III	Divided into stages IIIA, IIIB, and IIIC.
	In stage IIIA, the cancer either (1) is <5 cm (2 inches) and has spread to the axillary lymph nodes (in the armpit), which have grown into each other or into other structures and are attached to them; or (2) is >5 cm and has spread to the axillary lymph nodes, and the lymph nodes may be attached to each other or to other structures.
	In stage IIIB, the tumor, which may be any size, (1) has spread to the tissues near the breast (the skin or chest wall, including the ribs and the muscles in the chest); or (2) has spread to lymph nodes within the breast or under the arm.
	In stage IIIC, the cancer has spread to lymph nodes beneath the collar bone and near the neck and may have spread to tissues near the breast (the skin or chest wall, including the ribs and muscles in the chest) and to lymph nodes within the breast or under the arm.
Stage IV	Cancer has spread to other organs of the body, most often the bones, lungs, liver, or brain; or tumor has spread locally to the skin and lymph nodes inside the neck, near the collarbone.

Source: National Cancer Institute, *Dictionary of Cancer Terms* (http://www.nci.nih.gov/dictionary/).

doxorubicin-based neoadjuvant chemotherapy (preceding surgery) followed by lumpectomy, axillary dissection, and radiation therapy is an additional option.[1] However, nondoxorubicin regimens can sometimes be used, and endocrine therapy may sometimes be used rather than chemotherapy. For inoperable stage III breast cancer, initial primary treatment is doxorubicin-based neoadjuvant chemotherapy, which may be followed by total mastectomy with axillary dissection or lumpectomy with axillary dissection and radiation therapy. Stage IV metastatic breast cancer indicates the presence of distant metastases at the time of diagnosis. Recurrent breast cancers are divided into local and systemic recurrence. Local recurrence is further divided into cases previously treated with total mastectomy or by lumpectomy: the former cases are treated by surgical resection, if possible, and radiotherapy; the latter are treated by total mastectomy, although there are many exceptions. Both types of local recurrence are candidates for systemic chemotherapy and hormonal therapy, depending on hormone receptor status. For stage IV patients with systemic recurrence, hormonal therapy may be preferred because of fewer side effects. One factor driving the diffusion of HDC/ABMT was the perception that conventional treatment for stage IV breast cancer produced few good outcomes. However, some patients had very good outcomes, and breast cancer specialists were aware of this. But, the general perception by physicians and patients created great frustration among many physicians and substantial impatience among patients.

What's in a Name?

When first developed, HDC/ABMT was often described as BMT or ABMT (or sometimes AuBMT). In time, the procedure came to be referred to as HDC/ABMT. This acknowledges that treatment is HDC made possible by transplantation, a rescue procedure from an otherwise lethal dose of chemotherapy. *Autologous* refers to bone marrow from the patient herself; *allogeneic* bone marrow is donated by another individual. As the procedure developed, treatment was also described as HDC with peripheral blood (or hematopoietic) stem cell rescue or transplantation (PBSCR or PBSCT). This resulted from the discovery that stem cells could be obtained more easily from peripheral blood and substituted for bone marrow, which was typically harvested before chemotherapy. In this book, we use HDC/ABMT to emphasize that the procedure consists primarily of HDC enabled by transplantation. We use ABMT as shorthand for both autologous bone marrow transplantation and peripheral blood stem cell transplantation or rescue. When these differences matter, we make that clear.

Throughout this book, we refer to HDC/ABMT as a *procedure*. Strictly speaking, HDC/ABMT is not a procedure as it does not have a procedure code specified in *Current Procedural Terminology, Standard Edition*, published annually by the American Medical Association. But, we use procedure generically because no standard nomenclature exists for adequately describing all medical interventions, which are described by a family of terms (therapeutic and diagnostic products, medical and surgical procedures, medical technologies, and medical treatments or therapies). In this broader sense, the HDC/ABMT procedure involves the use of drugs in high-dose combination regimens, narrowly defined procedures, and supportive care. The operational distinction of consequence is that the Food and Drug Administration did not regulate the HDC/ABMT procedure. The drugs used in combination regimens had been approved previously as single agents, many for breast cancer. (Human growth factors were approved by the FDA in 1991 as the procedure began to be used widely.) Similarly, the agency did not regulate the high doses, which were being studied in clinical trials or used because of data from clinical trials. Some might view the HDC/ABMT procedure as a case of "off-label" use of drugs, a gray zone in which drugs approved by the FDA for one purpose are used by physicians for other indications. Again, such use is not regulated by the agency. The medical profession determined both the use and the evaluation of HDC/ABMT.

What does the HDC/ABMT procedure involve? Following primary treatment by surgery and radiotherapy and before induction chemotherapy, the procedure has these stages: harvesting the patient's bone marrow by aspirating bone marrow from the sacroiliac bone or obtaining peripheral blood stem cells through a blood-filtering process; storing the marrow or stem cells for later use; administering conventional chemotherapy to determine tumor responsiveness for metastatic disease patients; administering chemotherapy at doses several times that of standard treatment, killing both cancerous cells and normal cells, including the remaining stem cells in the bone marrow; reinfusing the patient with the marrow or stem cells to reconstitute the marrow and replenish white blood cells; monitoring and supporting the pancytopenic phase, in which infusion of platelets, red blood cells, and antibiotics may be required; managing early recovery, which is characterized by repopulation of hematopoietic cells from the transplanted marrow; and convalescence (Handelsman 1989).

Chemotherapy kills dividing cells, both normal and cancerous. High-dose regimens are extremely toxic to the blood-producing stem cells in the bone marrow, almost all of which are destroyed (myeloablation). Blood cells are required to transport oxygen, maintain immune function, and prevent bleeding. This degree of bone marrow depletion would normally be fatal, but the reinfusion of thawed stem cells or harvested bone marrow immediately after high-dose treatment allows marrow reengraftment. However, until white cells reappear in the blood in substantial numbers, which takes about 10 days, there is a high risk of opportunistic infections by bacteria, fungi, or parasites (Canales et al. 2000).

In addition to its myeloablative effects, HDC is extremely toxic to other tissues with dividing cells, such as the gastrointestinal tract, the skin, and the hair follicles. Acute toxicities include cramping and dysfunction in the gastrointestinal tract, mouth sores, nausea, diarrhea, rashes, and fatigue. Total hair loss is very common but varies with the type of chemotherapy used. Severe organ toxicity is less common but can be fatal. The lungs are particularly sensitive to some drugs (e.g., vincristine in the Solid Tumor Autologous Marrow Program I regimen), and life-threatening interstitial pneumonitis can occur, resulting in fluid accumulation and reduced blood oxygen. Other severe adverse effects may include liver damage and inflammation of the bladder. Cardiac events occur more often with HDC. For these reasons, patients who underwent HDC/ABMT were usually hospitalized for several weeks and sometimes for months if complications occurred. During hospitalization, patients were at risk of infection, were isolated, and were subject to situational depression. Long-term and possibly irreversible toxicities include damage to the auditory and other sensory nerves, infertility, premature menopause, chronic fatigue, impaired renal function, and neuropsychological disturbances. In addition, HDC appears to be associated with an increased risk of secondary malignancies, particularly bone marrow and blood disorders, such as leukemia (Rodenhuis 2000).

An oncology procedure, as we use the term, often consists of many elements, each with its own quite lengthy and independent history. In the case of HDC/ABMT for treating breast cancer, the elements included combination chemotherapy, HDC, BMT, adjuvant chemotherapy, and human growth factors. Some of these elements were firmly grounded on science, both conceptually and empirically; others defined hypotheses to be tested; still others developed after the procedure emerged and facilitated its wider use. We review briefly each of these elements.

Combination Chemotherapy

A basic limitation of cancer therapy is the *resistance* of tumors to cytotoxic drugs (I. C. Henderson et al. 1988). Combination chemotherapy developed as a way to overcome resistance. By the 1970s, it had been shown that metastatic breast cancer was moderately sensitive to single-agent chemotherapy (DeVita and Schein 1973). Several groups of cytotoxic agents were identified as active against metastatic breast cancer, including the alkylating agents (cyclophosphamide, thiotepa, L-phenylalanine mustard); the antimetabolites (5-fluorouracil, methotrexate); the vinca alkaloids (vincristine and vinblastine); and the antitumor antibiotics (doxorubicin, mitomycin, and others) (Hortobagyi 2000).

Soon after, the superiority of combinations over single-agent drugs was demonstrated. The *Cooper regimen*, consisting of cyclophosphamide, methotrexate, 5-fluorouracil, vincristine, and prednisone (CMFVP) and its derivatives (CMF and CMFP), were generally accepted as active and well tolerated. The antibiotic doxorubicin (known as Adriamycin) demonstrated marked antitumor activity and was also incorporated into combinations with cyclophosphamide and 5-fluorouracil (CAF, FAC). These combinations became established quickly as the most effective systemic therapies for metastatic breast cancer.

In patients with metastases, a number of clinical trials showed that CMF and similar regimens produced a 50% or greater regression in measurable tumors in 40%–50% of patients (Hortobagyi 2000). In separate trials, the FAC-type combinations produced partial or complete remissions in 50%–80% of patients. Eventually, these two types of regimens were compared in randomized clinical trials and meta-analyses, which demonstrated that regimens containing anthracycline produced objective tumor responses in a higher percentage of patients, that response duration or time to progression was longer for combinations with anthracycline than for those without, and that survival was improved. In part because of this increased efficacy and extensive experience with these combinations, FAC, CAF, and AC became the most commonly used chemotherapy regimens for metastatic and primary breast cancer. (Some high-dose regimens, as shown in table 1.2, were given entirely in the outpatient setting and were remarkably nontoxic.)

High-Dose Chemotherapy

The appropriate dosage for cancer chemotherapy has long been debated within oncology. In 1980, Frei and Canellos argued that the importance of the dose of chemotherapy drugs was "insufficiently appreciated." Chemotherapy drugs were so toxic that any suggestion that the dose–response curve was *not* steep or that lower doses were as effective as higher ones led oncologists to administer lower doses. They argued that the toxicity of antitumor agents was strongly dose related for *both* tumor and normal cells, and that the dose–response curve was steep for the majority of such agents.

A few randomized studies had examined dose as a variable, and most had found a dose–response curve, especially for Hodgkin's disease, non-Hodgkin's lymphoma, oat (small) cell carcinoma of the lung, and acute lymphocytic leukemia (Frei and Canellos 1980). Few of the studies in these sensitive cancers had established proof of principle. Even so, higher doses for these sensitive tumors were at most twice that of standard doses. Solid tumors that were only marginally sensitive to chemotherapy failed to respond to two- or threefold increases in dosage. Chemotherapy was also "much more effective" against minimal residual disease than against advanced

Table 1.2 Chemotherapy drugs and regimens commonly used for breast cancer

Abbreviation	Definition
Chemotherapeutic agents	
C	Cyclophosphamide
M	Methotrexate
F	5-Fluorouracil
A	Doxorubicin
T	Thiotepa
V	Vincristine
P	Prednisone, cisplatin, carboplatin, carmustine
Cooper regimen and its derivatives[a]	
CMFVP	Cyclophosphamide, methotrexate, 5-fluorouracil, vincristine, prednisone
CMF	Cyclophosphamide, methotrexate, 5-fluorouracil
CMFP	Cyclophosphamide, methotrexate, 5-fluorouracil, prednisone
Combination regimens	
CMF	Cyclophosphamide, methotrexate, 5-fluorouracil
CAF	Cyclophosphamide, doxorubicin, 5-fluorouracil
FAC	5-Fluorouracil, doxorubicin, cyclophosphamide
AC	Doxorubicin, cyclophosphamide
Solid tumor autologous marrow program (STAMP) regimens	
STAMP I	Cyclophosphamide, cisplatin, carmustine (BCNU)
STAMP II	Ifosfamide, carboplatin, etoposide
STAMP III	Cyclophosphamide, thiotepa
STAMP IV	(antibiotic protocol)
STAMP V	Cyclophosphamide, thiotepa, carboplatin

[a] The letter sequence in a combination regimen corresponds to the sequence in which the individual chemotherapy drugs are administered.

disease, suggesting that the dose–response curve would be steeper in the adjuvant (or early-stage) setting than in the metastatic setting. This appeared to be true for the CMF regimen in breast cancer treatment, but results differed for pre- and postmenopausal women (Hortobagyi 2000, p. 588).

Dose intensification received a powerful stimulus from several articles published in the mid-1980s. In 1984, Hryniuk and Bush lamented: "Combination chemotherapy has failed to cure advanced disease, patients who have received adjuvant chemotherapy continue to relapse, and chemotherapy has not dramatically increased survival in Stage IV disease. Manipulations of doses, schedules, and combinations do not seem to improve results. Combination chemotherapy of breast cancer appears to have reached an impasse" (1984, p. 1281). Their review of metastatic breast cancer studies suggested that the Cooper regimen "might improve results," but that the high remission rates achieved by its developers were not matched by others. They calculated that published doses in other studies appeared higher than actual doses. In their view, a clear relationship existed "between response rate and average relative dose intensity," which was "even more evident" when actual doses delivered were correlated with response rate (p. 1282). Their conclusion, derived solely from the literature, had not been tested directly in a randomized clinical trial. Nevertheless, they asserted that "dose intensity of drugs actually delivered can be measured and manipulated and *may* [emphasis added] be a major determinant of response and survival" (p. 1288).

In 1986, Hryniuk and Levine extended the analysis: Could adjuvant CMF therapy for stage II breast cancer also be correlated to dose intensity? A retrospective analysis of 13 trials involving 6106 women led them to a startling conclusion: "The relationship between 3-year relapse-free survival and projected dose intensity is highly significant. ... [and] appears to be linear" (p. 1163). These results were "particularly remarkable" because the analysis included a wide variety of chemotherapy regimens. The then-director of the National Cancer Institute (NCI), Vincent DeVita, greeted the article enthusiastically in an accompanying editorial: "The use of a standard calculated for dose intensity ... is a brilliant simplification of a complex problem" (DeVita 1986, p. 1157). The article generated substantial enthusiasm among oncologists for the dose intensity concept, not least because of its endorsement by the NCI director. Thus, Hryniuk and colleagues set the stage for use of HDC/ABMT against both metastatic and high-risk breast cancer.

Not everyone was as confident as Hryniuk or as enthusiastic as DeVita. Craig Henderson had recommended against acceptance of the 1986 paper. He and Gelman published a critique in an obscure Swiss journal and later, with Daniel Hayes, an extended critique in the *Journal of Clinical Oncology* (Gelman and Henderson 1987; I. C. Henderson et al. 1988). The dose response was fundamental to pharmacology, and the efficacy and toxicity of most drugs, including cytotoxic drugs, increased with dose. "The assumption of a steep dose-response underlies the experimental design of many current clinical trials," they wrote, "including those using autologous bone marrow transplantation to ameliorate the [toxic] effects of high-dose therapy. However, few studies have specifically and systematically evaluated this principle in the clinic" (I. C. Henderson et al. 1988, p. 1501). They reviewed the data from animal studies, from retrospective studies of patients unable or unwilling to tolerate initially prescribed doses, and from the retrospective studies of Hryniuk and Levine that emphasized dose intensity. These studies suggested a hypothesis about dose rate "but neither analysis provides data to firmly establish the hypothesis" (I. C. Henderson et al. 1988, p. 1508). In short, the clinical evidence for dose response was inferential, with virtually no evidence of dose response for conventional treatment. A "promising pilot approach" by Peters required confirmation "in an appropriately controlled trial." The data from very-high-dose studies, Henderson and colleagues argued, did not "justify the use of this approach *outside an experimental setting* [emphasis added], especially in light of the very substantial morbidity, mortality, and cost of this type of therapy," but did provide "sufficient rationale to initiate randomized controlled trials ... especially among women with newly diagnosed metastases" (I. C. Henderson et al. 1988, p. 1511).

Henderson's criticisms were acknowledged in the literature but did not persuade his oncology colleagues. The Hryniuk analyses reinforced an already strong disposition toward high-dose regimens that characterized oncology in the 1980s. The view that "if some chemotherapy works, more is better" carried the day.

Bone Marrow Transplantation

Bone marrow transplantation is an offshoot of whole organ transplantation.[2] *Allogeneic* BMT involves infusing marrow cells from an immunologically compatible donor to the patient being treated. It had been applied therapeutically mainly to hematologic disorders and was described as "curative" for severe immunodeficiency, aplastic anemia, thalassemia, and leukemia and lymphoma (Hansen et al. 1989). *Autologous* BMT involves extracting a patient's marrow, preserving it through a freezing process, treating the patient's cancer with HDC, and reinfusing the patient's marrow cells in the hope that the hematologic and immunological capability depleted by chemotherapy will be restored.

The success of allogeneic transplantation in dealing with acute leukemia resistant to standard chemotherapy led investigators to use autologous transplantation against other cancers responsive to chemotherapy and radiation. Canellos (1985) compared the relative merits of allogeneic versus autologous BMT for treating non-Hodgkin's lymphoma. The former was limited by the few donors, patients in "a gross state of relapse," infections from suppressed immune systems, the limiting effect of prior chemotherapy on whole-body irradiation, and graft-versus-host disease, a severe complication of allogeneic transplantation in which the donor cells attack the transplant recipient. Autologous BMT was "more practical"; it not only obviated dependence on a limited number of donors and eliminated graft-versus-host disease GVHD, but also involved "compromised stem-cell reserve and marrow contamination by malignant cells" (p. 1452). Canellos emphasized that the use of ABMT with combination chemotherapy against solid tumors was clearly experimental.

High-dose chemotherapy destroys both malignant and healthy tissue even more than standard chemotherapy. The most vulnerable tissue is bone marrow, the source of red and white blood cells, platelets to control bleeding, and the immune system's capacity to repel foreign invaders. For HDC to work, it was essential to find a way to restore the cellular elements of healthy bone marrow destroyed after the administration of HDC. ABMT was that method. Frei and Canellos (1980) viewed transplantation as opening the possibility of increasing the chemotherapy dose 5- to 10-fold above the maximum achievable without transplantation, in contrast to studies in which the difference between high and standard dose was 2-fold or less.

Adjuvant Chemotherapy

Historically, primary treatment of breast cancer by surgery, or surgery with radiation, assumed that the cancer was physically confined to the breast. But, high recurrence after treatment led clinicians to believe that submicroscopic or occult cancers typically spread from the primary tumor to other areas of the body "before diagnosis and primary treatment with surgery and radiotherapy" (I. C. Henderson 1985, p. 140). Adjuvant therapy—"the use of cytotoxic drugs after primary therapy"—developed as oncologists sought "to eradicate occult metastatic disease which otherwise would be fatal" (National Institutes of Health [NIH] 1980, p. 2).

Initially, the HDC/ABMT procedure was applied to women with metastatic breast cancer. Soon after, it began to be used in the adjuvant setting with patients at high risk of recurrence who, at the time of primary treatment, were found to have cancer cells disseminated to their axillary lymph nodes. Advances in adjuvant chemotherapy were deemed sufficient to justify using the procedure against early-stage breast cancer. By the time HDC/ABMT emerged in the late 1980s, adjuvant chemotherapy had developed to the point at which it was standard therapy for a small set of patients: premenopausal women with positive lymph node involvement. Its use in other women was under intense study (I. C. Henderson 1985).

The evolution of adjuvant chemotherapy was documented in a series of NIH consensus conferences.[3] A 1980 conference concluded that efficacy had been established for adjuvant chemotherapy "with any degree of certainty" only for stage II "premenopausal breast cancer patients with histologic evidence of lymph node metastases who have undergone local therapy by mastectomy" (NIH 1980, p. 3). For these patients, survival benefits "appear to outweigh the disadvantages of early toxicity" (p. 4), but more research was needed to determine those for whom it was applicable. A 1985 NIH consensus conference noted that a number of clinical trials had been conducted since 1980 (NIH 1985). Even so, a "significant benefit" could be demonstrated only for premenopausal women with positive lymph nodes, for whom "highly significant disease-free survival and a significant reduction in mortality" had been demonstrated and for whom adjuvant chemotherapy could be considered "standard care" (I. C. Henderson 1985, p. 140). It was generally not recommended for premenopausal women with negative node involvement, and the efficacy for postmenopausal, node-positive women was "less well established." Careful research was needed.

A 1990 NIH consensus conference on the role of breast-conserving surgery versus mastectomy for early-stage (node-negative) breast cancer reported in passing that "adjuvant therapy has become the standard of care for the majority of cases of breast cancer with axillary lymph node involvement" (NIH 1990, p. 2; also NIH 1991). Clear evidence existed that local and distant breast cancer recurrence was decreased by both adjuvant chemotherapy and adjuvant tamoxifen.

Growth Factors

Human growth factors, also known as colony stimulating factors (CSFs) were developed in the 1980s to stimulate the production of blood cells. These factors can help blood-forming tissue recover from the effects of chemotherapy and radiation therapy. Two forms of CSF were studied as Investigational New Drugs (INDs): granulocyte colony-stimulating factor (G-CSF) and granulocyte-macrophage colony-stimulating factor (GM-CSF). In the 1980s, these drugs were made available for clinical research under the Schedule C program of the NCI, which provided oncology-related IND drugs to investigators before FDA approval. Peters and colleagues studied both GM-CSF and G-CSF clinically at the Duke University Bone Marrow Transplant Program (Brandt et al. 1988; Peters 1989). They reported in 1989 that colony-stimulating factors

> possess the capacity to enhance proliferative capacity of myeloid progenitors in patients undergoing intensive chemotherapy and bone marrow support, resulting in a decrease in the time to leukocyte and neutrophil recovery and an associated decrease in infectious complications compared to historical controls. Prospective evaluation and randomized comparative trials are needed to evaluate the final import of such factors. (p. 22)

The called-for studies generated evidence of safety and effectiveness that satisfied the FDA. In its February 21, 1991, announcement of approval of G-CSF, the FDA said that this new genetically engineered drug "stimulates the production of infection-fighting white blood cells . . . [that are] reduced or destroyed during many kinds of cancer chemotherapy" (FDA 1991, p. 1). G-CSF, manufactured by Amgen and marketed as Neupogen, is administered to reduce the duration of neutropenia and neutropenia-related clinical effects of myeloablative chemotherapy followed by marrow transplantation. GM-CSF, developed by Immunex and later sold to Berlex Laboratories and marketed as Leukine, was approved by the FDA on March 5, 1991. The indications for Leukine relevant to HDC/ABMT include myeloid reconstitution after ABMT and mobilization before and reconstitution after autologous peripheral blood stem cell transplantation and after transplantation failure or engraftment delay.[4]

The FDA approval of human growth factors occurred after the introduction of HDC/ABMT into clinical practice. Growth factors were enabling technologies: They accelerated recovery of immune function, thus reducing toxicities; they enhanced the efficiency of peripheral blood stem cell collection; and they reduced the costs of treatment by making it easier to provide in outpatient settings. The availability of FDA-approved growth factors provided a powerful stimulus to the rapid diffusion of HDC/ABMT as a breast cancer treatment.

The HDC/ABMT procedure built on the prior demonstration of combination chemotherapy as more effective than single agents. The heart of the procedure, HDC, was made technically feasible by ABMT. Growth factors enabled the reconstitution of the patient's immunological capability following treatment, reducing mortality, lowering toxicities, and shortening length of hospital stays.

New breast cancer treatments, as was true for HDC/ABMT, are often used initially to treat women with metastatic (stage IV) disease. The disease is often terminal, surgical and radiological treatment is not possible, and conventional chemotherapy and hormonal therapies are relatively ineffective. Treatment is palliative, not curative. As conventional treatment offers limited hope to patients, the willingness to take risks is often much greater. Although conventional treatments for metastatic breast cancer exist, they are often based on phase 2 studies; treatments based on phase 3 randomized clinical trials are more recent. When a new breast cancer treatment emerges, the woman with metastatic disease becomes, in effect, the experimental subject on whom the new approach is tried. Complete or partial tumor response to treatment is an important outcome.

By contrast, new treatments in the adjuvant setting of high-risk breast cancer patients (those with stage II or III disease) have often been evaluated in randomized clinical trials before widespread use. But, the HDC/ABMT procedure was soon applied in the adjuvant setting before randomized trials had been conducted. Hudis and Munster (1999) showed that in 1989–1990 fully 88% of the HDC/ABMT procedures were applied in the metastatic breast cancer setting and 12% in the adjuvant or neoadjuvant setting; by 1995, the proportions had shifted to 50% and 49%, respectively. The fateful branching we describe above occurred in both cases: Widespread clinical use began and was sanctioned concurrent with the initiation of randomized clinical trials. The promising procedure merited evaluation in such trials, but in neither setting did evidence of effectiveness exist that justified its widespread clinical use.

How Does a Procedure Emerge?

How does a new treatment emerge from clinical research? How is it recognized? How is it evaluated? How is it granted legitimacy as a medical procedure? Who is responsible for its evaluation and diffusion to clinical practice? Medical specialists involved with a given procedure know the answers to these questions quite well, but the historical development of a procedure is far less transparent to others. The opaqueness of a procedure's history complicates the task of some who must evaluate its effectiveness. So it was for HDC/ABMT. Here, we consider the role of the BMT specialists within oncology and that of phase 2 studies.

The Transplanters

Surgeons dominated the treatment of cancer until recent decades. Radiologists came to play a supporting role after World War II. Hematologists developed a similar role for leukemias and lymphomas. Only in the 1970s did medical oncology emerge as the primary cancer-treating specialty. Each group had its own treatment technology (surgery, radiotherapy, and chemotherapy) that depended partly on the prevailing concept of cancer and partly on the empirical outcomes of treatment. As oncology developed as a specialty, it confronted the challenge of differentiating itself from both surgery and radiation therapy. Within internal medicine, it faced hostility from chairs of major departments and from the subspecialty of hematology. Chemotherapy was viewed by many with great skepticism as little more than the administration of toxic chemicals to patients with a barely understood disease.

Oncology grew up in specialized cancer treatment centers. The most prominent centers included Memorial Sloan Kettering in New York City, M. D. Anderson Cancer Center in Houston, and the Dana-Farber Cancer Institute in Boston. Other centers developed after the National Cancer Act of 1971 (Rettig 1977). In the ensuing 30 years, however, academic medicine accommodated itself to oncology partly because of the enormous funds being invested in research, partly because the understanding of the disease and its treatment improved, and partly because cancer treatment had become financially lucrative.

Bone marrow transplantation developed within oncology primarily in specialized cancer centers and later migrated to academic medical centers. The Fred Hutchinson Cancer Center in Seattle is perhaps the most prominent BMT center, and Dr. E. Donnal Thomas, its Nobel laureate, is perhaps the most visible transplant physician. The "Hutch" has emphasized allogeneic BMT over the years and has historically limited its activity in ABMT.

The prominence of the Dana-Farber Cancer Institute in Boston was due in large part to the presence there of Dr. Emil (Tom) Frei III. A Yale Medical School graduate in 1948, he went to the NCI in 1955, where he would become chief of medicine (Dana-Farber Cancer Institute 2004). He would spend 1965 to 1972 at the M. D. Anderson Cancer Center, moving to the Children's Cancer Research Institute, as Dana-Farber was once known, in 1972. He served as physician-in-chief at the Farber until 1991. Frei was a pioneer in chemotherapy of children's cancers, especially leukemia. While at NCI, with Dr. Emil Freireich and Dr. James F. Holland, he devised the first children's combination chemotherapy treatment that led to complete remission of pediatric leukemia. He also became an advocate of HDC. In 2004, he would receive the first Award for Lifetime Achievement in Cancer Research from the American Association for Cancer Research.

It was at the Farber that HDC/ABMT for breast cancer treatment received its major impetus. Frei recruited Dr. Ron Yankee, a former NCI colleague, and began some of the earliest work on ABMT (Tobias et al. 1977). The initial program, pronounced head-cams, was HDCAMS (high-dose chemotherapy with autologous marrow support), and the chemotherapy regimen used high doses of cyclophosphamide and doxorubicin. This led to the Solid Tumor Autologous Marrow Program (STAMP) and the STAMP I through STAMP V regimens. These regimens included cyclophosphamide, commonly used against solid tumors; cisplatin (platinum), which has waxed and waned in use over time; and BCNU or vincristine.

It was also at the Farber where the Breast Evaluation Center, one of the first disease-oriented clinics, was developed. Organized by Dr. Craig Henderson, the clinic began in 1979 as an effort to bring all disciplines (surgery, radiology, oncology, as well as supporting services) to bear on treating breast cancer. This approach would be replicated across the country over time. Henderson was involved in HDC/ABMT in the 1980s and 1990s: He headed the Oxford breast cancer review from 1985 to 1995; chaired the breast committee of the Cancer and Leukemia Group B cooperative oncology group from 1989 to 1995; served as a member of the FDA's Oncology Drug Advisory Committee 1989–1992 and chaired the committee in 1990–1992. He also became the first external member of the Medical Advisory Panel to the Technology Evaluation Center of the Blue Cross Blue Shield Association in 1990.

Much of the early BMT work at the Farber focused on ovarian cancer but soon came to be used for breast cancer. Henderson recalls Frei calling him in January 1982 to say, "Craig, We have the cure for breast cancer" (C. Henderson 2002a). He was proposing to use STAMP I, a regimen of cyclophosphamide, cisplatin, and BCNU. Henderson responded critically because at that time both platinum and BCNU were considered relatively ineffective agents for the treatment of breast cancer. "You should develop the treatment with real breast cancer drugs. Use alkylating agents, multiple alkylating agents that work against breast cancer," he said (C. Henderson 2002a).

To develop and apply the concept of HDC/ABMT as a breast cancer treatment, Frei would recruit and mentor first Dr. William Peters and then Dr. Karen Antman. William Peters is a graduate of Pennsylvania State University with bachelor of science degrees in biochemistry and biophysics and a bachelor of arts in philosophy. He received a doctor of philosophy in human genetics and viral oncology in 1976 and his doctor of medicine degree in 1978, both from Columbia University. He spent 1979–1984 in Boston doing a residency at Harvard's Peter Bent Brigham Hospital; he joined the Dana-Farber Cancer Institute in 1982, first as a clinical associate in oncology and then as a clinical fellow to Frei. As a result of his work with Frei, Peters became the foremost advocate for HDC/ABMT, initially in its use against a number of solid tumors and then focused on breast cancer. Peters would be recruited by Duke University in 1984 to establish a BMT program, which he directed until 1995. At Duke, he rose from assistant to full professor and would add a master of business administration degree to his list of educational accomplishments. He would go to Detroit in 1995 as professor of oncology and medicine at Wayne State University and president, director, and chief executive officer of the Barbara Ann Karmanos Cancer Institute.

After Peters left Boston, Frei recruited Karen Antman to work on BMT for breast carcinoma from her research on sarcomas. Antman had received her doctor of medicine degree from Columbia University College of Physicians and Surgeons and had joined the Harvard Medical School faculty in 1979. She would serve as director of the STAMP program at the Farber. Antman remained in Boston until 1993, when she moved to Columbia University College of Physicians and Surgeons, where she was professor of medicine and pharmacology and director of the Herbert Irving Comprehensive Cancer Center. She would serve as president of the American Society of Clinical Oncology in 1994–1995 and as president of the American Association of Cancer Research in 2003–2004. In 2004, she joined the NCI and become the deputy director for translational and clinical sciences. In 2005, Boston University appointed her provost of the Medical Campus and dean of the School of Medicine.

Peters and Antman overlapped at the Farber but were highly competitive. Yet, their de facto collaboration would be a major factor driving HDC/ABMT for breast cancer treatment. Peters would use STAMP I as his treatment regimen; Antman would later use STAMP V. Peters and Antman were accomplished clinical scientists engaged in BMT. Both became advocates within medicine for the use of HDC/ABMT for treating breast cancer and for coverage of clinical trials by health insurers. They provided leadership for transplanters interested in breast cancer. Over time, others (oncologists, hospital administrators, and entrepreneurs) would join them, all inclined to believe that the promising but experimental HDC/ABMT was better than conventional therapy for breast cancer. Henderson saw things differently. He had developed HDC regimens without ABMT in the 1970s but grew increasingly skeptical in the following decade as scientific evidence supporting HDC/ABMT failed to materialize.

Phase 2 Studies

Phase 1 studies in oncology seek to demonstrate the tolerable doses of chemotherapeutic agents. Phase 2 studies constitute an area of experimentation in which researchers examine promising new treatments. These studies provide the initial test of therapeutic benefit, further refine knowledge of toxicity and related issues of dosage, and basically generate the hypotheses for further investigation. Typically, phase 2 studies are conducted at single institutions, involve relatively few patients, and usually involve a comparison to historical cases. Phase 3 randomized clinical trials are designed to test the hypotheses of phase 2 studies.

In oncology, they involve comparing the effectiveness of an experimental treatment to standard therapy relative to a specified outcome. They typically involve a number of institutions, involve more patients, and rely on randomization to control for biases.

Peters laid out the rationale for using HDC/ABMT to treat breast cancer patients in 1985 in a study of various solid tumors, including breast cancer (Peters 1985). In May 1986, Peters, Antman, and Frei reported the results of a phase 1 study of high-dose combination alkylating agents with ABMT, involving 29 patients, of whom 9 were patients with metastatic breast cancer; the others had metastatic colon cancer, melanoma, lung cancer, various sarcomas, and testicular cancer (Peters et al. 1986). The purpose of the study was to determine the maximum tolerable dose of HDC: Doses 3 to 15 times standard doses were administered before dose-limiting toxicity was encountered. This study progressed to a phase 2 trial in breast cancer within a few months (Eder et al. 1986). Seventeen patients with metastatic breast cancer, 13 of whom had received prior chemotherapy, were treated with HDC/ABMT; among the 16 patients who could be evaluated were 14 responders, including 6 complete responses. Tumor regression was rapid. The Dana-Farber investigators reported their phase 1 and 2 experiences against all solid tumors in early 1987 (Antman et al. 1987). Among the 59 patients who had received HDC were 19 patients with metastatic breast cancer, all but 2 of whom had received prior chemotherapy; 16 of these could be evaluated, with 6 achieving a complete response and 9 a partial response.

Peters also reported the results of a phase 2 trial of HDC/ABMT as the initial treatment of metastatic breast cancer patients in September 1988 (Peters et al. 1988). The reality facing doctors and patients with metastases was that "no curative therapy is available for treatment of metastatic breast cancer" (p. 1368). But, Peters argued, a steep dose–response effect had been demonstrated in both metastatic and adjuvant breast cancer. Hryniuk and Bush (1984) had demonstrated "a consistent correlation" between administered dose and objective responses in metastatic breast cancer. Experimental and clinical data had shown that alkylating agents had a steep dose–response relationship and could be increased 5 to 20 times beyond standard doses before dose-limiting toxicity occurred. Consequently, a trial had been undertaken "to determine the effect of high-dose alkylating agents in the treatment of breast cancer patients who had not received chemotherapy for metastatic disease" (Peters et al. 1988, p. 1373). Among 22 patients, 12 had achieved a complete response, and another 5 had a partial response, for an overall response rate of 77%. But, 5 therapy-related deaths were also reported. Median time from treatment to disease progression was 7.0 months, and median survival for all treated patients was 10.1 months, although that for complete responders had not been reached at 18 months. "These data suggest," Peters wrote, "that the regimen reported here exceeds conventional therapy in the frequency of complete responses, is comparable to but not superior to conventional therapy in both disease-free and overall survival, and is clearly more toxic" (p. 1374). But a "direct comparison" to conventional chemotherapy was difficult due to differences in "design, patient selection, and evaluation" and because "reliable, comparable response and survival data for short-term unmaintained conventional chemotherapy" (p. 1373) were unavailable.

Peters's study stimulated the extensive study of HDC/ABMT for treating metastatic breast cancer among his fellow oncologists at other medical centers. Williams and Bitran at the University of Chicago studied women with metastatic breast cancer who had not received prior chemotherapy (Williams et al. 1989). Twenty-seven eligible patients were enrolled between July 1986 and May 1988 and were treated with standard induction therapy: 4 had a complete response and 15 a partial response for an overall response rate of 70%. Of these 27 patients, 24 were eligible for "intensification" treatment, and 22 received the high-dose therapy: 12 achieved a complete response, 7 a partial response. The contrast between the low complete response rate of induction treatment and the higher rate of high-dose treatment was encouraging. Intensified treatment also resulted in greater conversion of partial response to complete response in 9 of 14 patients. The median time to treatment failure was a disappointing 10 months for all patients in the study and 6.2 months for those receiving intensified therapy. Of the initial 27 patients, 4 died of "treatment-induced toxicity," including 3 who received HDC. Even so, the authors concluded: "We continue to believe that autologous marrow transplants might be curative in women with stage IV breast cancer and we plan to continue investigation of future programs that will increase the complete response rate of the induction program so that more patients can attain complete responses before high-dose induction therapy" (p. 1829). An extension of this study added more women and modified the drug regimen for both induction and intensified treatment, but encountered liver toxicity problems. Soberly, in 1992, the investigators concluded that "the high cost of this treatment approach both in terms of morbidity and mortality and actual hospital costs" requires modification and should be "reserved for clinical trials in high-risk patients who have obtained clinical remissions, either complete responses or partial responses, after [initial induction] therapy" (Williams et al. 1992, p. 1747).

Many other medical centers were also conducting phase 2 studies of HDC/ABMT; most studies focused on metastatic breast cancer. A list compiled in 1989 included Dana-Farber and Duke University as well as the following principal investigators and centers: Michael Kennedy at Johns Hopkins University; Gary Spitzer at the M. D. Anderson Hospital in Houston; John Glaspy at UCLA; William Vaughn at the University of Nebraska; City of Hope; Karl Blume at Stanford; Hillard Lazarus at University Hospital, Cleveland; Thomas Shea at the University of California San Diego; Peter Rosen at the University of Southern California; Sharon Coleman at the University of California San Francisco; and Axel Zander at Pacific Presbyterian, San Francisco.[5] At the time, none of these individuals was considered specialists in breast cancer management. What mattered was that prominent oncologists in major cancer centers were reporting in the scientific literature a promising treatment for breast cancer. But, the results were not overwhelming. The HDC/ABMT procedure had high treatment-related mortality, was very toxic, and was very expensive. These early phase 2 results argued for testing the clinical hypothesis that HDC/ABMT was superior to standard treatment in larger randomized phase 3 clinical trials. Would these oncologists advocate for phase 3 trials or for taking the new therapy directly into clinical practice? The latter course would dominate, as we shall see.

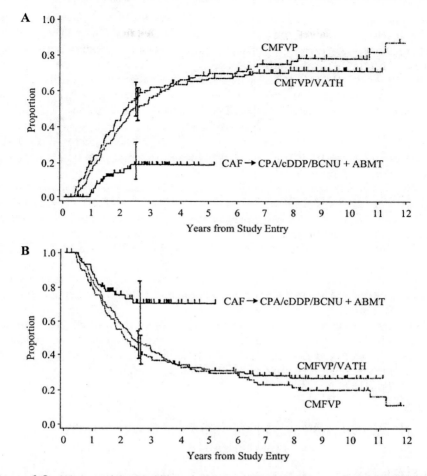

Figure 1.2. (A) Actuarial probability of relapse or (B) event-free survival for eligible and treated patients (CAF → CPA/cDDP/BCNU + ABMT) and for similar patients selected from two trials using adjuvant CMFVP (CALGB 7581) or CMFVP/VATH (CALGB 7581) or CMFVP/VATH (CALGB 8082). Vertical bars represent the 95% confidence intervals for each data set determined at 30 months. Tick marks indicate censored events. (See table 1.2 for definitions of drug abbreviations.) Reprinted from W. P. Peters et al. 1993 with permission from the American Society of Clinical Oncology.

Peters pioneered the use of the HDC/ABMT procedure, first in the patient with metastatic breast cancer, and soon applied it in high-risk patients. A widely cited 1993 article effectively sealed the discussion in favor of high-dose treatment for high-risk, poor prognosis—but not terminal—patients (Peters et al. 1993). Between February 1987 and January 1991, there were 102 patients who had been entered into a phase 2 trial, and 85 were treated with HDC/ABMT. Median follow-up was 2.5 years, with a range from 16 months to 5.2 years. Median age of patients was

38 years, with a range of 25 to 56 years. Ten patients had died of treatment-related mortality. Hospital charges, the authors indicated, ranged from $48,734 to $384,821, with a median of $88,836; these charges did not include harvesting bone marrow (median $6,276) or peripheral blood stem cells (median $5,100) or physician fees (~$8,500). Peters compared these patients with those receiving conventional adjuvant chemotherapy in two historical and one concurrent trial (figure 1.2). The figures showed dramatic differences in actuarial probability of relapse or event-free survival between the experimental treatment and the historical controls, sufficient to make the case for many that HDC was superior. It did not, however, present overall survival curves. This article, Henderson said, "drove the use of high dose chemotherapy more than any other" (C. Henderson 2002b).

We have, then, a promising new treatment for breast cancer applied first in the metastatic setting and soon after in the adjuvant setting. Use of HDC/ABMT in both settings called for evaluation in randomized clinical trials. But, rather than an orderly progression of scientific medicine before wider clinical use, evaluation and use began simultaneously. As the story developed, use would dominate evaluation.

In the next chapter, we examine how broad and conflicting general developments within oncology and health insurance set the stage for focused conflict regarding the HDC/ABMT procedure for treating breast cancer. Focused conflict in turn led to the fateful branching along two pathways: widespread clinical use of HDC/ABMT outside randomized clinical trials and the far slower but eventually more decisive path of clinical trials. Together, chapters 1 and 2 describe the initial conditions surrounding the emergence of the procedure and the course of events that characterized the decade of the 1990s.

2

Jumping the Gun

One easily believes what one earnestly hopes for.
—Terence

The inclusion of new treatments [in randomized trials] may legitimize them in [physicians'] minds as treatments worthy of trying in patients who have more severe forms of the target disease, who perhaps have failed to respond to other treatments, and who are viewed as having no alternative options. Existence of a national, peer-reviewed, funded trial signals that there is an enthusiastic group of practitioners who can provide the new treatment and whose patients may "deserve" to try it.
—W. F. Clark et al.

The high-dose chemotherapy with autologous bone marrow transplantation (HDC/ABMT) procedure, a promising but toxic new treatment for breast cancer, began diffusing rapidly into clinical practice just as randomized clinical trials were beginning, thereby "jumping the gun." Clark and colleagues in 2003 described a historical example of this phenomenon in a study of the early clinical use of apheresis, an experimental treatment. Use increased as the treatment was being evaluated in three randomized clinical trials, most of it outside the trials. Jumping the gun also characterizes the case of HDC/ABMT for breast cancer. How did the fateful branching to widespread clinical use occur just as randomized trials were beginning?

In this chapter, we describe the plate tectonic shifts that occurred in the 1980s in relations between medicine and health insurers and indicate how these set the stage for events bearing on HDC/ABMT. These shifts reveal oncology and health insurers moving at cross purposes relative to financing patient care costs of clinical trials, insurance coverage for experimental procedures, and criteria for evaluating effectiveness of new treatments. We describe the general developments that gave rise to conflict between health insurance and oncology. We then examine how oncologists, health insurers, and the National Cancer Institute (NCI), surprisingly, came together to initiate clinical trials of HDC/ABMT. Finally, we analyze how concurrent clinical use was legitimated by oncology, reinforced by the women's health movement, and reported by newspapers and television.

Health Insurance and Medicine in the 1980s

Health insurers have been challenged repeatedly in recent decades to respond to new medical treatments, technologies, and innovations. Slowly and haltingly they have developed institutions and strategies that ask for evidence of medical effectiveness as an input to coverage decisions. These developments have often brought them into conflict with medical innovators, as they did in the HDC/ABMT case.

Health insurance developed in the pre- and post-World War II period well before medical research began generating a continuing stream of new medical interventions. In recent years, insurers' response to new treatments has become a continuing challenge. "Medical necessity" provisions not only have anchored that response but also have revealed major problems with that reliance. Bergthold (1995) described medical necessity as "rarely defined, largely unexamined, generally misunderstood, and idiosyncratically applied in medical and insurance practice" (p. 181).

Historically, the term *medical necessity* has been a placeholder for health insurers that has served two functions over time. In the main, it has defined the medical services that are covered in insurance contracts under various benefit categories (i.e., hospital services, physician services, drugs, and durable medical equipment). In this respect, the term has essentially set the limits or boundaries of what is included or covered. In addition, typical medical necessity provisions, as defined in the evidence of coverage documents of insurers, have excluded coverage of experimental or investigational treatments a priori. Other provisions in a medical necessity definition that limit its scope under covered benefit categories include medical appropriateness for diagnosis, direct care, or treatment; standards of good medical practice; the most appropriate level of services (e.g., physician services, hospital services, drugs, durable medical equipment) that could safely be provided; and services not primarily for convenience (Bergthold 1995).

Elsewhere in health plan evidence of coverage documents, there are often additional exclusionary provisions that not only provide a general exclusion for experimental or investigational services (as specifically defined) but also exclude specific medical interventions or services, such as cosmetic surgery, dental implants, or in some cases during the 1990s, HDC/ABMT for breast cancer. A key point is that when coverage is excluded by benefit design (coverage categories) or by specific line item exclusions, medical necessity is irrelevant as coverage will always be excluded. Denials of specific services on the basis of the experimental or investigational exclusion or based on medical necessity, however, could be challenged on the basis of the process and the rationale for the decision. We discuss this in detail regarding HDC/ABMT litigation in chapters 3 and 4.

Notwithstanding medical necessity clauses and coverage exclusions of experimental or investigational treatments, these provisions were seldom invoked rigorously under fee-for-service medicine. Coverage of and payment for new procedures was often almost automatic among many insurers. Continuing double-digit growth in health expenditures in the 1980s forced change and stimulated a number of efforts to rein in health care costs. In 1983, Congress enacted a system for prospective payment for hospital services by Medicare and, by the decade's end, extended that to outpatient services. Private insurers began to follow, and there occurred a general movement away from fee-for-service medicine.

New medical technologies constituted a major factor in health care cost increases and became one driver of cost containment. A number of expensive new technologies had diffused rapidly before evaluation, including dialysis and kidney transplantation in the 1960s, computed tomography in the 1970s, and magnetic resonance imaging in the 1980s (Institute of Medicine 1985; Rettig 1991). This phenomenon drew the attention of health economists, who began to analyze the elements of increasing costs of health care. They concluded that roughly half of the annual increase in costs of health care could be attributed to the effects of new medical technologies (Newhouse 1992; Weisbrod 1991). Insurers were quite aware of these effects and the pressure they exerted on insurance premiums. Major corporations, as purchasers of health care, also became sensitive to new medical technologies as a source of increasing costs for employer-financed health insurance.

The awareness that many new medical procedures and technologies were not always evaluated for either their medical effectiveness or cost implications provided a major stimulus to technology assessment in medicine. An important Institute of Medicine (IOM) report published in 1985 enumerated the methods of technology assessment: randomized clinical trials, the series of consecutive cases, case studies, registries, sample surveys, epidemiologic studies, surveillance, meta-analysis, group judgment, cost-effectiveness and cost–benefit analysis, and mathematical modeling.[1] The appendix of that report and a later directory catalogued in great detail a large number of organizations engaged in technology assessment (IOM 1988).

One technology assessment approach emphasized group judgment and typically focused on the National Institutes of Health's (NIH's) consensus development conferences, which had begun in the mid-1970s. Consensus conferences raised the methodological questions of how physician experts make decisions about effective medical interventions when data are scarce or absent and about the validity of such decisions. A different approach developed in the mid-1980s, the systematic examination of the evidence of effectiveness as found in the medical literature. This movement toward evidence-based medicine would in time displace concern for the weaker methods of consensus development.

Technology assessment based on a systematic review of the evidence took hold among a number of insurers in the late 1980s and early 1990s as a way to make more informed coverage decisions (see chapter 7). The Blue Cross Blue Shield Association (BCBSA), representing 70-some independent Blue Cross plans, was a leader in this effort. In the mid-1980s, it established an internal analytical capability, the Technology Evaluation and Coverage (TEC) program, to evaluate systematically the effectiveness of medical interventions and advise the independent plans on coverage decisions. Assessments were available only to BCBSA member plans. A medical advisory committee, consisting entirely of Blue Cross medical directors initially, aided the program. (Craig Henderson was appointed as the first external member of this committee; other outside experts were added later.) Central to this effort were explicit and rigorous evaluation criteria (first established in 1985) for judging whether evidence of clinical effectiveness existed for a given intervention (see chapter 7, table 7.1). These developments would push the BCBSA into evaluating investigational procedures, which were becoming important for their coverage, reimbursement, and cost implications.

The TEC program was expanded in 1993 and renamed the Technology Evaluation Center. Kaiser Permanente joined as a sponsor of the program. The medical advisory committee was changed to include a majority of voting members with no Blue Cross affiliation, and Dr. Wade Aubry was named chairman. TEC ceased making coverage recommendations, restricting itself to determinations that an intervention did or did not meet the evaluation criteria. Assessments were made available to non–Blue Cross organizations by subscription. It has since generated a growing library of assessments of diagnostic and therapeutic interventions to assist member plans.

But, the BCBSA was not alone. Many other insurers and health plans developed technology assessment capabilities to aid in making coverage decisions. Similar efforts were initiated at Kaiser Permanente in southern and northern California that laid the foundation for joining the BCBSA effort. Group Health Cooperative of Puget Sound developed its own capability. In Minnesota, the Institute for Clinical Systems Integration, a collective effort of managed care organizations in that state, established both clinical guidelines and technology assessment efforts. Aetna created a technology assessment program, recruiting William McGivney from the American Medical Association (AMA). In addition, several analytical organizations, such as ECRI, began providing assessment services to smaller insurers (Rettig 1997).

For most of the health insurance industry, however, the inertia of medical necessity dominated coverage decision making well into the 1990s. The language of coverage was binary and blunt—either a procedure was covered or it was not. If experimental or investigational, then it was not covered. Not all insurers were committed to evidence-based coverage decision making. Policies, practices, and decisions varied greatly across insurers. In many cases, companies relied simply on the judgment of individual medical directors. As a result, the coverage decisions of individual health plans often appeared quite arbitrary at both the policy level and for individual patients (Newcomer 1990; Peters and Rogers 1994).

The evolution of technology assessment during this period allowed a number of major insurers and health plans to become much more sophisticated than they had been in making coverage decisions. The resulting increased scrutiny of new treatments often surprised both clinical researchers and community physicians, given the pattern that had existed under fee-for-service medicine. Some were aware of the development of technology assessment among health insurers. Many became aware of this development when a specific coverage request for a particular patient was denied. Many more were surprised at insurers asking for evidence of medical effectiveness.

Financing Oncology Clinical Trials

As health insurance was moving toward greater scrutiny of new treatments, medicine, especially the field of oncology, was moving in a somewhat different direction. In the mid-1980s, a number of forces were creating increasingly stringent resource constraints on medical research. Wittes in 1987 identified three powerful forces that threatened the progress of biomedical research: general health cost containment; the explicit exclusion by insurers of reimbursement for investigational treatments; and federal government deficit reduction, which limited all federal spending, including that for medical research. Cost containment pressures came from the federal government and private insurers. In 1983, Congress adopted prospective payment for Medicare hospital services. By early 1988, the Health Care Financing Administration (predecessor to the Centers for Medicare and Medicaid Services) was beginning to revise payment policies to price outpatient services prospectively, potentially affecting outpatient cancer centers. The oncology community expressed a fear that private insurers would follow the government's lead.

In addition, federal budget deficits were affecting all government agencies. Under President Ronald Reagan, the federal deficit grew to more than $200 billion annually (unadjusted) and ranged between 3% and 6% of gross domestic product in the two terms from 1982 to 1988. In the single term of President George H. W. Bush, the deficit ranged from slightly less than 3% of gross domestic product in 1 year to well over 4% in 2 years. These deficits produced intense pressures on the budgets of all federal government agencies. Congressional appropriations for the NCI hovered just under $1 billion from 1980 through 1983, breaching that threshold at $1,081,581 only in 1984 (NIH 1980–1989). Appropriations then grew from $1,183,806 in 1985 to $1,570,349 in 1989. Funding for the cooperative cancer groups, which conduct phase 3, NCI-approved clinical trials, was relatively stable. The *Cancer Letter* reported that 1989 funding for cooperative clinical research of $60 million faced a potential cut to $56.6 million if a Gramm-Rudman sequester (a draconian measure sometimes used to control federal budget deficits in this period) could not be avoided (*Cancer Letter* 1989).

In this context, the support of patient care costs of clinical trials by third-party insurers was raised as early as 1983 (Chalmers et al. 1983; Gelband and Office of Technology Assessment 1983). The issue was joined in earnest when Dr. Robert Wittes, then head of the NCI's Cancer Therapy Evaluation Program, asked rhetorically "Who is responsible?" for such costs (Wittes 1987). He framed the answer in a way that still dominates thinking: The value of biomedical research was axiomatic, the relief of suffering required no "elaborate justification," and the payoff from such research had been handsome. The three powerful countervailing forces mentioned above threatened research progress. His primary target was investigational exclusions by health insurers.

Clinical research—"the final common pathway for testing new treatments"—was jeopardized (Wittes 1987, p. 108). Clinical trials, which were "obviously necessary," were also expensive. Therefore, Wittes (1987) wrote that the "fostering of clinical trials research is a shared endeavor for which all interested parties must take explicit and purposeful responsibility" (p. 108). "What treatment can be classified as research?" Wittes asked, and he provided five answers: any treatment provided in a prospective clinical trial; a new treatment being compared to conventional care; any [drug] regimen not licensed by the Food and Drug Administration (FDA) for the use in question; any treatment not yet licensed by the FDA for any indication; and any regimen not yet considered standard medical practice (p. 108). Each definition had drawbacks for making reimbursement policy, but Wittes gave the benefit of doubt to new treatments. Experimental treatments were "generally less well characterized," he wrote, but usually "a substantial body of information [existed] indicating that the test treatment may have significant advantages compared to the [conventional] control" (p. 108).

Wittes called for shifting patient care costs of clinical trials from the public treasury to private insurers. Research sponsors such as the NCI, he argued, were in a weak position to assume full costs of such an episode of patient care. Phase 1 and 2 trials were often financed by NCI research grants, but the costs of phase 3 trials not financed by the pharmaceutical industry were borne by the NCI budget for the cancer cooperative groups, which had remained fairly stable for a long period of time. Therefore, the costs of phase 3 trials could easily create an unwelcome budget impact if unreimbursed by insurers. Wittes rejected as unreasonable the insurers' use of "investigational" as a criterion for excluding any payment. A more reasonable payment system would differentiate the costs of patient care from those of research. Investigational exclusion clauses that denied coverage for an entire episode of care hampered the rational allocation of resources between conventional and investigational treatments.

Wittes (1987) found it "easy" to outline a satisfactory solution to the problem. "A reasonable insurance system," he wrote, "ought to reimburse all medical care that is effective, whether investigational or not" (p. 110). "If there is only partially effective treatment or no effective treatment for a particular condition," he continued, "insurance ought to pay for the patient care costs of investigational treatment that has adequate scientific justification" (p. 110). He glided over the meaning of "effective" and "adequate scientific justification," implicitly suggesting that such determinations should be made by the NCI.

"Why should insurance cover the patient care costs of developmental therapy?" Wittes (1987, p. 110) asked. He advanced a moral argument that insurers should act in "the real interests of their constituency" (p. 110), namely, patients. Although trials might generate data on clinical and cost-effectiveness, "truth, justice, and societal responsibility" provided little financial incentive for any individual insurance company, he wrote, "to proceed alone along the lines we have outlined" (p. 111). An industrywide solution was necessary, which paid patient care costs through existing reimbursement mechanisms. Anything else would be "extremely disruptive" (p. 111).

Wittes' viewpoint was reiterated in July 1988 when Karen Antman, Lowell Schnipper, and Emil Frei III wrote that cancer clinical research was in jeopardy due to the combined effect of federal budget constraints, the increasing costs of care, and "the recent refusal of some third-party payers to support the cost of patient care as part of research trials" (Antman et al. 1988, p. 46). This was true, despite research advances of prior decades that had led to curative therapy for some cancers and improved palliative care for others. The problem was that "health insurance companies have refused to cover investigational therapy" for financial reasons (p. 46).

Who then should pay for clinical research? If patients were to pay, then access to new therapies would be limited to affluent patients. Including such costs in federal government research grants would create "unacceptable financial pressure" on the NIH budget (Antman et al. 1988, p. 47). Asking the pharmaceutical industry to assume more than the costs of drugs and clinical trial-related costs would be "a major financial disincentive" to drug research (p. 47). But "[i]n the appropriate clinical setting, investigational treatment should be equated with 'state of the art' care" and "the 'best' patient care should be covered by third-party payers" (p. 47). Although short-term costs of care might increase," the authors said, medical costs and productivity losses decrease when new treatments lead to "curative therapy" (p. 47). "In the long run," they claimed, "clinical investigation is cost-effective" (p. 47). The Dana-Farber investigators (Antman et al. 1988) concluded:

> The current system of refusing to pay the costs of hospitalization when patients receive investigational therapy is expensive to monitor, unfair to many patients, and arbitrary in distinguishing between best available patient care and investigative treatment. By refusing to cover the costs of investigational therapy, third-party carriers are in fact making decisions about the medical care of patients. In practice, they are equating investigational treatment with no treatment. If the health insurance industry does not cover investigational therapy, only affluent patients will have access to promising treatments, and both progress in clinical cancer research and, ultimately, treatment for all will be seriously compromised. (p. 48)

The argument would be repeated again in an October 1989 consensus statement issued by eight organizations recommending that "third party coverage be allowed for patient-care costs of all nationally approved (National Cancer Institute [NCI] or FDA) cancer treatment protocols" and for all protocols "not subject to national approval, provided [they] have been approved by established peer review mechanisms" (McCabe and Friedman 1989, p. 1585).[2]

In short, the NCI and academic researchers held that the refusal of insurers to pay for the patient care costs of experimental procedures constituted a major barrier to clinical research. Their viewpoint supported access to experimental cutting-edge treatments; shifting the costs of evaluation, especially patient care costs, from public to private sources; reliance on researchers to determine the meaning of effective medical care and adequate scientific justification; and a moral obligation of insurers to patients that embraced all NCI clinical trials (phases 1, 2, and 3), not just high-priority trials.

Not surprisingly, the argument that insurers should finance the patient care costs of clinical trials met stiff resistance. Insurers were moving in an opposite direction. Under increasing pressure from purchasers, especially large employers, they were moving rapidly away from fee-for-service reimbursement and toward cost containment, including reining in the costs of new treatments. Aubry (2002) described how insurers saw their traditional refusal to support procedures of unproven effectiveness:

> It was not the role of insurers to support research. Our role was to provide health coverage for accepted medical practice. Historically, this meant coverage of licensed professionals within the framework of their professional scope of practice. It then came to mean coverage of effective procedures based on data. It was the role of the government, of foundations, and of the drug industry, to pay for research. The payoffs to research went to developers, not to insurers. It was also important for insurers to establish consistency, equity, and fairness in their coverage policies. Why should there be special treatment of any given procedure? This would undermine our business position of fairness relative to everything else. (Aubry 2002)[3]

But, as some insurers were asking for evidence from randomized clinical trials in making coverage decisions, most were also asserting that financing research was not their business. They would not reap the benefits of research, they would incur additional costs, and they would underwrite higher charges for services billed to them later by physicians and hospitals as a result.

The Evaluation of New Treatments

Important segments of medicine, including oncology, were moving in a direction opposite that of insurers regarding the evaluation of new treatments. Although this movement focused on early access to new drugs, not procedures as we have described HDC/ABMT, the general principles shaped perceptions within the field of oncology and bore directly on HDC/ABMT.

The highly regulated process of new drug development begins with preclinical laboratory and animal studies and proceeds to extensive testing in humans. It requires FDA approval of a drug for safety and effectiveness before it can be marketed commercially. In general, phase 1 clinical studies test the toxicity of a new drug, typically in a small number of healthy volunteers. Phase 2 studies provide the initial test of therapeutic benefit, or effectiveness, in a larger number of patients having the disease in question; they further refine knowledge of toxicity and related issues of dosage and basically create the hypothesis for further investigation. Phase 3 studies, randomized clinical trials, seek to confirm the clinical hypothesis and establish the definitive safety and effectiveness profile of the new drug by comparing it to a placebo or standard therapy. Phase 3 studies require still larger numbers of patients, calculated by a statistical power analysis that is intended to determine whether a prespecified treatment effect (the difference between the experimental and control arms) is or is not attributable to chance.[4] Phase 3 trials are typically multi-center, both to obtain the needed number of patients and to rule out a treatment bias that might derive from a single site of care in a phase 2 study.

Phase 1, 2, and 3 drug trials are conducted under an FDA-approved Investigational New Drug (IND) application. Once the definitive trials have been completed, the data are submitted to the FDA in a New Drug Application (NDA) for review. If the FDA concludes that the new drug is safe and effective, then the drug is approved for marketing. Phase 4 studies, also known as postmarketing evaluation studies, are often conducted after the FDA has approved a drug. The FDA may require that the drug be studied in wider clinical practice to allay safety concerns identified in the review process. In addition, drug firms often initiate such studies to understand better the use of a drug in ordinary clinical practice or to expand the labeled indications for use.

Cancer chemotherapy drugs are evaluated somewhat differently from other drugs. Determinations about effectiveness require judgment about how much damage to normal cells can be tolerated in the effort to kill cancerous cells. Consequently, phase 1 studies in oncology, which test the allowable level of toxicity, typically involve patients with a cancer for which no effective treatment exists or for whom treatment has failed (or predictably will fail). Healthy volunteers are ruled out on ethical grounds as most chemotherapy drugs are toxic and cause harm. Phase 2 studies of new anticancer agents test for therapeutic effect, typically tumor response, in sick patients for whom standard therapy is known to be ineffective or nonexistent. Phase 3 studies in cancer, usually large, randomized trials, evaluate the risk–benefit relationship between toxicity and outcomes of treatment, which include tumor response (both complete response and partial response), overall survival, event-free or disease-free survival, and patient quality of life.[5]

One major issue driving change in this system has been the demand of patients and physicians for early access (i.e., before final FDA approval) to investigational new drugs. The treatment IND rule, proposed in 1983 and adopted by the FDA in 1987, responded to this demand (21 CFR § 312.34). It provided that a drug under investigation in a clinical trial might be made available to patients with "serious or immediately life-threatening" diseases for which "no comparable or satisfactory alternative" existed. The stated purpose of the rule was "to facilitate the availability of promising new drugs to desperately ill patients as early in the drug development process as possible, before general marketing begins, and to obtain additional data on the drug's safety and effectiveness" (21 CFR § 312.34a). For serious diseases, an investigational drug might be made available during phase 3 studies; for immediately life-threatening diseases, it might be made available during phase 2 studies.

The principles behind the treatment IND rule were extended in 1988. In that year, the FDA responded to the advocacy by gay men for early access to investigational drugs for treating acquired immunodeficiency syndrome (AIDS) by adding subpart E (21 CFR § 312.80–312.88) to the regulations governing drugs being reviewed under IND regulations. This new authority was intended "to expedite the development, evaluation, and marketing of new therapies intended to treat persons with *life-threatening and severely-debilitating illnesses* [emphasis added], especially where no satisfactory alternative exists" (§312.80). Life-threatening diseases were defined a having a high likelihood of death "unless the course of disease is interrupted" (§312.81(a)(1)) and severely debilitating diseases as those that caused "major irreversible morbidity" (§312.81(b)). The regulation called for early consultation between the FDA and sponsors of new drugs, including an "end-of-phase 1 meeting" (§312.82(b)). The primary purpose of this meeting was "to review and reach agreement" on the design of phase 2 controlled clinical trials, "with the goal that such testing will be adequate to provide sufficient data on a drug's safety and effectiveness to support a decision on its approvability for marketing" (§312.82(b)). In the regulation, the FDA acknowledged the need for a judgment on whether the benefits of a drug outweighed the "known and potential risks," especially in light of "the severity of the disease and the absence of satisfactory alternative therapy" (§312.84(a)). In short, the 1988 regulation was designed to allow for more rapid access of AIDS patients to investigational new drugs before phase 3 trials had been completed.

Subpart E generated pressures on the FDA to speed the approval of new chemotherapy agents. In 1988, Vice President George H. W. Bush, as chair of the Presidential Task Force on Regulatory Relief, asked the President's Cancer Panel to review issues related to the use of INDs in oncology. In response, the panel created the National Committee to Review Current Procedures for Approval of New Drugs for Cancer and AIDS, chaired by Dr. Louis Lasagna of Tufts University. This blue ribbon committee, representing the leadership of American oncology, examined the use of new cancer and AIDS drugs being studied under an IND application. The committee's report would lay down general principles and detailed recommendations about making new cancer treatments available to patients as early as possible.

The committee held 10 meetings across the country in 1989 and 1990 and submitted its report in August 1990 to Dr. Armand Hammer, chair of the panel; Dr. Samuel Broder, director of the NCI; and Dr. Louis Sullivan, Secretary of Health and Human

Services, and then presented it directly to then-President Bush on August 15 (*Cancer Letter* 1990b). The report was concerned primarily with the FDA issues: the need for more and better drugs for cancer and AIDS; expediting approval of important new drugs; the standard for effectiveness of new drugs; and the use of surrogate endpoints in clinical trials. Several actions intended to weaken FDA authority were recommended: a "permanent policy and oversight" committee to the Secretary of Health and Human Services to monitor the FDA; substitution of institutional review board approval for FDA approval to promote study in humans of potential drugs being investigated in phase 1 studies; institutional review board approval in lieu of FDA approval of phase 1 and 2 noncommerical clinical research aimed at finding new uses for marketed drugs; and outside review of NDAs (President's Cancer Panel 1990).

The committee noted that the FDA had the statutory authority to approve new drugs on the basis of one scientifically valid study and on the basis of phase 1 and 2 studies without the need for a phase 3 study. It recommended that the agency use this authority to approve drugs for marketing at the earliest possible time in their development and commended the FDA for its early approval of new AIDS drugs (President's Cancer Panel 1990).

The committee recommended that FDA's willingness to consider surrogate endpoints for AIDS drugs be extended to other disease areas. (Surrogate endpoints are biological outcomes, e.g., tumor response, that are believed to predict clinical benefit, such as increased survival and improved quality of life.) It called for research that would correlate surrogate and "ultimate" (i.e., clinical) endpoints, develop general principles for surrogate endpoints, and allow quality-of-life assessments to serve as a basis for regulatory approval. Since many years might be needed to demonstrate survival differences for slow-growing tumors, such as ovary, breast, colon, and other common tumors, it stated, "survival is in general an impractical and unethical endpoint for cancer drugs" (President's Cancer Panel 1990, p. 5). Few approved drugs had demonstrated an independent effect on survival; most produced tumor regression in certain cancers. When used in combination for selected tumors, "a major improvement in survival and cure has occurred" (p. 5).

The committee also expressed concern about insurance coverage. It recommended that coverage of investigational drugs be based primarily on their approval by expert government agencies (NCI approval of group C cancer drugs, FDA approval of drugs under treatment INDs or on their status in authoritative medical compendia namely, the American Hospital Formulary Service, U.S. Pharmacopeia–Dispensing Information, and American Medical Association Drug Evaluation) and not on decisions by insurers themselves. These decisions were more valid than FDA approval of an NDA, the committee stated. Coverage should be identical "under Medicare, Medicaid, and private insurance" and should not vary across states or regions or by [Medicare] carrier.[6] The committee further recommended that coverage be automatic once a drug had been approved in one of the compendia, and that individual carriers should have no discretion in the matter. Finally, it recommended that "the touchstone of drug coverage should be the medical judgment of the attending physician" (President's Cancer Panel 1990, p. 14).

The American Society of Clinical Oncology (ASCO) endorsed the committee's recommendations, both as directed to the FDA and to public and private health insurers. In a policy statement, it recommended that Congress "eliminate [Medicare] carrier discretion" on drug coverage issues and require that indications listed in the compendia or "supported in the peer reviewed medical literature" be covered. "Further, Congress should explore ways to compel individual private insurance companies—now free from federal regulation—to develop fair and rational coverage policies" (ASCO 1990, p. 1).

The recommendations of the Lasagna committee laid the basis for the FDA's accelerated approval regulations of 1992 for "serious or life-threatening illnesses" (21 CFR § 314.500–560). Subpart H, as these regulations were called, provided the FDA the authority to approve a new drug for marketing on the basis of an effect on a "surrogate endpoint that is reasonably likely . . . to predict clinical benefit" (§ 314.510) or on a clinical endpoint other than survival or irreversible morbidity (e.g., quality of life). Approval of a new drug under subpart H would subject sponsors to the requirement of further study to verify a drug's clinical benefit if uncertainty existed about the relation of the surrogate endpoint to clinical benefit or about the relation of the measured clinical benefit to "ultimate outcome" (§ 314.510).

The FDA's adoption of the treatment IND in 1987, subpart E in 1988, and subpart H in 1992 represented the success of efforts to make new drugs for AIDS and cancer available to patients as early as possible. These changes constituted a lowering of the bar of evidence required for FDA approval of new drugs. They clearly reflected the prevailing views within the leadership of oncology.

In the course of preparing its report, the Lasagna committee invited two representatives of the health insurance industry to meet with it. David Tennenbaum, who directed the BCBSA's Medical Necessity project, and Dr. David Plocher, of Prudential Insurance Company (representing the Health Insurance Association of America), encountered hostile questioning from the committee (*Cancer Letter* 1989). Tennenbaum had asserted that evidence of improved health outcomes was essential to good coverage decisions, and that cost was not a consideration in the assessment of new procedures. The dean of the University of Chicago School of Medicine, Dr. Samuel Hellman, rejected this: "You have just said that you require proof of efficacy for reimbursement . . . so you can protect subscribers' interest. But are insurance clerks more capable of determining treatment efficacy and quality care than a physician? You are confusing efficacy and quality of care with the cost issue—you're unable to pay and inadequate proof of efficacy is a mask for hiding the real reason" (Antoine 1989, p. 1766).

Tennenbaum clashed with NCI's director at that time, Dr. Samuel Broder. The BCBSA representative emphasized that "conclusive scientific evidence" of improved health outcomes "such as length of life, ability to function and quality of life" was necessary for coverage eligibility. He expressed concern that treatment IND drugs and NCI group C drugs had not been demonstrated as warranting full FDA approval. "Proposed coverage for treatment INDs brings to the forefront the broader issue of coverage for all investigational technologies, drugs, treatments, procedures and devices," he said (*Cancer Letter* 1989, p. 1). Neither treatment IND drugs nor Group C drugs were eligible for coverage. "We strongly object to your statement, strongly and vigorously," Broder retorted. "There is no way I can say how strongly we object to that . . . There's no scientific basis for that decision. This is an arbitrary decision" (*Cancer Letter* 1989, p. 1).

The broad principles that Wittes and others articulated about financing cancer clinical trials and those advocated by the Lasagna committee about the early use of investigational drugs made clear that oncology and health insurers were moving in opposite directions. Although focused on chemotherapy drugs, the views extended to procedures such as HDC/ABMT. The leadership of oncology had concluded that insurers should pay for patient care costs of all NCI trials; insurers were adamant that supporting research was not their business. Oncology was recommending that the FDA approve new cancer drugs on the basis of surrogate endpoints; insurers were emphasizing health (or clinical) outcomes, especially survival, as the basis for coverage. Oncology was proposing that the FDA demonstrate flexibility and approve new drugs on the basis of phase 2 studies; insurers were asking for data from phase 3 randomized clinical trials. Oncology claimed for itself the authority to determine medical effectiveness; insurers, in asking for clinical trial data, were challenging the authority of the individual physician to prescribe for an individual patient.

Not only did oncology and health insurers approach HDC/ABMT from quite different conceptual perspectives, they did so in the absence of an institutional framework for evaluation of procedures comparable to that for new drugs. All parties to the discussion of new drug review and approval—from the president on down—understood that oncology, including the leadership of the NCI, had to engage the FDA. No such framework exists for oncology to engage private health insurers. This meant that conflict over HDC/ABMT would play out against a larger background than either could control.

Outcomes of Conflict: Recognition and Randomized Clinical Trials

Conflict between health insurers and oncology regarding the HDC/ABMT procedure for breast cancer would produce two outcomes. Randomized clinical trials of HDC/ABMT would be initiated, and the procedure would be launched simultaneously on a path of wider clinical use. Before we address these developments, though, we consider how insurers and oncologists differed in their recognition of HDC/ABMT as a new treatment.

Recognition of a New Procedure

The recognition of a new drug follows a highly regulated and highly visible process. The progress of a new drug through clinical trials, the FDA's review, and the recommendation of an advisory committee are all followed closely in the trade press. The FDA approves or disapproves a drug on a date specific in a letter to the commercial sponsor, and announcement of that is also widely reported and often has an immediate effect on that firm's stock price. The marketing launch of a newly approved drug is often timed to coincide with publication in a leading medical journal of an article on the definitive trial by the principal investigator.

The highly structured recognition of a new drug stands in marked contrast to the poorly structured interaction between physicians and insurers regarding new procedures. Within medicine, a new procedure is first recognized in the cloistered confines of clinical research. It is often announced informally by an investigator through guest speaking engagements, at symposia and professional meetings (in both abstracts and posters), and only then formally in the scientific literature. As a procedure's use expands, patients become increasingly involved, and advocacy groups may promote its wider use. Seeking coverage for the new procedure, hospitals and physicians file claims and hope insurers pay without asking questions. If insurers require justification, then physicians will generally provide a rationale for medical necessity.

Recognition of a new procedure by insurers is less straightforward. They are strongly oriented to claims data and more attentive to the formal medical literature than to informal symposia and professional meetings. In fact, as HDC/ABMT emerged, insurers relied increasingly on the peer-reviewed journal literature to support medical necessity determinations. One consequence of this orientation to the published literature is that insurers typically lag the medical profession in recognizing a new procedure, thereby placing themselves at a disadvantage regarding the existing and developing body of scientific evidence.

In the case of HDC/ABMT for breast cancer, the new treatment became visible to insurers quickly as it was substantially more costly than existing treatments, and the number of potential patients was very large. As early as 1988, some patients, assisted by transplanters, had begun to seek insurance coverage for HDC/ABMT, and some physicians had begun to bill insurers for the procedure. As is often true for new procedures, billing used existing procedure codes or components of existing procedures. Often, there was legitimate confusion on how to bill. Some billings revealed to insurers that a new—and expensive—procedure was being used to treat breast cancer patients. Dr. Wade Aubry, then senior vice president and medical director for Blue Shield of California, recalls receiving the first requests for ABMT coverage in late 1988 (Aubry 2002). Initially, these requests were not recognized as ABMT: some were seen as high-dose chemotherapy, some as harvesting of bone marrow, and some as transplantation.

In mid-1989, however, the requests for ABMT coverage began increasing dramatically. Blue Shield of California received letters from physicians, mostly in southern California, associated with the Kenneth Norris Cancer Center, affiliated with the University of Southern California; City of Hope; University of California at Los Angeles; Stanford; Scrips; and University of California at San Francisco. Most requests were for harvesting of bone marrow, and some were for treatment, mostly for women with metastatic breast cancer who had failed other treatments. Blue Shield turned down these initial coverage requests as investigational, and these decisions were not initially challenged. They began to be challenged in late 1989, however, through internal grievance procedures but were not yet in litigation. Similar challenges to other Blue Cross Blue Shield plans were occurring nationally, with some plans being sued.

The conflict between oncologists and health insurers regarding coverage became very visible as the HDC/ABMT controversy unfolded. When the procedure was assessed initially, no data indicated persuasively that HDC/ABMT was as good as or more effective than conventional treatment in improving survival; it was also highly toxic, had a high treatment-related mortality, and was very expensive. Although explicit consideration of cost was not included in formal assessments of HDC/ABMT, this factor, when coupled with the absence of evidence of effectiveness, led most health insurers to deny coverage on grounds that the procedure was experimental or investigational. In turn, these denials raised the question of who should pay for the patient care costs of HDC/ABMT in clinical trials.

Health Insurers and Randomized Clinical Trials

Health insurers responded to the experimental, expensive, and visible nature of HDC/ABMT in three ways in 1988–1990. Many denied coverage for the procedure; some conducted formal technology assessments; still others financed randomized trials directly in 1990 or shortly after created new ways to do so. But, no matter how they responded, insurers were vulnerable to the charge of acting in their financial self-interest in their coverage denials, their resistance to paying for clinical trials, and their insistence on evidence of effectiveness. Physicians were usually very hostile to health insurers for these reasons.

Health insurers were not ambivalent about the need for randomized trials to provide the evidence that HDC/ABMT was effective treatment. Their assessments of the medical literature concluded that the existing data did not justify the provision of HDC/ABMT outside clinical trials. Most were adamant that they had no obligation to pay for patient care costs of such trials. Whereas costs for standard chemotherapy for metastatic breast cancer might run as high as $30,000 to $40,000 per patient, HDC/ABMT charges could easily run as high as $150,000, with a potential for going much higher if complications occurred, as they required weeks and sometimes months of hospitalization, more highly trained professional staff, and the complicated administration of bone marrow transplantation.

The issue of health insurers paying for clinical research was being actively discussed as HDC/ABMT emerged. The BCBSA found the discussion frustrating as disclosure was difficult on both sides. Sue Gleeson, director of medical and quality management for the BCBSA, who oversaw the development of the association's technology assessment program, recalled a late night discussion with Karen Antman about paying for clinical trials (Gleeson 2002). The question was how to decide what to pay for. "What about phase 3 trials?" Gleeson asked. "But you pay for all that anyway," Antman responded, suggesting that these studies were usually buried in existing fee-for-service billings. "Why don't you pay for phase 1 and 2 studies?" Antman asked, pleading for early-stage support. In such conversations, Gleeson said, the BCBSA learned from oncologists that the plans were paying for trials, but the plans could not admit that they were doing so. The plea for early-stage clinical trial support by researchers was also understandable as few patients were involved, and patient care costs typically differed little from standard treatment. Researchers also found it difficult to concede openly that managed care in the late 1980s was stripping away the cross-subsidy that academic medical centers had received through faculty practice and hospital fees and that had indirectly financed clinical research.

Gleeson (2002) described the issue this way: "If we were going to pay [for trials] in a public but discrete way, what would we pay for? The universe kept expanding.

The lists would go on and on—NIH trials, peer-reviewed trials, then center-based trials, then institute-based trials. This was a discussion in the abstract. We were always seeking a place to start. It was a theoretical discussion. If we could pilot something, perhaps we could go public". There was as much controversy among the Blues plans as there was between the BCBSA and the oncologists. Gleeson characterized it this way: "Paying for research was similar to abortion. It was very highly polarized. It would get the attention of health plan CEOs [chief executive officers] from time to time, who also had strong views from a business perspective about the precedent of research support."

Randomized Clinical Trials Are Authorized

Payment for clinical research was a discussion in the abstract until HDC/ABMT came into focus, Sue Gleeson of the BCBSA recalled (Gleeson 2002). A series of meetings in 1988–1990 forged a response to the specific issues raised by the new procedure. The medical directors of the Blue Cross Blue Shield plans met in fall 1988. Guests included Robert Wittes and Mary McCabe from the NCI and Karen Antman of Dana-Farber, who spoke about breast cancer and ABMT (Aronson 2002). Antman's message was that ABMT was an effective therapy that was not being covered and was thus unavailable to patients. Naomi Aronson, then a TEC staff professional and later its director, recalled Antman's presentation as "compelling."

The Blues, on the other hand, saw HDC/ABMT as a tremendous expense, unprecedented in promise, complexity, and cost. In 1986, the BCBSA TEC had begun to conduct systematic reviews of the literature, which reduce reliance on the opinions of medical specialists, to evaluate the effectiveness of new medical interventions. A general review of ABMT had determined that it was investigational. In that context, and after the 1988 meeting, Aronson sent Andrew Kelahan, another TEC professional, to the library for data regarding the effectiveness of HDC/ABMT. He found few data, all from small studies and none from randomized trials. Aronson repeatedly kept asking him, "Where are the data?" but definitive data did not exist. Kelahan's analysis would provide a point of departure for David Eddy's subsequent review (1992) of the literature (discussed in more detail below).

The individual Blue Cross plans in the meantime faced increasing patient and physician demand for coverage of HDC/ABMT, as well as increasing litigation, but evidence of the procedure's benefit was poor. They turned to the BCBSA for guidance; the association organized an August 1990 meeting at the Chicago O'Hare Hilton Hotel (Aronson 2002; Aubry 2002; Henderson 2002). The meeting, attended by about 60 people, included plan medical directors, advisors to the BCBSA, and leading researchers and transplanters, who had been invited to make the case for ABMT and show the BCBSA what the plans were missing. Why was standard therapy inadequate? Why should the Blues pay for the experimental procedure? Why was HDC/ABMT beneficial?

Presentations were made by Roy Jones of Colorado for Peters; Karen Antman of Dana-Farber; Gary Spitzer from M. D. Anderson; and William Vaughn, a University of Nebraska oncologist. Henderson recalled these as credible presentations: "All made the same pitch. 'This was proven therapy. It was superior to historical controls'"

(Henderson 2002). Henderson, however, compared the situation to the history of radical mastectomy, suggesting that the most aggressive therapy might not be the best, reminding participants of how long it took to get rid of the Halsted procedure, and arguing that a clinical trial was needed or there would be no answer to the question of superiority anytime soon. He also stated that if trials did not occur because of insurers either paying for the procedure entirely or denying coverage entirely, insurers would bear some moral responsibility for the failure to get an answer. David Eddy challenged Antman, "Doesn't a randomized trial need to be done?" (Aubry 2002). She and each researcher said yes, but that their current work was also valuable and should be supported.

Michael Friedman, who had succeeded Wittes as head of the NCI's Cancer Treatment Evaluation Program, participated by telephone. Aubry, who attended the meeting, recalled him speaking "in a measured way" that all the studies presented were interesting (Aubry 2002). A randomized clinical trial was needed, Friedman said, and the NCI was willing to sponsor such trials and collaborate with the BCBSA. Aubry saw this as a critical turning point, the beginning of collaboration among the researchers and between researchers and insurers.

The NCI was actually in something of a box. Unknown to the insurers, in late June the NCI had asked the cancer cooperative groups to formulate proposals for participation in a high-priority national clinical trial to test the effectiveness of tamoxifen in preventing breast cancer (*Cancer Letter* 1990a). At the same time, the cooperative group chairs had approved the addition of four more trials to the NCI high-priority list, which then included 10 trials, none of which dealt with breast cancer (*Cancer Letter* 1990a). Under the circumstances, it would have been difficult for the NCI not to add the breast cancer trials.

The BCBSA responded to the NCI's commitment to randomized trials by creating a way to support them that was the mirror opposite of traditional coverage (see chapter 7). A demonstration project was designed to protect the individual plans: Each participating plan would contribute to a central fund, so payment would be made by the BCBSA; reimbursement would be prepaid, not after the fact as is customary; and new contracts were created for this purpose. Beneficiaries of individual plans would be accepted into NCI-sponsored clinical trials and approved for payment under this project. The BCBSA office in Chicago, rather than the individual participating plans, administered the demonstration.

As a result of the 1990 BCBSA meeting, David Eddy (1992) reviewed the literature on HDC/ABMT for metastatic breast cancer to evaluate the evidence of its effectiveness and to estimate its benefits and harms.[7] Dozens of phase 1 and 2 studies had generated substantial controversy. Everyone agreed that the treatment was highly toxic but disagreed about whether it improved survival and "whether the benefits, if they exist, outweigh the harms" (p. 657). Controversy focused on whether HDC/ABMT was investigational, the traditional basis for insurers to exclude coverage. Opposing the insurers were "many patients, with the support of their oncologists" (p. 657), who had sued for payment.

In his review, Eddy (1992) argued that *health outcomes* (overall survival, relief of symptoms, risks of treatment, and side effects of treatment) were the appropriate bases for judging treatment effectiveness. These differed from *biologic outcomes* (such as complete and partial tumor response), which only provided "preliminary clues to effectiveness" (p. 658). Biologic outcomes were not health outcomes, in Eddy's view, and could not be the basis for decisions about treatment effectiveness. The benefits and harms of HDC/ABMT required comparison with conventional chemotherapy, he wrote, but there were "no published, randomized controlled trials" that compared any outcomes in patients with metastatic breast cancer to those treated with conventional-dose chemotherapy.

Tellingly, only 10 studies had more than 10 patients, reported some information on response rate duration or survival, and were published in peer-reviewed journals. Sixty-four other studies did not meet these criteria and were excluded from the analysis. Valid conclusions about HDC/ABMT were difficult to draw due to "the lack of any controls." Comparisons across these studies were also difficult due to differences in treatment regimens, patient selection criteria, measures for reporting results, index events for calculating survival and response duration, as well as incomplete reporting of patient characteristics, different definitions of such characteristics, multiple reporting of patients, incomplete measurement of health outcomes, and small sample sizes (Eddy 1992).

Eddy (1992) concluded his review by stating that complete and overall response rates were considerably higher in HDC/ABMT than observed with conventional chemotherapy; the conversion of partial responses to complete response by HDC compared with standard induction therapy was "impressive," but for neither complete nor partial response did the evidence suggest any longer median duration of response for HDC/ABMT than for conventional chemotherapy. For overall survival, existing evidence did not demonstrate that HDC/ABMT improved actual survival in women with metastatic breast cancer or support the conclusion that an increase in complete response rates indicated an improvement in survival. No studies of symptom relief or quality of life had yet reported on the effect of HDC/ABMT. On the key measure of acute toxicity and death, treatment-related mortality rates for the procedure ranged from 0% to 25% with a weighted average of 12%; by contrast, very few such deaths were reported for conventional chemotherapy. Finally, few investigators systematically reported the nonfatal side effects of HDC, and none compared such outcomes with conventional chemotherapy. For the health outcome of survival, Eddy wrote, there was no basis "for concluding that HDC with ABMT is superior to or worse than conventional-dose chemotherapy" (p. 666). The best that could be said on the basis of the available evidence was that the effect was unknown.

In Eddy's (1992) view, if phase 2 studies generated hypotheses that needed to be tested, then phase 3 randomized controlled trials were clearly indicated. However, if such studies generated data about the effectiveness of a new procedure when standard therapy was known to be of very limited effectiveness, such as metastatic breast cancer, comparing study results to historical controls might justify progression to wider clinical practice in the minds of clinicians. In addition, if such studies provided a "treatment of last resort" for women for whom nothing else was available, then the impetus to go from phase 2 studies to clinical practice was greatly reinforced. Although acknowledging that pressures on physicians and patients might drive the procedure into wider clinical use, he clearly believed that the phase 3 trials were needed. Small phase 2 studies done at single institutions, with few or no controls, could provide an important hypothesis for further examination, but they provided no basis for widespread clinical use of HDC/ABMT outside controlled clinical trials.

Dr. Nancy Davidson (1992), in an editorial on Eddy's article in the same *Journal of Clinical Oncology* issue, characterized HDC/ABMT aptly as one of the "more hotly debated" issues in breast cancer treatment. Its use for treating metastatic breast cancer had shown higher "overall and complete response rates" than conventional therapy, a first step toward a potentially curative treatment. She criticized Eddy's analysis on various grounds but conceded the limits of the review stemmed from the limits of the data, and that it was "indeed difficult to establish the unequivocal superiority of HDC over conventional-dose chemotherapy based on current treatment results" (p. 517). But even the "most ardent critic," she wrote, had to recognize the rationale for use of HDC, and that the "sufficiently compelling results" of phase 1 and 2 studies justified continued investigation of the treatment. She briefly reviewed the trials under way (the Philadelphia trial of metastatic breast cancer discussed in more detail below and the NCI trials) and anticipated that their successful completion "should begin to shed light on the true value of HDC, although we must be modest in our expectations that these trials will provide a definitive answer" (p. 518). Davidson noted that the reluctance of insurers to provide coverage had "hampered its critical evaluation," and that their continuing support of well-designed trials was "desperately needed." Although she mentioned the Philadelphia trial, she made no mention of US HealthCare's financing of it or of the BCBSA's decision to support NCI trials, both of which had occurred by this time.

Notwithstanding "publicity in the lay and medical press" (Davidson 1992), she was clear that even well-designed trials could not justify "the uncritical adoption of HDC for women with poor prognosis breast cancer" (p. 518). Neither physicians nor patients could assume that "the decision to study this approach [in high-risk patients] . . . gives them license" (p. 518) to use HDC outside a clinical trial. The expense of the procedure and uncertainty about its optimal use argued for application "in the context of a clinical trial." But this did not mean that third-party coverage should be denied because the treatment was experimental. She called for "a responsible collaboration between medical practitioners, patients, and third-party payers [that] will allow us to move the discussion . . . from the courtrooms and newspapers back into the clinic and medical literature where it belongs" (p. 519). In chapters 3 and 4, we shall see that court trials would loom even larger in the future than they had to that point.

The conflict between oncologists and insurers over the HDC/ABMT procedure turned in part on the appropriate endpoints for evaluating medical effectiveness. Clinicians were attracted to the procedure because of the complete and partial responses it induced in breast cancers. They believed that tumor shrinkage meant longer life and better quality of life. Insurers seeking evidence of effectiveness emphasized the clinical benefits or health outcomes of overall survival and quality of life, not tumor response, which was viewed as an intermediate outcome. Data on response were forthcoming early in the HDC/ABMT trials. Data showing a survival benefit failed to develop over time.

US HealthCare acted sooner and more directly than the BCBSA. In early 1990, Dr. Hyman Kahn, the organization's medical director, called Philadelphia breast cancer doctors and transplanters together and asked, "Who should we cover? What's the consensus?" (Stadtmauer 2002). "We don't know," replied the oncologists. "We won't know without an randomized clinical trial." Kahn proposed to cover the transplant and nontransplant arms of such a trial, including a data management center. So, US HealthCare gave an unrestricted educational grant of $1.5 million to finance a randomized trial of HDC/ABMT for metastatic breast cancer (Glick 2002). This trial, known as the Philadelphia trial, would later become the sole NCI high-priority clinical trial of HDC/ABMT for treating metastatic breast cancer. We return to an extended discussion of clinical trials in chapter 8.

Outcomes of Conflict: Clinical Use

Notwithstanding the NCI commitment to sponsor phase 3 trials of HDC/ABMT, developments in the 1988–1992 period led to a fateful branching along two pathways. Both began with the results of the phase 2 studies, but one pathway led to randomized clinical trials and the other to wider use in oncology practice. How did this happen? It happened because no central institution existed to insist on phase 3 studies before widespread use; because of ambivalence within oncology on the need for randomized clinical trials of HDC/ABMT; because the leadership of oncology legitimated the widespread use of the procedure; and because patient demands, reinforced by the women's health movement and how the media reported the story, drove developments along this path.

The Ambivalent Commitment of Medicine to the Gold Standard

Randomized controlled trials are often described as the gold standard by which reliable medical knowledge is validated. They constitute the most persuasive way to test the validity of hypotheses that emerge from phase 2 studies. Randomization is central to ruling out the confounding factors, especially patient selection biases that confound comparisons of an investigational therapy with historical controls, and treatment biases that may reflect practice at a single institution.

Oncology is noteworthy in its commitment to clinical trials, including phase 3 randomized trials. The NCI has the most developed system of clinical trial support of any of the institutes of the NIH. The NCI cancer cooperative groups have existed for 50 years. The NCI also supports clinical trials through its comprehensive cancer centers and through community cancer centers. ASCO has exercised leadership in the promotion of cancer clinical trials. Its annual meetings present the results of many clinical trials and include sessions on the organization and conduct of such trials.

It is essential, nevertheless, to recognize that deep ambivalence exists within medicine, including oncology, toward randomized clinical trials. Harry Marks (1997) provided a historical account of the struggle to establish the importance of randomized clinical trials in medicine after World War II. Barron Lerner (2001) documented the complex process by which randomized trials came to be adopted as a guide to clinical practice in oncology, especially in the challenge by Bernard Fisher to the Halstead radical mastectomy in breast cancer.

Phase 3 randomized trials are clearly difficult to mount (as we discuss in chapter 8). An oft-cited figure is that only 3%–5% of adult cancer patients are entered into randomized clinical trials. This is due to many factors, prominent among them patient resistance to randomization. On the one hand, ineffective standard therapy may encourage patients to seek experimental treatment outside of trials. Patients with a terminal illness, such as stage IV breast cancer, may say that they have nothing to lose from seeking access to new treatments, further complicating efforts to conduct randomized trials. On the other hand, some patients may be unwilling to risk exposure to the experimental procedure within a trial, viewing the untested negatively. Physician incentives to encourage patient participation in randomized trials are often weak or negative. Although some compensation for research is generally provided, the time required to persuade a patient to enter a trial is often substantial and seldom compensated. The costs of care for a patient who is randomized to the experimental treatment are often not compensated, further costing physicians money.

Ambivalence among many oncologists must be counted among the difficulties of organizing randomized trials. Belief in the value of trials may conflict with belief in the value of a treatment outside a trial. In 1991, Belanger et al. reported on a survey of 230 oncologists about "the impact of clinical trials" on their preferred methods of treating breast cancer. They found that preferred treatments for primary breast cancer and inflammatory breast cancer were supported by clinical trials; that adjuvant chemotherapy for node-negative breast cancer was not based on consistent improvement in survival; and that adjuvant chemotherapy for postmenopausal women with node-positive breast cancer was contrary to results from large randomized clinical trials. They suggested "that even large randomized clinical trials may have a minimal impact on practice if their results run counter to belief in the value of the treatment" (p. 7).

Oncology was divided about the need for phase 3 randomized clinical trials of HDC/ABMT. Skeptics believed such trials were essential to determine whether the procedure was superior to standard therapy. Believers, with varying degrees of enthusiasm, believed that the results of phase 2 studies justified wider clinical use of the procedure without trials. Some regarded phase 2 results as so persuasive that randomization was unethical. Others straddled both camps. Peters both acknowledged the importance of clinical trials and played a major role in organizing them but firmly believed that trials would confirm the superiority of HDC/ABMT. Simultaneously, he advocated that insurance companies should cover the procedure as effective treatment. Still others thought that the responsiveness of metastatic breast cancer to HDC/ABMT could be extrapolated to stage II high-risk breast cancer, even though the biology was different. These divisions within oncology were masked to patients and the general public. Many enthusiasts, in Henderson's view (2002), found themselves torn between their own uncertainty about the procedure and the need to defend it so claims to insurers would not be denied and so the medical profession, not health insurers, would decide its value.

Oncology Legitimates an Experimental Procedure

The limited commitment to randomized trials was reflected in several statements that emanated from the AMA. Its Diagnostic and Therapeutic Technology Assessment (DATTA) program solicited the opinions of clinicians rather than systematically reviewing the literature. In an early 1990 poll of 45 oncologists on ABMT, an "overwhelming majority" rated the safety and effectiveness of ABMT as "established or promising" (AMA DATTA 1990). Although the report limited itself to acute lymphocytic leukemia, acute myelogenous leukemia, and lymphoma, it would be used to support coverage for HDC/ABMT as a breast cancer treatment. The then-director of the DATTA program, Dr. Elizabeth Brown, would write: "In summary, the DATTA panelists considered the harvesting, cryopreservation and reinfusion of autologous bone marrow an appropriate method for managing bone marrow hypoplasia/aplasia in patients undergoing treatment for cancer" (Brown 1990a, p. 1). She would make no mention of those cancers for which the treatment was appropriate or inappropriate.

In a related letter, Brown (1990b) wrote that the "intense focus" on investigational procedures by insurers was problematic, especially when coupled with the requirement of evidence from well-controlled clinical trials published in peer-reviewed medical journals. This emphasis failed to account for publication lag, the absence of clinical trial evaluation of many procedures, and the fact that "medicine is always in a state of evolution." A "rigid interpretation" was especially problematic for terminally ill patients "who may have very limited treatment options" and for whom "a medical service is not investigational if there is no alternative." She encouraged third-party payers to "be flexible in their interpretation of the term investigational, to acknowledge that the medical literature did not always reflect current clinical practice, and to recognize the physician's and patient's perspective, particularly in the case of terminal illness, when making a coverage determination" (p. 1).

A lengthy and widely distributed document, "High Dose Chemotherapy and Autologous Bone Marrow Support for Breast Cancer: A Technology Assessment. Confidential Draft," provided a more explicit and extraordinary legitimation of HDC/ABMT for breast cancer and further sanctioned its wider use (Peters et al. 1990). Prepared in July 1990, the authors of this self-initiated technology assessment included William Peters of Duke; Marc Lippman, head of oncology at Georgetown University; Gianni Bonadonna of the National Cancer Institute of Italy; Vincent DeVita, former NCI director and then physician-in-chief of Memorial Sloan Kettering Cancer Institute; James Holland of Mount Sinai School of Medicine; and Gary Rosner, also of Duke. (Lawrence Rose, a prominent defense attorney for insurers, dubbed this group the "Dream Team" and its report as the "Dream Team document.")

The assessment, which used the BCBSA criteria to make its case, argued in its summary: "The use of high-dose chemotherapy and autologous bone marrow support for selected patients with breast cancer *should no longer be considered investigational* [emphasis added]" (Peters et al. 1990, p. 2). A higher frequency of objective response had resulted in all settings in which the procedure had been tested; some patients with poor prognosis patients had obtained long-term disease-free survival; HDC/ABMT produced results "equivalent to, and with certain regimens, superior to" (p. 2) conventional therapies for early and metastatic breast cancer; a treatment program that combined induction chemotherapy and ABMT produced "higher complete response rate, higher overall response rate, and usually an increased median duration of progression-free survival and median overall survival" (p. 2) when compared to those that did not. The evidence, the document argued, "strongly favors the conclusion" that HDC/ABMT, when used in stage II or III breast cancer involving large numbers of axillary lymph nodes, is superior to alternative currently available therapeutic approaches" (p. 2). Randomized trials would "strengthen the scientific position, [but] the magnitude of the therapeutic benefit evidenced already may raise in some patient's minds concern that such trials would be unethical if they denied access to the high dose therapy" (pp. 2–3). Therefore, both randomized and nonrandomized trials should be encouraged "wherever feasible and ethical" (p. 3) to increase understanding of the various elements of treatment.

It was well known that this document had been submitted for publication to various medical journals. A 2002 Medline search failed to indicate that it had ever been published. Written a month before the August 1990 BCBSA meeting, it was not discussed on that occasion. It was available to the BCBSA Medical Advisory Panel members at their February 1991 meeting but received only cursory attention. David Eddy (2003) was caustic in his view of it. The document was widely cited by plaintiffs' lawyers in litigation but without the scrutiny applied to the medical journal literature (Rose 2002).[8] It signaled to treating oncologists that the procedure was established therapy, not only for metastatic breast cancer but also for early-stage, high-risk breast cancer. Some very senior, very prominent oncologists had stated on the record that HDC/ABMT for breast cancer was "no longer experimental."

Additional indication that many, if not most, oncologists viewed HDC/ABMT as no longer experimental was provided in a series of letters obtained from the litigation of the 1990s. A Seattle law firm (Culp, Guterson, and Grader), in 1992, had solicited the opinions of oncologists across the country on the status of HDC/ABMT.[9] A careful reading indicates clearly that the opinions expressed established policies and practices. Scripps Clinic and Research Foundation wrote that the procedure was "generally accepted medical practice in our community for the treatment of certain patients" (McMillan 1992, p. 1). The University of Michigan Medical Center wrote: "Sufficient data has accumulated to make us believe that high dose chemotherapy with autologous bone marrow transplantation for metastatic breast cancer which remains sensitive to chemotherapy, is an effective therapy. This therapy is generally accepted medical practice in the State of Michigan and is one of a number of standard therapies for the treatment of this disease" (Silver 1992, p. 1). The writer enclosed a position statement of the Michigan Society of Hematology and Oncology, which said: "Sufficient data has accumulated to make us believe it [HDC/AMBT] is an effective therapy" (n.d, p. 1). The H. Lee Moffitt Cancer Center and Research Institute in Tampa, Florida, wrote that the procedure was "generally accepted by the medical oncologists of our state" (Elfenbein 1992, p. 1). Emory University responded: "It is becoming clear that it is effective therapy for certain patients with advanced breast cancer and is an acceptable medical practice" (Vogler 1992, p. 1). The Ohio State University responded that HDC/ABMT was "generally accepted medical practice in our community" (Tutschka 1992, p. 1). The University of Nevada indicated that the procedure "is accepted in our community and we believe that it may be cost effective" (Ascensao 1992, p. 1).

Insurers came in for a drubbing. The University of Utah Medical Center wrote: "The majority of these women needed to seek legal counsel in trying to obtain authorization from their insurance company for this life-saving therapy. . . . Recent literature, especially those written by Dr. Karen Antman as well as Dr. Bill Peters, show us that this treatment modality is becoming an appropriate treatment option for patients with advanced recurrent breast cancer" (Artig 1992, p. 1). The University of Louisville's James Graham Brown Cancer Center wrote that the procedure "was generally accepted practice in our area. . . . [However] not all insurance carriers will include coverage. . . . It is my opinion that exclusion on the grounds that such treatment is experimental or investigational is inappropriate" (Herzig 1992, p. 1). The respondent from New York Medical College commented that a "number of Blue Cross/Blue Shield companies would like to embark on a randomized controlled study. . . . None of these companies have ever required a randomized controlled study" (Ahmed 1992, p. 1). Why now? was the clear implication. The director of clinical oncology at Albert Einstein Cancer Center wrote that they offered HDC/ABMT both in cooperative clinical trials and "directly" to those patients who wished it:

> Many of my colleagues and I *do not* [emphasis in original] consider autologous BMT as an experimental form of treatment since we believe there is sufficient literature evidence that high-dose chemotherapy and autologous BMT is clearly superior to any other treatment approach when used in the adjuvant setting and that 10–29% of women with metastatic breast cancer can be place in long term progression-free status using this high-dose treatment. (Ciobanu 1992, p. 1)

Other letters supporting HDC/ABMT were received from California (University of California, Los Angeles; Stanford University Medical Center, Stanford), Delaware (Christiana Hospital, Newark), Massachusetts (Tufts University School of Medicine, New England Medical Center, Boston), Michigan (Detroit Medical Center, Bone Marrow Transplantation Program, Detroit), Missouri (Hematology-Oncology Associates of Columbia), New Jersey (St. Joseph's Hospital and Medical Center, Paterson), New York (Mt. Sinai Medical Center, New York, NY; University of Rochester, Rochester), Oklahoma (Cancer Care Associates, Tulsa), Pennsylvania (Temple University Comprehensive Cancer Center), Tennessee (The University of Tennessee Medical Center at Knoxville), and Wisconsin (Marshfield Clinic, Marshfield).

Some respondents to the Culp, Guterson & Grader request were more clearly guarded. The director of bone marrow transplantation at Case Western Reserve University wrote: "The great majority of women treated with this regimen are enrolled in one of several clinical trials . . . designed to compare the efficacy of bone marrow transplantation with that of conventional therapy" (Lazarus 1992, p. 1). The clinical director of bone marrow transplantation at the University of Nebraska wrote that it had "specifically defined protocols in which patients must meet eligibility requirements," which allowed it "to better evaluate" the role of HDC in breast cancer treatment (Reed 1992, p. 1). The director of the program at the University of Minnesota wrote that women were accepted for HDC/ABMT treatment "only if they meet the eligibility criteria outline in prospectively designed clinical trials approved by the Committee on Human Research." While the treatment was "promising in some subsets of breast cancer patients, our role is to determine this efficacy through properly designed clinical trials" (McGlave 1992, p. 1).

In general, the clear majority of respondents to the law firm's solicitation supported the clinical use of HDC/ABMT for metastatic and early stage breast cancer and regarded the procedure as standard of care. A minority had committed themselves to providing the treatment only within randomized clinical trials.

Enthusiasm for HDC/ABMT was also demonstrated in a press release of ASCO at its 1992 annual meeting (ASCO 1992). "Bone Marrow Transplants Increase Survival for Breast Cancer Patients" read the lead.[10] Dr. Rein Saral of Emory University School of Medicine was quoted as saying: "It is clear from these studies that high-dose chemotherapy supported by bone marrow transplantation is superior to current conventional treatments for high-risk breast cancer patients" (p. 1). He was referring to two studies, one a trial by Dr. A. M. Gianni of Milan, Italy, involving 85 patients, with 93% of those receiving HDC/ABMT relapse free after a median time of 2 years compared to 43% of those in the conventional treatment historical control group. The other was Peters's Cancer and Leukemia Group B study at Duke, also of 85 patients; 72% of those receiving HDC/ABMT were event free after a median follow-up of 2 years compared to 30% in the historical control group. "The results of these studies are in line with current thinking that dose intensification, using higher doses of chemotherapy and ABMT, appear, at least in short term follow-up, to be associated with a lower recurrence rate" (p. 2), according to Saral. The press release indicated that the Duke study had also measured quality of life after 1 year and reported only that it was "acceptable," which Saral characterized as "similar to" that of patients receiving conventional treatment. Diminished interest in sexual activity and pain during intercourse were mentioned as requiring attention in patient rehabilitation.

The legitimation of HDC/ABMT in 1988–1992 was complete. The oncology leadership had argued that the procedure was clearly superior to conventional treatment. The need for validating superiority was not clear, but the need for treating patients was clear. Concurrent, then, with the initiation of clinical trials to evaluate the procedure, the leadership of oncology, challenged by skeptical oncologists and by insurers, encouraged the wider use of the procedure before adequate evaluation had taken place.

The Women's Health Movement

Two other factors—the women's health movement and its breast cancer patient advocacy offshoot and the role of the print and broadcast media—drove events along the path of wider clinical use. In 1970, the Doctor's Group, forerunner to the Boston Women's Health Book Collective, published a successful underground booklet, *Women and Their Bodies* (Doctor's Group 1970), which led to the first edition of the book *Our Bodies Ourselves* in 1973 (Boston Women's Health Book Collective 1973). The purpose of the Boston group was to provide "clear, truthful information about health, sexuality and reproduction from a feminist and consumer perspective" and to "vigorously advocate for women's health by challenging the institutions and systems that block women from full control over our bodies and devalue our lives" (Boston Women's Health Book Collective 2004, p. 1). It was followed in 1975 by the creation of the National Women's Health Network, a membership organization committed to advancing women's health through self-determination "in all aspects of reproductive and sexual health," changing the cultural and medical perception of menopause and establishing a universal health care system to meet the needs of women (National Women's Health Network 2006). The nonprofit network fused two ideas: a permanent Washington, D.C., lobby and an information clearinghouse.

By the late 1980s and early 1990s, these developments had given rise to general dissatisfaction with the limited attention to women's health issues. Women argued that a medical gender gap had created an atmosphere of stigmatization and bias against research on women's health. Women's groups protested that not enough was being done for women's health, especially medical research. In response, Congress enacted the 1990 Women's Health Equity Act, which mandated equal funding for research on women, including participation in clinical trials, and created the Office on Women's Health Research at the NIH. In 1991, the NIH launched the Women's Health Initiative, a $625 million program to study the prevention of heart disease, osteoporosis, and breast cancer in 160,000 women aged 50–59.

The broader movement stimulated more focused, disease-specific efforts, one of which was the breast cancer patient advocacy movement. This movement, anchored in the personal experiences of women with breast cancer, includes strong local efforts of patient support, fundraising, education, and information. Local organizations in turn are connected to the national scene by networks, coalitions, alliances, and organizations. Issues included mammography, lumpectomy versus mastectomy, medical research, and the integrity of clinical trials.

Susan Love, M.D., a University of California at Los Angeles surgeon and author of a popular book on breast cancer, wrote that breast cancer patient advocacy began in 1952 with the Reach to Recovery program (women with breast cancer helping other women) of the American Cancer Society (Love and Lindsey 2000). This organization in turn stimulated the formation of other support groups. In the 1970s, Shirley Temple Black, Betty Ford, and Happy Rockefeller publicly disclosed their breast cancer diagnoses, which helped move the disease from "a private and shameful secret" to one that finally could be addressed in public. In 1975, Rose Kushner published the first lay guide to breast cancer, initially *Breast Cancer: A Personal History and Investigative Report* (Kushner 1975), later published as *Why Me? What Every Woman Should Know About Breast Cancer* (Kushner 1977). A tireless advocate for patients, she wrote about her encounter with breast cancer; described the disease and its treatment; emphasized early detection, including breast self-examination; challenged the quality of mammography; asserted the freedom of women to choose the type of surgery they received, challenging the one-step mastectomy procedure in the process by insisting that surgeons discuss a woman's disease with her, how it would be treated, and her options, all before surgery; highlighted the importance of staging; reviewed chemotherapy in a balanced way; and emphasized the importance of a good prosthesis after surgery. Dr. Thomas L. Dao, writing the foreword to the 1977 book, wrote of Kushner that she "draws every woman reader into the sisterhood of fear and suffering" (p. x).

A number of new organizations appeared on the national stage. Y-ME National Breast Cancer Organization (its name was taken from Kushner's book), dedicated to peer support of women with breast cancer, was established in 1978. Nancy Brinker organized the Susan G. Komen Foundation in 1983 to raise money for breast cancer research; the foundation pioneered the now-familiar Race for a Cure. The National Alliance of Breast Cancer Organizations (NABCO), of which Kushner was a cofounder, was created in 1986 to serve as a coordinating and central resource for breast cancer organizations and to promote awareness and education about the disease. Later, it would provide information for women with suspected or confirmed breast cancer and conduct programs to increase public awareness, influence medical and regulatory policy, and support outreach to medically underserved women (Langer 2004).

Four distinct activities characterize the movement: support, information, education, and advocacy (Langer 2004). Support, whether from peers or trained psychosocial professionals, involves helping a woman with breast cancer cope with her diagnosis, treatment, and follow-up and its emotional and personal aftermath. Y-ME was one of the earliest support groups, but SHARE, a support organization for women with breast and ovarian cancer in New York City (www.sharecancersupport. org), also has a long history. Information involves either putting medical, practical, or support information in a woman's hands or directing the woman to sources of information about all aspects of breast cancer. NABCO engaged in this early in its existence and had the first national Web site in 1995. Education addresses the broader issue of public information and awareness, typified by the Avon Foundation with its Walks for Breast Cancer.

Advocacy, which is addressed to various parts of the health care system, expresses the needs of women with breast cancer and seeks to improve their care. Within advocacy, three trajectories can be identified: political advocacy for more money for breast cancer research; regulatory advocacy for early access to experimental treatments, especially if conventional treatment is not very good; and support for evaluation of experimental treatments through randomized clinical trials. The Susan G. Komen Foundation supports efforts to raise money for cancer research, as does the Avon Foundation.

In the late 1980s and early 1990s, a number of cancer and breast cancer support groups began to organize forces toward advocacy. These included Breast Cancer Action in San Francisco, the Women's Community Cancer Center of Oakland, and You Are Not Alone in southern California. Dr. Susan Love, on tour in 1990 for the first edition of her book, *Dr. Susan Love's Breast Book* (1991), "began to realize how deep women's anger was, and how ready they were to do something" (Love and Lindsey 2000, p. 591). She, Amy Langer, who was executive director of NABCO, and a group that included Y-ME, the Women's Community Cancer Center of Oakland, and CanAct of New York, called for a planning meeting for early 1991. It was attended by 100 individuals from 75 organizations, the National Breast Cancer Coalition (NBCC) was formed, and its initial board was selected. NABCO served as the fiscal agent, and Langer chaired the initial board meetings until bylaws were written and officers chosen. Fran Visco, a Philadelphia lawyer, was elected president in 1992 and remains in that position today.

In the prior decade, gay men with human immunodeficiency virus/acquired immunodeficiency syndrome (HIV/AIDS) had become powerful advocates for expanded medical research, regulation of drugs, insurance coverage, and care (Epstein 1996). The lessons of that effort were not lost on breast cancer advocates. Susan Love would write the following:

> All of these [breast cancer] groups were aware of the work the AIDS movement had been doing. For the first time we were seeing people with a killer disease aggressively demanding more money for research, changes in insurance bias, and job protection. Women with breast cancer took note of that—particularly those women who had been part of the feminist movement. They were geared, as were the gay activists with AIDS, to the idea of identifying oppression and confronting it politically. (Love and Lindsey 2000, p. 591)

Langer said: "We took inspiration from gay men and the HIV/AIDS movement, not necessarily their tactics, but we gained confidence that an organized effort could change how the health care system responded" (interview with Langer 2004). Visco said: "AIDS showed us it could be done and helped create an atmosphere that fostered our success" (Boodman 1994, p. E1). Imitating the AIDS red ribbon, breast cancer activists adopted a pink ribbon. "Unlike previous congressional lobbying efforts mounted by cancer groups, the new generation of breast cancer activists ... adopted an approach that was more 'in your face' than 'hat in hand'" (Boodman 1994, p. E1).

The issue that generated intense interest and energized breast cancer patient advocates was breast cancer research. In the fall of 1991, NBCC brought droves of breast cancer survivors and supporters to Washington, held a candlelight vigil on the Capitol steps, and launched a massive letter-writing campaign. The campaign generated 600,000 letters to Congress in just 6 weeks (Marshall 1993). NBCC held hearings on research in February 1992 to determine what the price tag was for enough research to break medicine out of its standard regimen of surgery, radiation, and chemotherapy. Prominent oncology researchers supported more funds for breast cancer research. Then, representatives of NBCC, NABCO, and others visited congressional offices, testified before appropriations committees, and called the allocation of only 13.5% of the NIH budget to women's issues a travesty (Kadar 1994; Stabiner 1995).

The criticism that too few women were enrolled as subjects in federally funded clinical trials prompted a response from the NCI. Referring to a General Accounting Office report that concluded that the NIH had inconsistently included women, two officials from the NCI's Division of Cancer Treatment responded (Ungerleider and Friedman 1991). They presented data on trial accrual of women to the NCI's clinical cooperative groups; showed that nearly 40 phase 2 and 3 breast cancer trials were under way in 1989, following only the leukemias and lymphomas; and examined treatment trials by cancer site or type, by gender, for new cases, estimated deaths, and accrual to trials. "We conclude," they wrote, "that women are not underrepresented as subjects in federally funded studies conducted by NCI's Clinical Trials Cooperative Group Program" (p. 17).

Advocates scored a stunning success in 1992 in persuading Congress to increase the NCI budget for breast cancer research from $133 million to $197 million and to create a new program within the Department of Defense administered by the U.S. Army, which received $210 million (Marshall 1993). Senator Tom Harkin (D, Iowa), who lost two sisters to breast cancer, was responsible for this Department of Defense appropriation, the only avenue available to him at the time. Surprisingly, the U.S. Army Medical Materiel and Research Command, designated to administer the Department of Defense program, did not transfer the funds to the National Cancer Institute. The continuing efforts of advocates resulted in Congress enacting a sustaining appropriation of $25 million in fiscal year (FY) 2004, $150 million in FY05, and another increase of $75 million in FY06.

How did breast cancer patient advocates respond to HDC/ABMT, which emerged as a promising treating in this formative period? In general, local and regional breast cancer advocacy groups across the country supported access to HDC/ABMT without regard to clinical trials and saw insurers as the enemy of women in the denial of coverage. National organizations in the 1988–1992 period were supportive of early access, cautious or silent, or preoccupied with other issues. Few challenged the oncology establishment on whether the data supported the use of the procedure outside clinical trials. Some were among the strongest proponents of early access.

Some organizations took a cautious approach. Diane Blum, executive director of Cancer Care, at a June 1991 medical conference about the initial HDC/ABMT randomized trials (see chapter 8) identified four questions important to patients: "What is a clinical trial? Is it for me? What will it cost? How will I cope long term?" (Forum on Emerging Treatments for Breast Cancer 1991, Blum, p. 101 These questions arose in the context of a potentially fatal disease, the need to decide about entering a trial "in a life and death context," and the uncertainty about eligibility, informed consent, and randomization. The ABMT patients she had consulted had wanted to know where they would be treated, how long they would be there, who would be with them, what the side effects would be, how much pain they would experience, and which physician would follow them long term. Information seekers were perhaps more likely to enter clinical trials, but a lot of women were not information seekers. Ideally, information was provided by a primary physician, she said, but "there are a number of community physicians who might not believe in a particular clinical trial or want their patients to get a certain treatment" (p. 102). She identified the NCI Cancer Information Service, the media, conferences, consumer groups, and the patient's family as other sources of information about clinical trials.

NABCO adopted a wait-and-see stance toward HDC/ABMT, seeking to provide realistic information about the treatment, its experimental nature, and its side effects (NABCO 1992). In 1990, in response to plaintiffs' lawyers asking for *amicus curie* briefs in suits against insurers, NABCO adopted a policy of refusing such requests (Langer 2004). "We discovered," Langer, NABCO's executive director, would say, "there were a lot of non-reputable law firms out there. And many of the patients seemed less than rational" (Langer 2004). Individual women also asked NABCO for help in appealing insurance denials. NABCO provided both medical and practical information to these women and to insurers but took no position in any given case. As a result, NABCO was "misunderstood," according to Langer, as being anti-ABMT rather than neutral.

NABCO did produce a video in 1992 that sought to provide balanced information about the procedure, its practical difficulties, treatment-related mortality, side effects, and its investigational nature. Langer, introducing the video, said that HDC/ABMT "holds promise but it is relatively new and it is not for everyone." The physicians featured were William P. Vaughn, University of Alabama; Stephanie Williams, University of Chicago; and Larry Norton, Memorial Sloan Kettering Cancer Center. Six patients were profiled regarding their treatment, hospital stay, side effects, and uncertainty about the future. Although the promise of the unproven treatment was made clear, the importance of ongoing research was emphasized. Patients indicated their preferences clearly. One (Mary Schumaker) said: "This was the only thing for us. Aggressive, and that's what we wanted. We wanted to get rid of the cancer." Another (Mary Carrara) declared: "I asked my doctor. I asked him squarely. 'What are my chances without this?' He replied, 'Without it you're dead.' No matter what the cost, I had to go for it. It was really my only alternative." The husband of one woman said: "This treatment buys time for the next thing that comes along."

NBCC, which had promoted increased federal government appropriations for breast cancer research, discussed the issue at a January 1993 board meeting. It debated vigorously whether HDC/ABMT should be available only within a randomized clinical trial. The question was tabled and then folded into a motion that insurers should pay for the costs of clinical trials. Given that all the drivers of widespread use had been deployed by 1993, it is noteworthy that NBCC did not endorse access to HDC/ABMT outside randomized clinical trials. By the end of the decade, NBCC would develop a very strong policy commitment to the thorough evaluation of new breast cancer treatments by randomized clinical trials.

What lay behind the demand for unrestricted early access pressed by many advocates? Amy Langer, in retrospect, interpreted it this way:

> There was a shift in breast cancer advocacy, which was legitimated by the media. Women needed to be actively involved in their own treatment and had begun to understand that research in breast cancer had been woefully underfunded. These good and correct media messages, taken to extreme, become less about process and more about entitlement. The approach to cure by the breast cancer movement was "We have been denied in the past and now we're going to get it." We had engaged in aggressive shopping as medical consumers and voters and now were beginning to engage in the political process of funding for breast cancer research. Women tended to be unengaged until becoming energized by anger and concern about their personal breast cancer experience. Part of the story, then, was the advocacy claim, "You cannot deny women this [ABMT] treatment." In 1991–1992, there was an interlacing of several things—entitlement, anger, and aggressive approach to treatment. This intimidated a lot of doctors, who proceeded to make the treatment available. There has been a mission morphing [within the breast cancer movement]. Then it was still a bunch of angry women. The sophisticated technical knowledge and commitment to evidence-based medicine by advocates had yet to evolve; it had not evolved at this time. (Langer 2004)

In general, the breast cancer patient advocacy movement would support access to HDC/ABMT without regard for randomized trials until the mid-1990s. Insurers were the enemy. Only later would some organizations advocate for access that was restricted to randomized trials. Even then, they risked the anger of women with breast cancer who were willing to risk this treatment.

The Media

The media (newspapers, magazines, and television) were also a major force in the use of HDC/ABMT for breast cancer. They reported the story as women being denied access to lifesaving treatment by insurance companies interested only in financial considerations. Langer (2004) recalled how that organization had attempted to influence the general reporting of breast cancer in the late 1980s and early 1990s.

> The overlay to all of this is that huge tensions were created by the advent and growth of the advocacy movement and the media interest in breast cancer. Before 1991, the media treated breast cancer as women's personal stories and ran them on the women's page. They described them as victims, the procedures as mutilation; it was scary reporting. NABCO wanted to address this issue. We tried to educate the media about how to talk about breast cancer. We urged the media to write about women, not victims, but women with breast cancer. The media were coming around just as the ABMT story provided opportunity to backslide. The drama returned. We talked a lot to the media; but made little headway. The media did a job on ABMT. The timing was not propitious. It was concurrent with 1993–1994 when our breast cancer movement had taken hold. The write-in campaign for medical research had been successful. Networks of breast cancer patients had been created, and the grass roots effort was mobilized. (Langer 2004)

The media played a central role in both shaping the debate about HDC/ABMT and encouraging women with breast cancer to demand it. The first story appeared on successive days, April 6 and 7, 1988. Daniel Haney, long-time science writer of the Associated Press, pegged his story to a *New England Journal of Medicine* article reporting the use of growth factor to reconstitute a functioning immune system after HDC. The Duke University study had been done at the Bone Marrow Transplant Program, headed by William Peters. The newspaper account lagged by more than a decade the initial research at the Sidney Farber Cancer Center, stimulated by Dr. Emil Frei, which had studied 17 patients with metastatic carcinoma, 3 of whom had carcinoma of the breast (Tobias et al. 1977).

Elizabeth Rosenthal, of the *New York Times,* in 1990 captured all the pieces of the story that put HDC on the map for both reporters and patients. Her article, "Patient's Marrow Emerges as Key Cancer Tool," quickly conveyed the sense of hope that would characterize nearly all of the hundreds of newspaper, magazine, and television stories of the next decade. Her piece appeared on page 1 of the Science Times section on March 27, 1990; at 1904 words, it was long even by the science section's standards. By the third paragraph, Rosenthal made the case for the treatment, saying, "Although such autologous bone marrow transplants were first used experimentally over a decade ago as heroic treatments for hopeless cases, researchers have only recently accumulated enough data to prove definitively that they work."

Rosenthal (1990) outlined the rationale for the treatment: the idea that cancer could be killed if only doctors could administer high enough doses of chemotherapy.

She also described some of the harrowing symptoms, the bleeding and daily fevers during the nadir period, when the body has little functioning bone marrow left after the chemotherapy and virtually no capacity to fight infection. But, as she portrayed it, the risk was offset by the potential reward of a cure or at least 5-year survival: "Some of the initial patients have long outlived the time they were expected to survive with their fatal diseases" (1990, p. 1). "And, although the risk of dying in the procedure is still 5% to 15%, autologous transplants have taken off."

What Rosenthal could not have known was that her story, and the hundreds that followed, would help autologous transplants "take off." By year's end, at least 15 stories about HDC had appeared in major newspapers, including the *Wall Street Journal, Washington Post,* and *Los Angeles Times.* That Rosenthal's piece appeared in the *New York Times* helped push the story forward, according to Shannon Brownlee (2004), a former medical writer for *U.S. News & World Report.* "There's a saying in newsrooms, to the effect that a story isn't a story until it appears in the *New York Times,*" she said. "And once a story has appeared there, you can bet your editor is going to want to know why you aren't covering it" (Brownlee 2004). Rosenthal gave HDC/ABMT a visibility that would interest other reporters in their writing stories.

It was not just the venue of the *New York Times;* it was also the content of Rosenthal's story that made other reporters prick up their ears, the saga of combating a desperate disease treated with desperate measures. All of the stories that followed that year, with one significant exception, retraced the format laid out by Rosenthal. They relayed the hopelessness of the diagnosis—late-stage breast cancer—and contrasted that with the hope offered by the new treatment. In a 1990 *Washington Post* piece, for instance, writer Lisa Leff quoted the husband of a breast cancer patient as saying, "We feel if she doesn't get this operation now, she's going to die" (Leff 1990, p. B1). In the *Atlanta Journal Constitution* in 1991, Diane Loupe reported that two breast cancer patients who were seeking the treatment "shared a common fate ... they had only months to live" (p. A1). At the same time, the stories also highlighted the risks of the treatment, just as Rosenthal had done, while explaining the rationale, which boiled down to the idea that more chemo is better—if only it didn't tend to kill the patient.

The most critical part of Rosenthal's story, the one piece of information that would serve to enrage reporters, breast cancer patients, and advocates over the coming years, focused on the fact that most insurers, including Medicare and Medicaid, were refusing to pay for the procedure. The only thing missing from Rosenthal's piece that would become a staple of later stories was a patient whose tragic tale could dramatize the need for the new treatment.

Combined, these elements made for great copy, the kind of tale that reporters instinctively want to tell. "People like to tell stories about heroism, about overcoming the odds," said Gina Kolata of the *New York Times* (Kolata 2004). Medical reporters have also learned that editors—and presumably readers—are most easily drawn in to the science of medicine if they are told a human interest story first. HDC/ABMT was a ready-made allegory of good versus evil, of heroism in the face of overwhelming odds. A young woman with advanced breast cancer, typically in her 30s or 40s, married with two children, faces almost certain death unless she braves a harrowing procedure. She is desperately seeking a lifesaving treatment, a fight for her life of Homeric proportions, only to be denied insurance coverage by a hard-hearted, financially self-interested insurance company. Litigation, though costly, would be viewed as a last resort as the treatment would be seen as one's only hope. Bake sales and other community fund-raising efforts to pay for the HDC/ABMT procedure were frequently highlighted, furthering a negative perception of insurers.

While the patient played the victim, the doctor was often cast as the hero, a savior who took the patient almost to the brink of death, only to snatch her back with a lifesaving dose of bone marrow. Indeed, transplanters were often viewed that way by their fellow doctors, as Craig Henderson, quoted in *Discover Magazine,* would say: "Transplanters became gods at hospitals" (Brownlee 2002, p. 76).

The villain in the story, of course, was not only breast cancer itself, but also frequently the insurance companies that refused to pay for the procedure. This was the view of many doctors treating breast cancer, and many reporters simply followed their lead, letting the doctors set the tone for the story rather than giving the insurance industry equal footing. In a 1990 front-page story in the *St. Petersburg Times,* for example, reporter Carol Gentry quoted oncologist Dr. Gerald Elfenbein, director of the H. Lee Moffitt Cancer Center, in Tampa, who said about an insurer who was denying coverage: "I cannot believe that a potentially life-saving treatment can be denied. It's just inhumane" (Gentry 1990, p. 1A). By 1994, nearly 200 stories a year on high-dose chemotherapy were appearing in magazines and newspapers around the country, the vast majority touching at least briefly on the alleged perfidy of insurers.

All this was happening at a time when women were pouring into newsrooms, taking positions as reporters and editors, changing the face of journalism. Between 1989 and 1999, the decade when the number of bone marrow transplants skyrocketed, the number of female reporters and editors in newsrooms was also increasing rapidly, especially in medicine and science. The top science and medical writers in the country today were just beginning their careers in the 1980s, and more and more of them were women, many of whom left the study of medicine or basic science to enter journalism. Elisabeth Rosenthal, for instance, is a doctor of medicine. Gina Kolata spent the early years of her career at the journal *Science.* Brownlee, who left the study of marine biology to write for *Discover* magazine, recalled, "When I began writing in 1982, there were two women in a staff of eight writers. Five years later, the split was 50–50. That wasn't the case for other areas of journalism, like sports" (Brownlee 2004). No longer relegated to the lifestyle section of papers and newsmagazines, female medical writers soon were getting their stories on the front pages, and increasingly, their stories covered issues that concerned women.

No medical issue of the 1990s concerned women more than breast cancer. In 1985, a mere 592 stories about breast cancer appeared in newspapers and wires around the country. A decade later, more than 1000 stories on the topic were appearing each month.[11] By then, women's health, especially breast cancer, had become not only a medical or lifestyle story, but also a hot political issue.

As the issue of insurance companies denying coverage for HDC heated, breast cancer advocacy groups pushed state legislatures to mandate coverage for the procedure. This made HDC/ABMT even more appealing to reporters, especially medical reporters, who were always searching for ways to make their stories worthy of front-page play.

Now, the story combined not only the pathos of young victims and the heroics of doctors, but also political controversy. The media also loved stories about women who took their insurers to court. Plaintiffs called on doctors to back up their claims that HDC was the only thing that could save them. The doctors delivered: They told judges and juries that HDC was proven to be effective. Reporters accentuated the seeming greed of the insurers with quotes from doctors and the families of patients. In her 1990 account in the *St. Petersburg Times,* for example, Gentry quoted from a letter Bill Bentzer wrote to the insurer that had denied coverage to his wife: "Coping with the anguish of my precious wife's breast cancer is bad enough without having to fight with Aetna for the coverage she needs. You have made a terrible nightmare worse" (Gentry 1990, p. 1A).

That HDC/ABMT had not yet been shown to be lifesaving was lost on most reporters, including medical reporters, who failed to grasp the difference between a randomized controlled trial and the historical controlled trials that were being used to justify the treatment. They also failed to see the "story behind the story," the fact that patients were now demanding HDC in the absence of good evidence that it worked, and that hospitals and doctors were profiting from the procedure. The general reporters who wrote human interest stories about the ordeal women went through often had no background in medicine. Laura Kiernan, a longtime reporter at the *Boston Globe,* in 1991 wrote about several women challenging their insurers in court. That year, she also wrote about a volunteer firefighter suspected in an arson case, the upcoming presidential debates, and baseball card collectors. Political reporters who wrote about the insurance debate in state legislatures saw only the politics, and they simply repeated as a matter of course the unsubstantiated claims being made by the treatment's proponents in medicine. On May 6, 1990, for instance, *Boston Globe* reporter Brian McGrory wrote that insurers were refusing to pay for a treatment that "some doctors say represents [the] only hope against the fatal disease" (p. 44). He would go on to become the *Boston Globe's* White House correspondent and a columnist.

One of the few reporters to grasp the real story was Robert Bazell, chief science correspondent for NBC. He became interested in the procedure in 1990 after a friend of his wife's died soon after undergoing a transplant. "Then I found some people in the insurance industry," he recalled, "who said, 'There is this amazing thing happening, we are losing all these court cases, being portrayed as villains, but we don't know if this [treatment] works' " (Bazell 2004). In the December 31, 1990, issue of *The New Republic,* he had pointed out that the insurers might actually be right to question the use of HDC. He quoted Craig Henderson, one of the few oncologists willing to critique the procedure, as saying that the bone marrow transplanters who were treating breast cancer patients "think they are performing miracles" (p. 10). Bazell also wrote that HDC was hugely profitable for doctors and hospitals, which charged insurers many times what the procedure cost.

The print and television reports dealing with HDC/ABMT for breast cancer are shown for 1989 through 2000 in figure 2.1. These data were obtained by a Lexis-Nexis guided news search of full-text major papers and news transcripts, which were searched for "breast cancer" and "high dose chemotherapy." Inclusion criteria included relevance to HDC/ABMT for breast cancer. The results included brief

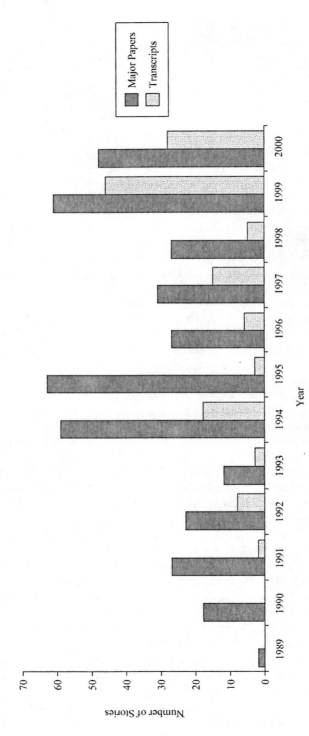

Figure 2.1. Number of stories published about HDC-ABMT published or aired per year between 1989 and 2000.

segments in news programs and full stories. This is not comprehensive as Lexis-Nexis does not have full-text records for all U.S. major newspapers, television, or radio programs.

Conclusion

In the 1980s, HDC/ABMT emerged from clinical research. By the end of that decade, attention focused increasingly on its use as a promising new treatment for breast cancer. A constellation of forces drove the procedure along the path of widespread clinical use just as rigorous evaluation in randomized clinical trials was beginning. In the next two chapters, we review one of the most powerful of those forces: courtroom trials involving patients, physicians, insurers, and lawyers.

Part II

Drivers of Clinical Use

3

Court Trials

Diseases desperate grown,
By desperate appliance are relieved,
Or not at all.
—William Shakespeare

Illness is the night-side of life, a more onerous citizenship. Everyone who is
born holds dual citizenship, in the kingdom of the well and in the kingdom
of the sick. Although we prefer to use only the good passport, sooner or later
each of us is obliged, at least for a spell, to identify ourselves as citizens of that
other place.
—Susan Sontag

It is not surprising that the controversy over high-dose chemotherapy with autologous bone marrow transplantation (HDC/ABMT) ended up in the courts. Regardless
of their institutional capacity to resolve such disputes, the courts have long been central to resolving contentious social policy debates. In fact, it would have been quite
unexpected if an alternative forum had emerged to settle the matter. This is illustrated clearly by the following account by Musa Mayer:

> Nine years ago this spring [2003], I sat in a Long Island courtroom with the rest of my
> breast cancer support group. We had come in solidarity for our friend Pat, whose
> insurance company had refused coverage for a second bone marrow transplant, after
> the first had failed, on the basis that this was an experimental treatment.
>
> Experimental? Surely not, I thought. The insurance company didn't care about
> patients; its only concern was the bottom line. When Pat's doctor took the witness
> stand, he offered testimony that seemed persuasive to me. At the time, I couldn't have
> told you the difference between a phase 2 study and a phase 3 randomized clinical trial.
> All I knew was that many oncologists were recommending this promising treatment to
> their high-risk and metastatic breast cancer patients.
>
> Pat felt that the transplant was her only hope. It would be cruel to take away
> that hope, I thought. Members from the local advocacy group turned out in force that
> day. The press was there, working on yet another story of a young woman fighting for
> her life.
>
> The judge, a cancer survivor himself, was clearly moved. Pat got her transplant. Six
> months later, however, she was dead—not from her metastatic breast cancer, but from
> treatment-induced damage to her bone marrow.

Then a second friend died following her transplant a few months after that, and I began to read the research myself, and to piece together what the studies actually showed—and what they didn't show.

Looking back now, I can trace my radicalization as a patient advocate to the troubling discovery that in the case of high-dose chemotherapy with bone marrow or stem-cell transplant in high-risk and metastatic breast cancer, the tools of science had been subverted by the rush to embrace the treatment. Most disturbing to me was the role that advocates had played in guaranteeing broad access to an unproven and highly toxic treatment, effectively sabotaging enrollment in the randomized trials that would have provided a definitive answer years sooner. (Mayer 2003, p. 3881, reprinted with permission from the American Society of Clinical Oncology)

Advocacy for the HDC/ABMT procedure entered the courtroom before randomized clinical trials (RCTs) were initiated. Musa Mayer's recollection captures the dynamic interaction of patients' hopes and fears, the witness of patient advocates, the advice of physicians (to both patients and judges), health insurers' denial of coverage of the experimental, and the press. In this chapter, we analyze the context and issues of HDC/ABMT litigation and in the next chapter address the litigation strategies of plaintiffs' and defense attorneys.

The HDC/ABMT treatment for breast cancer had not been proven through RCTs to be a safe and effective alternative to standard chemotherapy. From a scientific perspective, evidence from RCTs should have preceded its widespread use. Absent evidence of effectiveness from such trials, insurers balked at reimbursing what was a very expensive procedure. Naturally, women brought litigation to compel insurers to pay. Judicial trials, which are not well suited to resolving scientific controversies, were every bit as important as clinical trials in determining the use of HDC/ABMT. They certainly dominated the initial years.

The mixed, and sometimes startling, results and consequences of the court cases have received considerable public and scholarly attention (Mello and Brennan 2001). In particular, the jury verdict in *Fox v. HealthNet* to award the plaintiff $89 million (including $77 million in punitive damages) not only shook the insurance industry but also generated a wave of subsequent media attention to HDC/ABMT.[1] Although the specifics of each case will differ, the facts in the *Fox* case (if not its outcome) seem reasonably representative of the difficult decisions facing both the insurer and the patient at a time when little hope for survival remains.

At the age of 38, Nelene Fox was diagnosed in 1991 with breast cancer and underwent two modified radical mastectomies. After the cancer spread to her bone marrow, she underwent conventional chemotherapy. When the conventional therapy did not work, her two treating physicians recommended HDC/ABMT and supported her attempt to obtain the procedure at the University of Southern California Norris Cancer Center, which declared her eligible for the treatment. Fox's insurer, HealthNet, nevertheless denied coverage, arguing that the procedure was experimental/investigational and therefore contractually excluded from coverage, despite the fact that HealthNet's Evidence of Coverage booklet seemed to cover bone marrow transplants.

According to Fox, HealthNet then put pressure on one of her treating physicians to reverse his recommendation. Instead, HealthNet requested a second opinion from another medical center. Fox refused and then attempted to raise the cash on her own.

After raising the money, Fox underwent the procedure at the University of Southern California in August 1992. She died shortly after the procedure, and her husband filed suit in the California state courts for breach of contract, bad faith breach of contract, intentional infliction of emotional damages, and punitive damages. After a very contentious trial, the jury awarded plaintiff the large punitive damages noted here.

For this study, we examined three separate aspects of the legal system's role in HDC/ABMT: litigation trends involving HDC/ABMT (this chapter); strategies used by both plaintiffs and defense attorneys (chapter 4); and one state's legislative mandate requiring insurers to pay for the procedure (chapter 6). We first describe the litigation context and the issues raised in the judicial process. After discussing our methodology for examining the legal issues, we describe our results. We conclude with a discussion of the litigation trends and the lessons learned.

The Litigation Context

Health insurance coverage determinations and challenges revolve around two questions.[2] Is the recommended clinical treatment covered under the insurance benefit contract? If so, are the benefits medically necessary for the particular patient? Inevitably, these will be case-by-case determinations and will form the backdrop for HDC/ABMT litigation.

To simplify a complex set of relationships, most people purchase health insurance through their employer. Most large employers offering health benefits have encouraged patients to enroll in managed care plans. Managed care combines the financial (insurance) and medical care under one entity. Plan physicians recommend treatment (such as HDC/ABMT), but plan administrators determine whether the benefit contract includes coverage for it. The problem is that there is considerable variability on how coverage decisions are made. Dissatisfied patients, especially those with little hope remaining, often turn to the courts to order the plan to provide the benefits.

Establishing Liability

At its simplest, tort law (civil wrongs such as negligence) establishes standards of reasonable behavior that individuals are expected to meet. Based on notions of what is reasonable (often using a risk–benefit analysis), the tort law of negligence is the legal standard of care that the community establishes to set appropriate rules of conduct. When a person's or an institution's conduct falls below the minimum standard of care expected, the injured party (the plaintiff) may sue the wrongdoer (the defendant) for appropriate damages.

In general, tort law is based on showing that the defendant was at fault for the injuries.[3] To meet the burden of proof for a damage award, the plaintiff must prove the following four elements by a preponderance of the evidence (i.e., that one side's arguments tip the scales, even if ever so slightly): (1) that a duty of due care exists; (2) that a breach of that duty has occurred; (3) that the conduct caused the injuries; and (4) that the injury produced actual damages.[4] Each state court system establishes its own body of negligence law, although all states use this basic framework. This means that legal doctrine will vary across states, so that what may be negligent in one state will not necessarily be negligent in another.

In ordinary negligence, a breach of duty occurs when the defendant's actions fall below the standard that a reasonable person would maintain. Courts usually look to industry custom to determine whether the defendant's conduct was reasonable.[5] Establishing medical liability also involves each of the four elements, with one important difference from nonmedical cases. Unlike the situation with general negligence, for which the standard of care is determined by what is reasonable under the circumstances (usually based on industry custom), the medical profession itself largely sets the standard of care in medical liability litigation. In medical liability cases, the standard of care is based on what is customary and usual practice as established through physician testimony and medical treatises. A typical statement of the law is that each physician must "exercise that degree of skill ordinarily employed, under similar circumstances, by the members of [the] profession" (*Lauro v. The Travelers Insurance Co.*).[6] In effect, this means that the same level of care must be provided to all patients, regardless of resource constraints.[7] The primary reason why medical liability diverged from general negligence is that courts did not feel capable of second-guessing customary medical practice. Courts held that nonphysicians do not have sufficient training to establish customary and reasonable medical practices.

Each physician must exercise the degree of skill ordinarily practiced, under similar circumstances, by members of the profession. Physicians with special knowledge, such as cardiologists, will be held to customary practices among those of similar skill and training. If, however, there is more than one recognized course of treatment, most courts allow some flexibility in what is regarded as customary treatment, known as the respectable minority rule. Also known as the two schools of thought doctrine, it is designed to deal with situations for which there are two or more recognized and accepted clinical strategies. The doctrine is most useful as a defense to a malpractice claim but may have some applicability to the HDC/ABMT cases in setting the standard of care (Cramm et al. 2002).[8] In relatively rare instances, courts will allow a plaintiff to challenge the adequacy of customary medical practice, resulting in a higher standard of care than determined by the profession.[9]

When these rules were originally established, courts relied on customary practice within the physician's local area. Only physicians familiar with local practices could testify on behalf of an injured patient, but many physicians were unwilling to testify against local friends and colleagues. Most state courts have abandoned the locality rule to avoid the harshness of its results and because medical schools now use a uniform national curriculum. The customary practice standard is now based on national practices. Physicians from anywhere can testify regarding the national standard of care. In most states, an expert witness must have sufficient expertise about the type of care provided to testify. For example, a radiologist would be expected to testify whether another radiologist properly read a computed tomographic scan. A general practitioner would not ordinarily or be assumed to have enough knowledge about radiology to testify.

Courts are reluctant to substitute their judgment for that of the medical profession, even when a new, safer technology is being considered (Jacobson 1989; Jacobson and

Rosenquist 1996).[10] Despite this deference to medical professionals, the tort system operates as a quality control mechanism over medical care in providing incentives for meeting the standard of care and sanctions for providing substandard care.

An important aspect of the trial process is the distinction between the admissibility of evidence (whether someone is allowed to testify) and the weight of the evidence (how the jury treats each witness relative to other evidence introduced during the trial). The judge has sole discretion to determine the admissibility of evidence. Under recent U.S. Supreme Court rulings, judges are authorized to exclude testimony lacking an adequate scientific foundation (Shuman 2001).[11] Once the judge permits the witness to testify, however, it is then the jury's responsibility to weigh an individual's testimony against that of any other witness or piece of evidence introduced.

Employee Retirement Income Security Act Preemption

Traditionally, health care litigation, such as patients suing physicians or hospitals to recover monetary damages for medical injuries, is resolved by state courts. Before the rise of managed care, health insurance cases were litigated in state courts, often to decide whether an insurer should pay for care already provided. Managed care changes the policy and litigation context in two respects. With the integration of financing and care delivery under managed care, refusing coverage means denying care altogether. Then, if a plan subscriber challenges a denial, the health plan can invoke protection from liability under the Employee Retirement Income Security Act's (ERISA's) preemption provision.

Congress enacted ERISA in 1974 primarily to regulate pension plans, but also included health benefit plans within its scope.[12] ERISA's goals are to establish uniform national standards; safeguard employee benefits from loss or abuse; and encourage employers to offer those benefits. To achieve these objectives, ERISA imposes strict requirements on pension plan administrators for reporting and disclosure,[13] participation and vesting,[14] funding,[15] and performance of fiduciary obligations.[16] ERISA does not mandate that employers offer benefit plans but provides a structure for national uniformity of administration once such plans are extended. Only a few of these requirements apply to health benefit plans, in part because Congress did not pursue the implications of regulating both pension and health benefit plans under one statute. Congress could not have anticipated the dominance of the managed care model. As a result, ERISA provides almost no federal regulation of health plans.

ERISA governs private employer-sponsored employee benefit plans, including health care benefits offered by self-insured firms, covering approximately 65% of the insured population. Legally, ERISA preempts state laws, including personal injury claims that relate to an employee benefit plan. In this context, preemption means that state courts cannot decide the litigation. When a law or legal action involves the administration of plan benefits, such as a state law mandating certain benefits or a patient's challenge to denial of a plan benefit, ERISA preemption is triggered. In essence, ERISA preemption creates a regulatory vacuum in which states cannot act and there is no comparable federal regulatory presence, and it blocks individual litigation against health plans. Even though a patient could still sue in federal court if the state lawsuit is preempted, ERISA only permits recovery for the amount of a claimed benefit, leaving the patient with no adequate remedy, especially for economic and noneconomic (i.e., pain and suffering) damages if the care was wrongly denied. In the Nelene Fox case, for example, Fox was covered by her school health plan, which was not an ERISA-covered plan. Therefore, a state court jury could award much higher damages. Had she been in an ERISA-covered plan, she could have only recovered the amount of the denied benefit.

Until recently, courts have interpreted the phrase *relates to* very broadly, preempting most challenges to managed care cost containment programs. Courts have consistently held that challenges to the quantity of care, including delayed or denied care resulting from cost containment initiatives, will be preempted as involving the interpretation of plan benefits. Recent cases have established the principle that challenges to the technical quality of care (i.e., claims against managed care organizations [MCOs] for their role in substandard clinical care) do not involve the administration of plan benefits and will not be preempted, allowing state courts to resolve the litigation. In practice, the quantity/quality distinction is difficult to maintain, as many clinical decisions involve both aspects. Discharging a patient 2 days early, for instance, may represent a clinical decision, or it may be a based on a benefits determination.

The quality/quantity distinction and similar incremental changes to ERISA preemption case law have opened the possibilities of successfully challenging cost containment initiatives, although ERISA remains a major hurdle to challenging MCO benefit denial decisions. In response to highly publicized horror stories resulting from ERISA preemption, Congress has considered, but not yet enacted, patients' rights legislation that would permit patients to sue MCOs in state courts.

Understanding ERISA is important for litigation over HDC/ABMT for two reasons, with one favoring the defendant, and the other partially favoring the plaintiff. First, an ERISA-covered plan can have the case removed from the state courts and have it decided in the federal courts. By itself, removing state courts from considering liability litigation against MCOs and transferring the case to federal court would not mean very much if patients could still seek the same range of damages. The problem is that ERISA greatly restricts the patient's available remedies in federal court. Second, an ERISA-covered patient can seek an injunction barring the insurance plan from denying coverage. If an injunction is issued, it almost always requires the insurer to pay for the care. Yet, the legal standard for issuing an injunction favors the defendant.

In evaluating coverage determinations under ERISA-governed plans, the courts use two standards of review: arbitrary and capricious and de novo.[17] The arbitrary and capricious standard applies when the health insurance plan has specifically conferred discretionary authority on its plan administrator to determine eligibility for benefits and to interpret the terms of the plan.[18] Under the arbitrary and capricious standard, courts are to defer to the decision of the plan administrator unless the decision constituted an abuse of discretion.[19] The de novo standard applies if the plan has not conferred such authority on the plan administrator.[20] Under this standard, courts interpret the policy as they would any other non-ERISA contract, applying the traditional rules of contract law.[21] For obvious reasons, many commentators claim that the arbitrary and capricious standard favors the insurer, while the de novo standard favors the policyholder (Kennedy 2001, p. 374).

Contract Interpretation

Contract law is primarily concerned with establishing and enforcing promises that are freely arranged by competent adults who understand the nature of the agreement. Contracts constitute voluntary agreements for mutual benefit between parties and specify in advance what services will be provided and what the consequences (i.e., damages) will be for breach of contract. By designing rules that protect freedom of contract, individuals are able to bargain with others to purchase or sell goods and services under mutually agreed terms and circumstances. In the language of economists, contracts establish the expectations of the parties *ex ante* (from the beginning). When the contract is signed, people agree to be bound by its terms. An *ex ante* analysis binds the parties to what they understood regarding benefits, rights, and responsibilities when entering into a contract, even if their personal circumstances and desires change.

For our purposes, the most important contractual arrangement is between patients and health plans. The selection of a health insurer or a health plan is a contractual arrangement that sets the scope and limits of expected health care coverage. In return for a set premium, the health care benefits defined by the contract will be provided. That contract forms the basic understanding of what benefits will be provided (the benefit package); how decisions regarding coverage are made (medical necessity); what alternatives exist regarding out-of-network coverage; the gatekeeper role of the primary care physician; how patients can challenge the denial of medical care (grievance procedures); and available remedies to resolve any disputes (arbitration). The available benefit packages for employees of most large firms (more than 100 employees) are relatively similar, with insurers and MCOs competing on price. There is much greater variation in the benefit package for employees of small firms (fewer than 50 employees) or those purchasing individual health insurance coverage from a commercial insurer.

With either type of employer, patients usually sign a standard contract, negotiated between the employer and the health plan, setting forth the terms and conditions on a take-it-or-leave-it basis.[22] In theory, the employer negotiates the best available package of benefits and price, but the employer and employee have different interests and incentives as we discuss in this chapter. A major problem for employees is that it is difficult to define important terms, including limits on benefits such as experimental therapy, with enough detail to avoid arguments over what is covered.

When interpreting contracts, courts first look to determine whether there was a meeting of the minds (that is, mutual assent to the terms and obligations in the contract) between the contracting parties. As long as the terms of the agreement are clearly stated and there was reasonably equal bargaining power, courts will not overturn the contract reached. To determine whether a meeting of the minds occurred, courts will look to the parties' intent, as indicated by the plain language of the agreement. As one court noted recently: "[T]he objective in construing [a contract] is to ascertain and carry out the true intentions of the parties by giving the language its common and ordinary meaning as a reasonable person . . . would have understood the words to mean."[23]

An important concept in contract interpretation is that contractual ambiguity will be resolved against the party who drafted the agreement, known as the doctrine of *contra proforentem*. This doctrine has been especially important in cases challenging the denial of experimental treatments. Since it is difficult to specify every conceivable health care contingency up front, health insurance/coverage contracts exclude coverage for most experimental treatment but do not attempt to list or define all treatments likely to be excluded. Some courts have required coverage if the exclusion is not specific, leading some scholars to complain about judge-made insurance (Abraham 1981).

When parties to a contract disagree about its terms or meaning, courts are asked to determine whether a promise contained within the contractual agreement has not been performed or whether the agreement has been breached. Here, courts must ask whether the injured party has been deprived of a benefit that he or she reasonably expected. In the health care context, potential contractual breaches arise when patients allege that a health plan failed to provide benefits included in the patient's benefit package or failed to provide medically necessary care as recommended by the treating physician, out-of-network coverage, or experimental therapies. To determine whether the plan breached the contract, a court will examine the terms of the agreement and interpret them according to the parties' intent and common meaning of the terms.[24] In the context of HDC/ABMT, the issue is whether the contract specifically excluded the procedure as experimental or investigational and whether the patient knew about the exclusion.

If a court finds a breach of contract, then the next step is to assess how to compensate the injured party adequately. The basic remedy for breach of contract in the Anglo-American legal system involves awarding damages to compensate an injured party for the loss. In certain cases, courts could compel specific performance of the contract, meaning that a plan would be required to provide a benefit that was otherwise denied. In HDC/ABMT cases (especially under ERISA), a court might enjoin the insurer from denying the procedure. Specific performance is an equitable remedy that is available when monetary damages would not be adequate. If, for example, a plan denies a bone marrow transplant and thereby breaches the health insurance contract, then a court could order the plan to provide the transplant because monetary damages would not be adequate if the patient's life could be saved (especially under ERISA, for which monetary damages are not available).

Another type of remedy is that of punitive or exemplary damages. Such damages are designed to punish the offending party and to deter similar conduct in the future; they are reserved for cases for which the defendant's conduct is tantamount to fraud, malice, or oppression. Punitive damages are not available for breach of contract in most jurisdictions (and not at all in ERISA cases) but may be appropriate when a defendant acts in bad faith.

Bad Faith Claims

One area where tort and contract law overlap is with the concept of bad faith breach of contract or bad faith coverage denial. Suppose, for example, that a patient presents with anorexia nervosa, with insurance coverage for 70 days of inpatient psychological treatment. If the plan has no comparable inpatient eating disorder program, then the treating physician may recommend referral to an out-of-network program. The health plan may approve a total of 6 weeks of inpatient therapy but then discontinue coverage over the treating physician's objections. In response, the patient may sue the plan for bad faith breach of contract.[25]

The claim emerges from an alleged breach of contract but has a different legal basis. Unlike the traditional suit for breach of contract, bad faith is a tort claim separate and apart from the breach of contract allegation: "The rationale underlying a bad faith [claim] is to encourage fair treatment of the insured and penalize unfair and corrupt insurance practices. By ensuring that the policyholder achieves the benefits of his or her bargain, a bad faith [claim] helps to redress a bargaining power imbalance between parties to an insurance contract."[26]

To win, the plaintiff must show that the refusal to provide coverage was malicious or recklessly disregarded the terms of the contract. If bad faith can be shown, then the patient can recover both compensatory and punitive damages. The import of bringing a tort action for bad faith as opposed to a breach of contract case (where it is not subject to ERISA preemption) is in the damages allowed and in forcing the MCO to show a reasonable basis for its actions to avoid liability.

The Issues

Litigating HDC/ABMT cases involves a number of intersecting and contentious legal issues. First, how should the judge interpret the contract? Did the health plan clearly explain that there would be no coverage for HDC/ABMT because it was considered experimental or investigational? Did the patient understand the contractual limitations? Did the definitions of HDC/ABMT and investigational or experimental occur in the same part of the contract, or were they in different sections? In short, did the patient knowingly consent to the coverage exclusion?

Second, what is the current state of the scientific knowledge? At the time of the treatment recommendation, was HDC/ABMT considered experimental? Did judges and jurors comprehend the nature of the scientific controversy? In particular, did judges and jurors understand that the positive evidence favoring HDC/ABMT came from phase 2 studies that were not necessarily definitive for high-risk or metastatic breast cancer patients, as opposed to RCTs, which have greater scientific validity and reliability?

Third, what constituted the standard of care when the treatment recommendation was made? In weighing expert testimony, what weight should the jury allocate to the treating physician or community oncologist relative to the plan's medical director or a university-based clinical researcher? Is the treatment medically appropriate for the patient?

Aside from the legal issues, nonlegal considerations played a role in the litigation. Most significantly, what role did sympathy for a dying patient play in the cases? Were jurors (or judges) overly sympathetic to the plaintiff given the lack of effective medical alternatives? In addition, what role did costs play in deciding the cases?

Were judges and jurors insensitive to the economic consequences of ordering insurers to pay for HDC/ABMT? Did the courts ignore technology assessments revealing the procedure's high cost and lack of effectiveness?

Finally, what were the effects of how the case was framed? Defendants portrayed the cases as being about science and the lack of proven effectiveness, while plaintiffs framed the case as being about a women's right to choose given a set of poor options and alternatives. Did the case framing affect judicial trial results?

These HDC/ABMT cases were also litigated within a health care policy context that was very much unsettled. When the litigation began in the late 1980s, the concept of managed care was still battling with fee-for-service providers for dominance over the health care delivery system. Although cost containment was a central public policy goal, patients had little understanding of how managed care operated and what the tradeoffs were likely to be between access to care and cost containment. The public was accustomed to receiving basically everything the treating physician recommended without interference from the insurer. Operating on a different conceptual model, managed care was designed to impose cost constraints where none existed before. To be sure, traditional health insurers also confronted this issue and might not have authorized HDC/ABMT in the less cost conscious fee-for-service environment. In the managed care era, the procedure was certain to be much more closely scrutinized.

Methods

For this study, we conducted two separate analyses of the litigation. First, we analyzed the reported litigation. In conducting this analysis, we used the standard electronic legal research tools such as West Law and Lexis-Nexis. Although the published litigation is usually just the proverbial tip of the litigation iceberg, we believe that reliance on the reported cases is justified in this instance. It is clear that the reported cases and jury trials in our sample were the key factors in the insurance industry's response to patient challenges to denial of HDC/ABMT. We also have no reason to believe that the issues litigated differ from those cases that were either settled or resolved internally.

In traditional legal scholarship, commentators analyze a large number of cases for trends or focus on a few leading cases to suggest both the doctrinal implications of the decisions or ways in which the decision could be improved. In litigation, not all cases are created equal. Some cases, by virtue of the reputation of the particular court or judge, because they may set precedent, are the subject of extensive scholarly commentary, or are cited by other courts, become more important than other cases. We used both methods in our analysis, in part because of *Fox v. HealthNet's* large influence and public prominence.

We also reviewed the law review literature and the published health services literature to learn about cases that might not have been available through an online search. To capture cases that might not have been reported, we contacted people involved in the litigation and other stakeholders.

Beyond the 75 unique reported cases, we have identified only four jury verdicts in HDC/ABMT cases. Each side won two cases, but the large award in *Fox v.*

HealthNet dominates the field. Many, if not most, of the cases resulted in settlements or were decided on requests for injunctive relief. Unfortunately, we have not been able to obtain reliable data on the settlements.[27]

For the judicial case analysis, Stefanie Doebler read and reread all of the cases and compiled a list of case themes and descriptive data. To corroborate the analysis, Peter Jacobson independently read and analyzed several leading cases. Together, the authors discussed the recurring case themes.

Litigation Issues and Trends

After their health insurers refused to pay for HDC/ABMT on the grounds that there was no evidence that HDC/ABMT was superior to standard-dose chemotherapy, many women responded by seeking insurance coverage of the procedure through the judicial system. In most cases, they filed a motion for a preliminary injunction to compel their insurer to provide coverage in advance of the treatment. In other cases, the women underwent the therapy, and then they—or, all too often, their estate—sued their insurer to recover the cost of the procedure. Most cases were settled out of court to avoid the expense and publicity of a jury trial, but numerous others were litigated to the appellate level.

The remainder of this chapter reviews the HDC/ABMT cases, highlighting the major issues facing those courts called on to adjudicate a coverage dispute between a breast cancer patient and her health plan. It explains how the cases differed depending on the type of policy at issue (ERISA, non-ERISA, Civilian Health and Medical Program for the Uniformed Services [CHAMPUS], Federal Employees Health Benefits Act [FEHBA]) and depending on whether a federal or state court heard the case. Finally, this chapter identifies trends in the litigation: Were courts that found for the patient more likely to consider the scientific evidence than courts that found in favor of the insurer? Were courts that found for the insurer more likely to interpret the contract language strictly? Although some such trends are evident, perhaps the most accurate conclusion that can be made is that the outcomes were maddeningly unpredictable.

Even with the benefit of being able to review the entire spectrum of cases, it is still difficult to discern the factual or legal distinctions between cases that led the courts to come to such inconsistent results. Perhaps most surprising is the fact that the 1993 jury verdict in *Fox v. HealthNet* had essentially no effect on a patient's chances of winning her case. From 1988 to 1993, insurers prevailed in 17 cases and patients in 16 cases, but from 1994 to 2002, insurers prevailed in 26 cases and patients in 28 cases. Thus, the roughly 1 : 1 ratio of patient to insurer victories established in the pre-*Fox* cases unexpectedly continued in the post-*Fox* cases. Surprisingly, the *Fox* jury verdict was not mentioned in a single reported case—not even in passing.

As a cautionary note, the discussion that follows is not an exhaustive analysis of all of the 86 HDC/ABMT cases but highlights a set of representative cases, including those that are particularly significant for one reason or another. Also, courts generally treat HDC/ABMT and HDC/PSCR (peripheral stem cell rescue) as the same, although they recognize the differences between these procedures.[28] This analysis also includes HDC/PSCR under the HDC/ABMT umbrella.

Summary of the Cases

All of the reported HDC/ABMT cases are listed in table 3.1, including the four jury trials identified during our interviews. In reviewing those cases, it is important to remember that the chart is necessarily incomplete because data are not available on the many cases that were settled. In addition, we have excluded a list of cases compiled by Blue Cross Blue Shield that were not reported, either because they eventually were settled or were withdrawn or because their outcome is otherwise unknown.

Table 3.2 is a brief summary of the HDC/ABMT cases decided between 1988 and 2002. The number of reported cases peaked in 1993–1994. Of note is the small resurgence of cases beginning in 2000, which is surprising given that the procedure was essentially disproved that same year.

Table 3.3 is a summary of the outcome of the few cases decided in state court. Although state courts overwhelmingly favored the plaintiff in these cases, a number

Table 3.1 All of the reported HDC-ABMT cases

	Trial court[a]		Court of Appeals[b]		
	Patient wins	Insurer wins	Patient wins	Insurer wins	Total cases[c]
1988		1			1
1989		1			1
1990	1	1			2
1991	5				5
1992	3	3	1	1	8
1993	5	7	1	3	16
1994	10	3	2	2	16[d]
1995	2	4	3	2	11
1996	3	3		2	8
1997	2	2		2	6
1998			1	1	2
1999					0
2000			1	1	2
2001		1		3	4[e]
2002	1		3		4
Total	32	26	12	17	86

[a] Cases listed in this category include those that were later affirmed or reversed by an appellate court.

[b] Only reported appellate decisions are included in this category. Unreported decisions are not included (although they are indicated in the table of cases).

[c] As noted in the text, this figure includes only reported cases. This figure includes only cases in which the court addressed substantive legal questions, not those in which the court decided procedural issues.

[d] In *Hawkins v. Mail Handlers Benefit Plan*, the court found in favor of the patient in her suit against CHAMPUS but in the insurer's favor in her suit against FEHBA. As a result, there are only 16 cases in 1994 but 17 total "wins" (12 for patients and 5 for the insurers).

[e] Note that all four of these cases were part of the *Zervos v. Verizon New York* lineage.

Table 3.2 Summary of the HDC-ABMT cases

	ERISA		FEHBA		CHAMPUS		Non-ERISA (group or individual)		
	Patient wins	Insurer wins	Patient wins	Insurer wins	Patient wins	Insurer wins	Patient wins	Insurer wins	Total cases
1988		1							1
1989		1							1
1990	1	1							2
1991	5								5
1992	3	1	1	2				1	8
1993	4	3		7			2		16
1994	5	4	1	1	5		1		16[a]
1995	3	4			1	1	1	1	11
1996	1	3			1	1	1	1	8
1997	3	2					1		6
1998	1	1							2
1999									0
2000	2								2
2001		4							4
2002	3						1		4
Total	31	25	2	10	7	2	7	3	86

[a] In *Hawkins v. Mail Handlers Benefit Plan*, the court found in favor of the patient in her suit against CHAMPUS but in the insurer's favor in her suit against FEHBA. As a result, there are only 16 cases in 1994 but 17 total "wins" (12 for patients and 5 for the insurers).

of cases were decided in federal court under state law, at least one of which favored the insurer.

In federal court, 35 district courts ruled on HDC/ABMT cases, but most decided only 1 or 2 cases. In contrast, the Eastern District of Michigan and the Northern District of Ohio decided 3; the Southern District of New York decided 4 (although 3 of the 4 were related cases); the Eastern District of Virginia decided 5; and the Northern District of Illinois decided 10 cases. At the appellate level, each of the circuits ruled on at least 1 case, but the Seventh Circuit led with 5 cases (not surprising given the volume of cases in the Northern District of Illinois). The Second, Fourth, and Eighth Circuits each ruled on 4 cases.

Table 3.3 Outcome of cases decided in state court

State	Patient wins	Insurer wins
Arkansas	1	
Colorado	2	
Illinois		1
Michigan	1	
Total	4	1

Analysis of the Litigation

The Courts' Initial Response

The first cases challenging insurers' refusal to cover the procedure were filed in the late 1980s, shortly after HDC/ABMT initially attracted interest as a therapy for breast cancer but before much was known about it. Consequently, it is not surprising that in these early cases (before 1990) courts supported the insurers' determination that the treatment was experimental.[29] These relatively short opinions focused on the fact that HDC/ABMT was still in phase 3 clinical trials (in which the efficacy of the treatment is studied), and that it had not yet been generally recognized throughout the medical profession as an appropriate treatment for high-risk or metastatic breast cancer.

For example, Janice Thomas was diagnosed with breast cancer in 1984.[30] After a chest x-ray revealed that the cancer had spread to her lungs, she began chemotherapy—to no avail. Her oncologist referred her to Vanderbilt University Medical Center, where doctors recommended HDC/ABMT. Before Ms. Thomas was admitted to the hospital to have her bone marrow harvested, her insurer, Gulf Health, Inc., precertified coverage of the harvesting procedure only (but not the HDC) as "medically necessary" and later paid the claim in full. On her admission, Ms. Thomas signed a consent form, which stated the following:

> At this time, your consent is being obtained only for the removal, freezing, and storage of the bone marrow. This consent is not for higher dose therapy. At the time that high-dose therapy may be recommended, you will be asked to read and sign another form which tells about the high-dose treatment. Having your bone marrow collected does not mean that you will have to undergo high-dose therapy.[31]

A year and a half later, Ms. Thomas requested that Gulf Health precertify coverage of HDC/ABMT. Gulf Health denied the request on the grounds that the treatment was still considered experimental or investigative and thus not covered. In court, Ms. Thomas sought an injunction that would prohibit Gulf Health from denying coverage, but the Southern District of Alabama held that Gulf Health's denial was "rational and supported by the evidence" (*Thomas v. Gulf Health Plan, Inc.,* 688 F. Supp. 590 (S.D. Ala. 1988)).[32]

The court commented that it was "undisputed that, as relates to the treatment of breast cancer, high-dose chemotherapy with bone marrow transplantation is experimental."[33] According to the court, the fact that Gulf Health had paid for the harvesting of Ms. Thomas's bone marrow did not create any obligation on the part of the insurer to pay for the HDC/ABMT procedure.

Although the courts in these early cases deferred to the decisions of the health insurers, they were not unsympathetic to the plight of the patients. In *Sweeney v. Gerber Products Co. Medical Benefits Plan,* the court noted that

> [a]s much as this Court sympathizes with the plaintiff, and understands her desire to undergo the treatment which is the subject of this lawsuit in hopes of prolonging her life, the Court cannot order the defendant medical benefits plan to do that which it is not legally obligated to do. There is no question that high dose chemotherapy accompanied by autologous bone marrow transplantation as a treatment for breast cancer remains today a treatment which is in an experimental and investigational stage.[34]

Despite their sympathy for the plaintiff, courts were unwilling, at least at first, to find in her favor simply because the treatment was her last hope of escaping death.

Consideration of Scientific Evidence and Medical Experts

As new evidence emerged to support the claim that HDC/ABMT was a legitimate treatment for breast cancer, courts in the early 1990s became more willing to find for the plaintiff and to order coverage. Unlike the initial cases, courts began to review the scientific literature in support of the treatment and to consider the opinions of expert witnesses. In *Pirozzi v. Blue Cross–Blue Shield of Virginia,* the court engaged in a lengthy review of the scientific evidence supporting HDC/ABMT as a safe and effective treatment for breast cancer and ultimately concluded that the treatment was not experimental.[35] In particular, the court relied on the testimony and research of Drs. Peters and Antman, noted cancer researchers whose studies demonstrated that "high-dose therapy and bone marrow autotransplants can produce remissions in patients with advanced breast cancer unresponsive to conventional therapy" (Antman and Gale 1988, p. 570).[36] The court noted that "this [finding] fits plaintiff's case perfectly as she is a patient 'with advanced breast cancer unresponsive to conventional therapy.'"[37]

In that case, plaintiff Pamela Pirozzi was a 35-year-old premenopausal woman with three children. She was insured, through her husband's employer, under a Blue Cross Blue Shield group health policy issued in Virginia. Her oncologist prescribed HDC/ABMT for treatment of her stage IV breast cancer as the "best chance for any type of meaningful survival."[38] A physician from Montefiore Hospital in Pittsburgh, where the HDC/ABMT was to be performed, contacted Blue Cross on Ms. Pirozzi's behalf seeking preauthorization. The plan's medical director refused to authorize the treatment on the grounds that the plan excluded coverage for "experimental or clinical investigative" procedures. The insurance contract between Blue Cross and the Pirozzis did not define an "experimental or clinical investigative" procedure, so Ms. Pirozzi sought a declaratory judgment that the plan did indeed cover HDC/ABMT. District Judge Ellis granted her request for an expedited trial due to the rapid progression of her condition and ultimately concluded that HDC/ABMT was covered under her contract. Judge Ellis cautioned, however, that his decision was not intended to signal a broad expansion of coverage under policies such as Ms. Pirozzi's but rather was anchored in the testimony of cancer specialists: "Purveyors of quack remedies and fringe therapies should derive no comfort from this decision. HDC-ABMT is neither of these. It is, instead, medicine's state of the art treatment for certain stage IV metastatic breast cancer patients."[39]

In *White v. Caterpillar, Inc.,* the court reviewed a number of studies, including the Diagnostic and Therapeutic Technology Assessment from the American Medical Association, as well as the findings of a number of peer-reviewed studies.[40] The court concluded that the insurer had erred in refusing to cover the treatment by relying on outdated data and granted the plaintiff's request for a preliminary injunction, commenting that the "plaintiff will probably suffer the greatest harm possible, loss of life, if she is denied coverage for the prescribed treatment."[41]

Rather than review the literature directly, many courts instead relied heavily on the testimony of expert witnesses to interpret the data for them. In doing so, the courts generally deferred to the plaintiff's expert witnesses, usually cancer researchers or the patient's treating physician, who argued that medical research had demonstrated that HDC/ABMT was no longer an experimental treatment for breast cancer. In *Kulakowski v. Rochester Hospital Service Corp.*, the plaintiff offered only the testimony of her personal physician, who described the procedure and its efficacy relative to standard treatments in great detail.[42] In contrast, the insurer presented testimony from the medical director of the plaintiff's insurance plan, as well as from a registered nurse employed by the plan, the vice-president for medical affairs of Blue Cross Blue Shield of the Rochester area, and an oncologist recognized for his expertise in the field of breast cancer, but the court was not convinced. It said, "In choosing to give more weight to the opinion of [the treating physician], I am persuaded by the decisions of a number of other district courts which, in considering this very issue, and relying upon expert testimony, have stated without qualification that conventional chemotherapy cannot cure metastatic breast cancer."[43]

In another case, *Jenkins v. Blue Cross Blue Shield of Michigan,* the director of the Cleveland Clinic Bone Marrow Transplant Program and an oncologist at the Cleveland Clinic testified that the treatment was a nationally accepted treatment for breast cancer.[44] The court, impressed by the credentials of the witnesses, held that reasonable minds could have concluded that HDC/ABMT was an accepted treatment for breast cancer.

Of note in *Pirozzi* and *Jenkins* is the fact that, in both cases, the insurer relied exclusively on its medical director to rebut the testimony of the plaintiff's expert witnesses. The *Jenkins* court noted that the opinion of Blue Cross's medical director that HDC/ABMT as a treatment for breast cancer is experimental "constitutes no more than a scintilla of evidence in support of Blue Cross's contentions, the mere existence of which is insufficient to avoid summary judgment."[45] During our interviews, a defense attorney in at least two jury trials explained that insurers were often forced to rely on their medical directors because it was difficult to line up expert witnesses willing to testify for the defense, a problem that placed the insurers at a "distinct disadvantage."

Not all courts were so easily persuaded by the plaintiff's evidence and experts. In particular, the Seventh Circuit noted in *Smith v. CHAMPUS* that it had considered the issue on several occasions and reaffirmed its earlier findings that then-current data did not suggest that HDC/ABMT produced better outcomes than conventional therapy.[46] In a footnote, the court commented that it "could attempt to argue with these conclusions, [but that doing so] simply would be taking sides in a medical dispute about which [it had] no independent expertise."[47]

Other courts linked their skepticism of the scientific research to the fact that the plaintiff had signed an informed consent document stating that the treatment was experimental or investigational. For example, the Fifth Circuit emphasized in *Holder v. Prudential Insurance Co.* that the plaintiff's deceased wife had signed a consent form describing the purposes of the study exclusively in experimental terms.[48] Thus, the procedure could only be classified as experimental. The court also commented that "[h]ad Mrs. Holder undergone a similar treatment more recently under an accepted protocol, this case may have turned out differently."[49]

Interestingly, the fact that the plaintiff had signed an informed consent before undergoing the procedure was not always persuasive to the court that the treatment was actually experimental. Frequently, courts were willing to dismiss the informed consent entirely on the grounds that many accepted treatments are routinely performed under research protocols.[50] In one case, the court dismissed the fact that the treatment was provided on protocol at a research hospital, noting that "physicians deliver many of today's accepted medical treatments at major teaching hospitals, whose practice it is to collect data on the patients they treat."[51] In another case, both the research protocol and informed consent contained research-related language, including the stated purpose of "'defining the proposed therapy's toxicity and efficacy.'"[52] Even so, the court held that the "evidentiary materials submitted [led] to the conclusion that the treatment was not research-related, but rather, was provided as the only alternative for saving plaintiff's life."[53] The court noted that as of the trial, the plaintiff was still cancer free, which may have influenced its unwillingness to rule that the treatment was experimental.

Contractual Ambiguity and Deference to the Medical Community

While courts recognized the inherently experimental nature of science, some were still willing to hold that HDC/ABMT did not fall under contractual exclusions for experimental treatments because the medical community had accepted the procedure and because many physicians were regularly performing it. Essentially, courts allowed widespread use to substitute for evidence of clinical effectiveness for purposes of satisfying the experimental exclusion. In *Pirozzi*, the court interpreted the widespread usage of HDC/ABMT for breast cancer at major medical centers across the country as evidence that the treatment had "scientifically proven value."[54] In *Adams v. Blue Cross/Blue Shield of Maryland*, the court noted that a consensus of Maryland doctors considered HDC/ABMT to be accepted medical practice despite the fact that it was not scientifically proven.[55] The court disregarded the testimony of several oncologists on behalf of the insurer because they testified only peripherally about the opinion of the Maryland oncological community.

Adams involved two plaintiffs, Alexandra Adams and Kelly Whittington, both of whom were diagnosed with advanced breast cancer in 1990. Both women were under age 35, had two children, and had had a mastectomy. Their physicians judged them to be at high risk for recurrence due to their age and the fact that their cancer was described as estrogen receptor negative. The women each contacted their insurance carrier, Blue Cross Blue Shield of Maryland to seek preauthorization for HDC/ABMT, but Blue Cross denied their requests, relying on a policy provision that excluded experimental treatments from coverage. Blue Cross acknowledged that the policy did cover HDC/ABMT as a treatment for other diseases (Hodgkin's lymphoma, non-Hodgkin's lymphoma, acute leukemia, testicular cancer, and neuroblastoma) but claimed that the treatment was still experimental for breast cancer.

In holding that Blue Cross's decision was "incorrect and unreasonable," the federal district court noted that the insurer had ignored the consensus of opinion of Maryland cancer specialists. At trial, Blue Cross had argued that its evaluation of the procedure reflected a national consensus that mirrored the consensus in Maryland. The insurer introduced testimony from five experts, most notably Dr. David M. Eddy, in support of its belief that HDC/ABMT was still experimental, but the court was unwilling to accept the opinion of a biostatistician rather than a practicing oncologist: "Instead of focusing testimony on the opinion of members of the Maryland oncological community, the Blue Cross experts concentrated on their own independent evaluations of the scientific data."[56] Interestingly, at least two of Blue Cross's witnesses were in fact practicing Maryland oncologists, but both admitted that given the appropriate patient, they also would have suggested HDC/ABMT.

The *Adams* court's unwillingness to trust the testimony of a research scientist over that of a practicing physician was not unique. A Colorado district court that directed the insurer to cover the plaintiff's treatment noted that all of the practicing oncologists who testified agreed that HDC/ABMT was no longer experimental.[57] Only Dr. Ronald B. Herberman, a nontreating research oncologist who testified for the insurer, stated otherwise, but the court noted that he had not treated a patient in years, and that his testimony was less credible than that of the practicing oncologists who testified for the patient.

Similarly, in *Healthcare America Plans, Inc., v. Bossemeyer*, the court noted that the plaintiff had marshaled substantial evidence (letters from 56 cancer centers, a letter from the American Medical Association, and 17 abstracts from peer-reviewed medical literature) that HDC/PSCR was generally accepted in the medical community despite the lack of evidence indicating its scientific effectiveness.[58] The court noted that "the nature of cutting-edge medical technology is that opinions may differ as to whether a certain procedure has crossed the threshold from experimental, investigational, unproven, or educational to general acceptance by the medical community and demonstrated efficacy."[59]

Clear Exclusions by Insurers

In response to the rulings in favor of breast cancer patients seeking coverage for HDC/ABMT, insurers quickly began to draft their policies in ways that made the exclusion of the treatment hard to dispute, even under the de novo standard (as described in the section "ERISA Standards of Review"). By 1993, circuit courts had faced a number of so-called clear-drafting cases (*ERISA Litigation Reporter* 1996). In one case, the plan did not include breast cancer in its list of specific cancers for which HDC/ABMT was covered and stated that "[s]ervices or supplies for or related to surgical transplant procedure for artificial or human organ tissue transplants not listed as specifically covered" were excluded from the policy.[60] The court held that the Office of Personnel Management's (OPM's) exclusion of HDC/ABMT was "the only logical interpretation of the policy."[61] In another case, the plan excluded coverage for treatment provided as part of a phase 1, 2, or 3 clinical trial; because the plaintiff's proposed treatment was the subject of a phase 2 clinical trial, it was excluded from coverage.[62] Thus, a plaintiff challenging this type of clear exclusion was essentially destined to fail by virtue of the contract language alone.

In *Bechtold v. Physician's Health Plan of Northern Indiana, Inc.*, the health plan at issue provided

- "Experimental or Unproven Procedures" means any procedures, devices, drugs or medicines or the use thereof which falls within any of the following categories:
- Which is considered by any government agency or subdivision, including but not limited to the Food and Drug Administration, the Office of Health Technology Assessment, or HCFA Medicare Coverage Issues Manual to be:
    1. experimental or investigational;
    2. not considered reasonable and necessary; or
    3. any similar finding;
- Which is not covered under Medicare reimbursement laws, regulations or interpretations; or
- Which is not commonly and customarily recognized by the medical profession in the state of Indiana as appropriate for the condition being treated.
- PLAN reserves the right to change, from time to time, the procedures considered to be Experimental or Unproven. Contact PLAN to determine if a particular procedure, treatment, or device is considered to be Experimental or Unproven.[63]

The plaintiff argued that the language, "PLAN reserves the right to change, from time to time, the procedures considered to be Experimental or Unproven," suggested that the plan would revise its classification of treatments as experimental as science advanced. The court determined that the plaintiff was attempting to create an ambiguity in the policy where no ambiguity existed, and that the plan had no obligation under the contract language to cover HDC/ABMT. Consequently, the denial of coverage was proper.

In another case, the insurance policy provided only for coverage of "medically necessary" care, defined as follows:

required and appropriate for care of the Sickness or the Injury; and that are given in accordance with generally accepted principles of medical practice in the U.S. at the time furnished; and that are approved for reimbursement by the Health Care Financing Administration; and that are not deemed to be experimental, educational or investigational in nature by any appropriate technological assessment body established by any state or federal government; and that are not furnished in connection with medical or other research.[64]

In that case, the plaintiff, Grace Fuja, had been told by her physician that continued treatment with standard-dose chemotherapy would provide her with only a negligible chance of survival. Following a hearing in 1992, the district court issued a decision ordering Ms. Fuja's insurer to pay for the treatment. She underwent the procedure at the University of Chicago shortly thereafter but unfortunately died 3 months later. The insurer, Benefit Trust Life Insurance Company, appealed the district court's judgment, arguing that the procedure was not medically necessary as defined in the contract because it was provided in connection with medical or other research.

The Seventh Circuit found not only that the contract language was unambiguous, but also that the evidence that the treatment was experimental was overwhelming.

To receive the treatment, Ms. Fuja had signed an informed consent that identified the treatment as "research" and "experimental. The research protocol stated that the studies at the University of Chicago "have been one of the first in this area of investigation," and Mrs. Fuja's treating physician informed her prior to the procedure that the treatment would be "furnished in connected with medical research." [65] The court concluded that because the procedure clearly fell within the plan exclusion of coverage for experimental therapies, the district court's holding that Benefit Trust was liable was erroneous. Writing for the court, Judge Coffey also noted that the courts are not equipped to handle cases that present these types of troubling social and ethical questions.[66] Although he said that such problems of public policy are best handled by the political branches, he also suggested that some sort of collective task force might be convened to reach a consensus on the definition of experimental procedures and to determine which procedures are so cost prohibitive that requiring insurers to pay for them would lead to the collapse of the health care industry.[67]

Employee Retirement Income Security Act of 1974 Standards of Review

Because most employed individuals obtain their health insurance coverage from their employers, the vast majority of cases involving denial of coverage for HDC/ABMT were subject to ERISA.[68] In many of the HDC/ABMT cases, the courts devoted the bulk of the opinion to determining the appropriate standard of review, with the discussion of the merits of the case at times playing almost a secondary role. Judicial review of denial of coverage cases under ERISA turned at least partially on the standard of review adopted by the courts.

Courts were particularly likely to find for the plaintiff when given the opportunity to review the plan's denial of care under the de novo standard, which affords the courts an independent review of the insurers' decision. Conversely, the arbitrary and capricious standard requires courts to affirm the plan administrator's decision unless it was "arbitrary, capricious, or made in bad faith, . . . not supported by substantial evidence" (*Harris v. Mutual of Omaha Cos.*, 992 F.2d 706 (7th Cir. 1993)).[69] The Supreme Court has held that courts should review a denial of benefits under the de novo standard unless the health insurance plan specifically confers discretionary authority on the plan administrator to determine eligibility or to construe the terms of the plan.[70]

In cases such as *Pirozzi* and *Scalamandre v. Oxford Health Plans, Inc.*,[71] for which courts adopted the de novo standard, the judges looked closely at the findings of fact, particularly evidence relating to the efficacy of HDC/ABMT, and gave no deference to the insurer's decision to deny coverage. In evaluating the denials, the courts applied common law rules of contract interpretation and interpreted ambiguities in favor of the policyholder. For example, in *Simkins v. NevadaCare,* the court held "that a person of average intelligence and experience would interpret the terms of the plan to include coverage" and reversed the district court's finding for the insurer.[72] In these cases, courts found that the insurers failed to offer a "consistent, reasonable explanation" for denying coverage of HDC/ABMT.[73]

On the other hand, courts that reviewed the denial of coverage under the arbitrary and capricious standard were more likely to find for the insurer. Under this standard, the insurer's denial of care should be upheld unless it was "clearly erroneous."[74] In 1993, a district court held that the health plan's denial of coverage was not an abuse of discretion because it followed a standard for determining what procedures it would pay for.[75] Likewise, the Seventh Circuit affirmed a district court's holding that the insurer did not act arbitrarily and capriciously because the policy unambiguously precluded coverage for HDC/ABMT.[76]

Under the arbitrary and capricious standard, if the insurance company was able to introduce any credible evidence that the treatment was experimental, the court was obligated to find for the plaintiff even if it would not have found that way under a de novo review. Frequently, the courts expressed their displeasure at having their hand forced in this manner: "Although the Court sympathizes deeply with plaintiff's situation and may well have decided the issue differently based on the substantial evidence which plaintiff presented to [her insurer] in support of her claim for coverage, the Court cannot find on this record that [the insurer's] decision was arbitrary and capricious."[77]

While the arbitrary and capricious standard did provide some protection for insurers, that protection was far from absolute. In *Bucci v. Blue Cross/Blue Shield of Connecticut,* the court held that the exclusion of HDC/ABMT was arbitrary and capricious because the insurer did not provide a set standard to define when a medical procedure was nonexperimental and accepted.[78] In *Kulakowski v. Rochester Hospital Service,* the court held that HDC/ABMT was "not experimental, not unsafe, and not inefficacious" and thus could not fall under the experimental exclusion.[79]

In some of these cases, there probably was a legitimate argument that the insurer acted arbitrarily and capriciously. For example, in *White v. Caterpillar,* the insurer relied on an outdated version of a report as the basis of its decision to deny coverage.[80] In other cases, however, it is questionable whether the insurer really acted arbitrarily and capriciously or whether the court was perhaps motivated by some other concern. In most, though not all, cases for which the court held that the insurer had acted arbitrarily and capriciously, it did so because the insurer was also the plan administrator. This dual role creates a potential conflict of interest between the plan's economic interests and action on behalf of the patients. When this type of conflict of interest exists, the court may review the claim with a reduced level of deference, but there is no prescribed method of reviewing these cases. As such, courts reviewing denials of HDC/ABMT could essentially circumvent the coverage specified in the contract and find for the plaintiff in instances when the facts of the case do not support such a finding (Brostron 1999).

In *Bucci,* for example, the court found irrelevant the fact that the plan had applied a five-factor evaluation test to determine that HDC/ABMT was not a covered procedure because the criteria were subjective in nature and because the plan was subject to a conflict of interest.[81] Similarly, in *Killian v. Healthsource Provident Administrators,* the insurer made its decision that the procedure was not medically necessary based on the advice of three independent medical reviewers, but the court found the insurer to have acted arbitrarily and capriciously because it was acting under a conflict of interest.[82]

Arbitrary and Capricious Standard in FEHBA and CHAMPUS Cases

The FEHBA authorizes the OPM to contract with private insurance companies to provide health benefits to all federal employees.[83] The OPM has final authority to decide benefits and exclusions in all FEHBA plans. CHAMPUS is a health benefits program established by Congress to provide coverage to retired military personnel and their dependents.[84] CHAMPUS, which is financed through funds appropriated by Congress, contracts with MCOs to provide coverage for its beneficiaries.[85]

In reviewing coverage decisions made by the OPM and CHAMPUS, courts apply the same arbitrary and capricious standard as they do in ERISA cases. The outcome of the cases challenging denial of HDC/ABMT depended in part on whether the patient was covered by a FEHBA plan or CHAMPUS.

Courts interpreted the arbitrary and capricious standard more strictly in FEHBA cases than in ERISA cases, perhaps because most of the insurance plans provided by carriers with which the OPM contracts explicitly excluded coverage of HDC/ABMT for breast cancer. As a result of this strict interpretation, courts consistently upheld the OPM's denials of coverage. (Of the two cases in which courts found for the plaintiff under a FEHBA policy, one was reversed on appeal, and the other was a state court decision.) In *Caudill v. Blue Cross & Blue Shield of North Carolina,* the court upheld the district court's decision granting summary judgment to the insurer, noting, "[t]here is nothing to suggest that OPM's interpretation of the contract at issue here was irrational. But even if the court would have come to a different conclusion, it must not substitute its judgment for that of the administrative agency with a decision under review." [86] Even in cases in which the OPM made no explicit factual findings in its letter of decision, courts still found the decision to be neither arbitrary nor capricious. In *Harris v. Mutual of Omaha Cos.*, the Seventh Circuit noted, "Ms. Harris is correct that the final decision issued by OPM is less than an exacting account of its review process and conclusions. Nonetheless, it is adequate." [87]

In 1995, a new OPM policy took effect that required all plans to cover HDC/ABMT for breast cancer. At minimum, plans were required to cover non-RCTs, but the OPM's policy did allow some limitations for women receiving treatment through RCTs. Predictably, litigation regarding FEHBA policies all but ceased after OPM mandated coverage.

In contrast to the courts' deference to the OPM, they were far less deferential to CHAMPUS in determining whether CHAMPUS's action in denying coverage for HDC/ABMT was "arbitrary, capricious, . . . or otherwise not in accordance with the law." [88] The distinction seems to be that the OPM policies included specific provisions regarding coverage of HDC/ABMT, so by virtue of the plain meaning of the plan language, the courts could not conclude that the treatment was covered. Conversely, the CHAMPUS policies included only a provision excluding procedures "not in accordance with accepted standards, experimental, or investigational." [89]

In *Bishop v. CHAMPUS,* the court reviewed in great detail the materials CHAMPUS used to determine that HDC/ABMT is experimental and concluded that "[HDC-ABMT] is generally accepted and therefore covered under CHAMPUS policy." [90] In *Mashburn v. Mail Handlers Benefit Plan,* the district court found that CHAMPUS had acted arbitrarily and capriciously because the treatment did not fall under any of CHAMPUS's definitions of experimental and because CHAMPUS had failed to consider the opinion of the medical oncological community.[91]

Only the Seventh Circuit found that CHAMPUS did not act arbitrarily and capriciously in denying coverage of HDC/ABMT, overturning a lower court holding in *Smith v. CHAMPUS*.[92] The court commented that "[w]idespread disagreement among qualified medical experts over a medical issue virtually precludes a reviewing court from concluding that an agency decision that agrees with one side is arbitrary or plainly wrong even if the court finds other views more persuasive."[93] (This statement seems to apply to all cases decided under the arbitrary and capricious standard, including ERISA cases.)

Cases Subject to State Law

Only policies negotiated directly between the patient and an insurance underwriter are governed by the law of the state in which the agreement is consummated. State courts have traditionally viewed health insurance policies as contracts of adhesion rather than negotiated agreements and therefore have construed ambiguous coverage provisions in favor of the policyholder (Giese 1996, pp. 215–216). As such, state court decisions reviewing denial of coverage for HDC/ABMT tended to favor the policyholder. For example, in *Taylor v. Blue Cross/Blue Shield of Michigan,* a Michigan appellate court held that the exclusion clause in the policy was ambiguous because the terms *experimental* and *research in nature* could be interpreted in different ways.[94] Furthermore, the plaintiff had introduced evidence that HDC/ABMT was an effective treatment for breast cancer and thus not experimental. Likewise, in *Tepe v. Rocky Mountain Hospital and Medical Services,* a Colorado appellate court held that the exclusion clause was ambiguous regarding which services were covered and which were not and affirmed the trial court's decision granting the plaintiff's motion for summary judgment.[95]

When a federal court heard the case but applied state law, decisions still favored the policyholder seeking HDC/ABMT.[96] For example, in *Dahl-Eimers v. Mutual of Omaha Life Insurance Co.,* the court applied Florida law to determine that the phrase *considered experimental* in the policy was ambiguous.[97] In *Nichols v. Trustmark Insurance Co.* (Mutual), the Northern District of Ohio applied state law and ultimately found in favor of the policyholder.[98] Similarly, in *Frendreis v. Blue Cross Blue Shield of Michigan,* a federal court found that it was reasonable for the insured to believe that coverage was provided.[99]

Nevertheless, a finding for the plaintiff is not automatic under state law. In *O'Rourke v. Access Health, Inc.,* an Illinois appellate court upheld the trial court's finding that the experimental exclusion clause was not ambiguous because it explicitly vested the Access medical staff with the authority to determine whether a procedure was experimental.[100] In *Wolfe v. Prudential Insurance Co.,* a federal court applied Oklahoma law to find for the insurer.[101]

Unfortunately for many plaintiffs, state claims brought against self-funded plans were often preempted by ERISA. ERISA's preemption clause states that "[e]except as provided in subsection (b) of this section, the provisions of this subchapter and subchapter III of this chapter shall supersede any and all State laws insofar as they may now or hereafter relate to any employee benefit plan described in section 1003(a) of this title and not exempt under section 1003(b) of this title."[102] Therefore, courts had no choice but to hold that actions based on contract, tort, and other theories were preempted by ERISA, leaving the plaintiff without an effective remedy. ERISA limits recovery to the amount of the benefit, which as noted is often far below what a jury might award for economic and noneconomic (pain and suffering) loss.

For example, in *Bast v. Prudential Insurance Co.,* Roger Bast and his son Timothy filed a complaint against his late wife's insurer alleging breach of contract, loss of consortium, loss of income, emotional distress, breach of the duty of good faith and fair dealing, violation of the Washington Consumer Protection Act and the Washington Insurance Code, and ERISA.[103] Rhonda Bast, who was diagnosed with breast cancer in 1990, had sought preauthorization for HDC/ABMT. After 6 months of haggling, the insurance company finally authorized the procedure, but a month later magnetic resonance imaging showed that the cancer had spread to Ms. Bast's brain, making her ineligible for HDC/ABMT. She died less than a year later.

The Ninth Circuit held that ERISA preempted all of the plaintiff's state law claims. As noted, because extracontractual, compensatory, and punitive damages are not available under ERISA, the court held that the only possible remedy was equitable relief (i.e., providing the procedure), which was not appropriate because the plaintiff had already died. Under ERISA, plaintiffs may only recover the amount of the benefit. The court noted that "without action by Congress, there is nothing we can do to help the Basts and others who may find themselves in this same unfortunate situation."[104] Similarly, in *Turner v. Fallon Community Health Plan* (127 F.3d 196 (1st Cir. 1997)), the First Circuit held that ERISA does not provide a damages remedy for denial of rights under a benefits plan, and that ERISA preempted state law claims.

Other Claims for Relief

A few plaintiffs tried more creative approaches in their efforts to enjoin their insurer from denying coverage, albeit not with great success. In *Reger v. Espy,* the plaintiff argued that denial of coverage of HDC/ABMT violated Title VII of the Civil Rights Act of 1964 in that exclusion of the treatment has a disparate impact on females.[105] The court rejected that argument, noting that "[i]t is clear from the language of the Plan . . . that HDC-ABMT benefits are not available for most types of cancers, only one of which is breast cancer."[106] The court also found the exclusion to be facially neutral and "the decision not to provide HDC-ABMT benefits for all but the five listed diagnoses affect[s] both men and women equally."[107]

In *Dodd v. Blue Cross & Blue Shield Association,* the plaintiff claimed that excluding coverage of HDC/ABMT for breast cancer runs afoul of the Rehabilitation Act of 1973 and the Americans with Disabilities Act of 1993 (ADA) because the treatment is provided for some other forms of cancer.[108] The court rejected the Rehabilitation Act claim because it was the OPM's responsibility, rather than the insurance company's, to comply with the act, so the plaintiff had no claim against the insurance company. The court also rejected the ADA claim because "the Association is not an employer of federal employees enrolled in the Service Benefit Plan" and hence "may not be sued under the ADA."[109]

However, in *Henderson v. Bodine Aluminum, Inc.*, the Eighth Circuit reversed a district court's denial of injunctive relief on the grounds that her plan's refusal to cover the procedure constituted a violation of the ADA.[110] Karen Henderson's oncologist had suggested that she enter a clinical trial for breast cancer patients that randomly assigned half of the participants to a regimen of HDC/ABMT. Her insurer refused to precertify her enrollment in the program because of the possibility that she could be placed in the experimental group. The appellate court, which entered its order the day after the district court denied Ms. Henderson's request for injunctive relief, held that she had a legitimate chance of proving at trial that HDC/ABMT is an accepted treatment for breast cancer. Because her insurance company covered HDC/ABMT for other types of cancer, denying treatment for breast cancer could be a violation of the ADA.

Resolution and Postscript

In 1999, several randomized controlled studies reported that HDC/ABMT was no more effective than standard-dose chemotherapy (e.g., Stadtmauer et al. 2000; see also chapter 8). An editorial accompanying one study concluded as follows: "[T]o a reasonable degree of probability, this form of treatment for women with metastatic breast cancer has been proved to be ineffective and should be abandoned in favor of well-justified alternative approaches" (Lippman 2000, p. 1120). Predictably, requests for the procedure declined, as did the attendant litigation, although a few courts are still dealing with the issue.

Most recently, a federal district court in Michigan held that the insurer's denial of coverage for HDC/PSCR or HDC/ABMT for stage II breast cancer for which fewer than 10 lymph nodes were affected was arbitrary and capricious.[111] In that case, *Reed v. Wal-Mart Stores, Inc.*, Wal-Mart denied the plaintiff's request for coverage of the treatment because " '[b]ased on the medical information provided, the proposed procedure for this patient's diagnosis of stage II breast cancer with only six positive nodes is considered experimental/investigational and is therefore not covered under her medical plan.' "[112] The plan covered only patients at high risk of relapse, including those with 10 or more positive nodes or stage IIIB or IV breast cancer. Based on its interpretation of the expert testimony, the court concluded that the plaintiff's condition was biologically equivalent to a 10-node disease and therefore that the insurer acted arbitrarily and capriciously in denying her request for treatment. Conspicuously absent from *Reed* was a discussion (or even acknowledgment) of the contentious litigation over the previous 14 years. In fact, the court cited only two HDC/ABMT cases in its opinion, *Sluiter v. Blue Cross and Blue Shield of Michigan* and *Pirozzi v. Blue Cross–Blue Shield of Virginia*, and did not refer to the 1999 scientific studies discrediting HDC/ABMT.

Litigation Trends and Lessons Learned

The following discussion of the trends present in the HDC/ABMT cases requires several caveats. The definition of a *trend* is somewhat loose. Some trends are very clear, such as the fact that almost all of the cases discuss the language of the insurance policy at issue. Others involve only a handful of the cases; for example, among those cases favoring the plaintiff, several emphasize the fact that the treatment was generally accepted by oncologists. Second, as noted, many of the opinions focused largely on the proper standard of review (de novo vs. arbitrary and capricious) rather than on the merits of the case. Finally, the fact that these cases were driven largely by the specific facts of the case, such as the exact policy language at issue, makes it somewhat difficult to compare the cases. In many instances, virtually the only constant between two cases is that they both involved HDC/ABMT as a treatment for breast cancer. As Judge Sweet of the Southern District of New York noted, many courts have addressed the "'experimental' nature of HDC-ABMT for the treatment of Stage IV breast cancer," but "[t]hose cases provide little assistance since, by virtue of the task, they each are specifically focused on the particular contract language at issue."[113] Those qualifications aside, there are a number of themes present in many of the cases that favor the plaintiffs not present in those that favor the insurers and vice versa. Each is discussed in turn.

Contract Language

In virtually every case involving a denial of coverage for HDC/ABMT, the court reviewed the policy language, often in some detail. The primary difference between the cases that favored the insurer as opposed to those that favored the patient is the manner in which the court interpreted that language. In the cases that favored the patient, the courts were almost certain to find that the contract language was ambiguous: An average policyholder would not be able to determine whether the procedure was covered. When contract language is unclear, the court construes the contract against the drafter, in these cases, the insurer. For example, a Michigan appeals court held that the policy language was ambiguous because the plan did not define the terms *experimental* or *research in nature,* which was particularly troublesome because medical experts had divergent definitions of each of the terms.[114] A federal district court noted, "Judges need not check their common sense at the door when interpreting insurance policies and the plain language within them."[115] The court went on to explain that if an insurer wanted to limit coverage via an exclusionary provision, then that "language must be direct and specific."[116]

Even in cases in which the contract language was specific, some courts insisted that the policies use plain, readily understandable terminology. The Ninth Circuit held that a policy provision that limited tissue transplant coverage to allogeneic bone marrow only was ambiguous because the "average person would not understand the term 'tissue transplant' to encompass HDC/PSCR, because she would not understand stem cells to be 'tissue.'"[117] Here, there was not really an ambiguity in the contract language; the term *allogeneic* clearly refers to a transplant in which the donor and the recipient are not the same person. Hence, an autologous bone marrow transplant would not be covered. Yet, the court was unwilling to overlook the fact that the contract used language the average subscriber might not understand.

Conversely, in opinions that favored the insurer, the courts were likely to find that the plan language explicitly excluded HDC/ABMT. In *Bossemeyer,* the court determined that exclusion 11 was unambiguous because the policy used everyday English language. Exclusion 11 provided that the following were not covered by the plan: "Medical, surgical, psychiatric procedures, organ transplants and pharmacological regiments, and associated health procedures which are considered to be experimental, unproven or obsolete, investigational or educational as determined by Health Plan. 'Experimental' means those procedures and/or treatments which are not generally accepted by the medical community."[118] The court added that "[t]o pretend that their meanings are inscrutable to policy beneficiaries because the policy fails to set forth a legal definition of each term, would be to exercise inventive powers for the purpose of perverting the plain meaning of the exclusion."[119]

In many cases, courts based their decision entirely on the contract language, without consideration of any other factors.[120] Many of these cases involved federal employees; as noted, the courts were extremely deferential to the OPM's denials of care. In other cases, even when the contract did not explicitly define terms such as experimental, courts recognized that the grant of discretion to the plan administrator under the arbitrary and capricious standard provided the administrator with the authority to resolve any ambiguities. Furthermore, they were sensitive to the plaintiffs' attempts to have the policy construed in their favor by portraying the policy as less clear than it actually was. On a number of occasions, courts noted that plaintiffs had attempted to "create an ambiguity where none exists" and found in favor of the insurer.[121]

Although judicial interpretation of the contract turned on whether the policy was ambiguous, there is little consistency across cases regarding what language constituted an ambiguity. Absent a specific exclusion such as those in the clear-drafting cases discussed in the section "Clear Exclusions by Insurers," it is nearly impossible to determine how the courts would rule based on the wording of the policy alone. The fact that a number of cases were reversed on appeal further illustrates the elasticity of the ambiguity inquiry. In a case decided under Florida law, the policy at issue provided for coverage of medically necessary services or supplies and defined a medically necessary service as one that was "not considered experimental." [122] The Northern District of Florida found that, because the term experimental has a "plain and ordinary meaning" defined by *Webster's Dictionary,* the term was unambiguous in the contract.[123] The Eleventh Circuit, however, found that the same language was ambiguous, in part because the policy did not define the term and in part because it did not explain the basis for a determination that a treatment was experimental.[124]

Science/Expert Testimony

In the cases in which the courts overruled the insurers' denial of coverage, they generally relied heavily on the scientific evidence supporting the procedure. In a number of cases, the courts engaged in a lengthy review of the scientific literature, but in others they depended on expert witnesses to present and interpret the information for them. Generally, courts seemed to consider anyone with a medical degree to be a suitable expert witness. Most persuasive, however, were those experts who not only could explain why the treatment was appropriate for the individual plaintiff but also could discuss HDC/ABMT in a broader context by reviewing the relevant scientific literature.[125] Often, the result was a battle of the experts, with both the insurer and

the patient offering compelling physician testimony and scientific evidence supporting their belief that HDC/ABMT was or was not, respectively, experimental. In these
cases, courts were frequently unable to explain persuasively how they differentiated
between the experts and how they determined who was most credible.

Courts cited studies by Drs. Peters and Antman on only a few occasions but gave
them a fair amount of deference when they did. The source of this deference is unclear,
however, because the courts did not analyze the strength of the studies themselves or
spend a great deal of time summarizing the scientists' credentials. (They did note that
Peters was an oncologist at Duke, which seemed to carry some weight.)

In contrast, consideration of the science was often completely absent in those
cases in which the courts supported the insurers' denial of coverage, particularly in
the cases decided before 1994. As additional studies evaluating the HDC/ABMT
were published, courts became increasingly willing to consider the fact that not all
of the evidence overwhelmingly supported the procedure. In *Whitehead v. Federal
Express Corp.*, the court recognized that there was support for and against performing the procedure but upheld the plan's refusal to cover the treatment because it had
not violated its fiduciary duty.[126] The court added that the evidence need not be
overwhelming or compelling, but rather it must simply be sufficient to reach a
rational decision.

Standard of Care/Widespread Acceptance (or Lack of Acceptance)

Opinions that found for and against the patient considered whether HDC/ABMT was
widely used and accepted. Not surprisingly, a significant portion of those cases in
which the court found for the patient emphasized the fact that the treatment was used
at many hospitals nationwide, that numerous clinical oncologists and transplanters
recommended the procedure, and, to a lesser extent, that some insurers also covered
the procedure. On the other hand, several cases that favored the insurer stressed that
there was in fact no such consensus, and that the procedure was only performed at
large research hospitals and therefore could not be a community standard.

Informed Consent/Research Protocol

As noted, some courts used the fact that the patient had signed an informed consent
as evidence that the HDC/ABMT was still an experimental procedure. Those courts
that found for the patient often did not discuss the informed consent or research protocol and, in the few instances when they did, dismissed them as mere formalities.

Precedent

A number of cases in which the court found for the plaintiff stressed the fact that previous courts had also found for the plaintiff. For example, one state court commented
as follows: "The majority of courts that have considered the propriety of an insurer's
denial of coverage for HDC/ABMT treatment for breast cancer have concluded that
the treatment is not experimental and that benefits relating to that treatment may not

be denied based on policy exclusions based on policy exclusions for experimental or investigative treatments." [127] The court followed that statement with a string cite of supporting cases and only two cases with contrary holdings. Similarly, the case of *Duckwitz v. General American Life Insurance Co.* is essentially snippets of previous cases pieced together to form an opinion requiring coverage of HDC/ABMT.[128] This emphasis on precedent is predictably most evident in cases decided toward the end of the period of HDC/ABMT litigation. Certainly, cases favoring insurers are not devoid of any references to previous cases, but they rely far less heavily on precedent than do those that reached the opposite result.

Policy Arguments

In about half a dozen cases in which the court supported the denial of coverage, its opinion stressed the policy implications of the decision. In particular, courts were concerned about the rising costs of health care and the inability to provide all patients with all of the services their physicians might suggest. In a decision that was later upheld by the Fourth Circuit, the Eastern District of North Carolina explained that the public interest weighed against issuing a preliminary injunction: "To impose upon [OPM] the cost of benefits specifically excluded by its negotiated contracts jeopardizes the scope and extent of health insurance coverage otherwise available to federal employees as a whole, and, of course, imposes a fiscal burden upon all citizens, regardless of their occupation." [129] Likewise, the Northern District of Indiana suggested that "[p]erhaps the question most importantly raised about this case, and similar cases, is who should pay for the hopeful treatments that are being developed in this rapidly developing area of medical science." [130]

In contrast, several of the courts that ultimately found for the patient recognized the fact that these cases have greater policy implications but dismissed them. One court chastised the parties for "treat[ing] the public interest prong as if it were a debate on health care." The court concluded that

> [t]he public interest in this case is served by ensuring that the notice requirements of ERISA are complied with, that employers are enabled to make timely and informed choices regarding the benefits they provide their employees, and that insurance plans are interpreted fairly, free of conflict, and in a manner that preserves rather than removes coverage.[131]

Thus, the court was clearly not willing to consider the impact of its decision beyond its consequences for the patient in front of the court.

Sympathy for the Patient

Some commentators speculated that many of the HDC/ABMT case outcomes resulted from judicial (or juror) sympathy for the dying patient and a concomitant unwillingness to refuse to order a potentially lifesaving treatment (Morreim 2001).[132] As noted, it seems that de novo review of the denial of coverage provided the courts with a relatively straightforward way to issue a ruling in favor of the plaintiff. In other instances, the courts, to some degree, may have manipulated the arbitrary and capricious standard of review to find in favor of the dying plaintiff. Those courts that explicitly expressed sympathy for the patient or discontent with their decisions were those that found for the insurer. The decision of *Harris v. Mutual of Omaha Co.* began with a lengthy discussion of the tragedy of cancer and the fact that the plaintiff deserved any and all treatments that might offer relief from her "horrid disease." The court added:

> Despite rumors to the contrary, those who wear judicial robes are human beings, and as persons, are inspired and motivated by compassion as anyone would be. Consequently, we often must remind ourselves that in our official capacities, we have authority only to issue rulings within the narrow parameters of the law and the facts before us. The temptation to go about, doing good where we see fit, and to make things less difficult for those who come before us, regardless of the law, is strong. But the law, without which judges are nothing, abjures such unlicensed formulation of unauthorized social policy by the judiciary.[133]

In another case, in which the Eastern District of Texas denied the plaintiff's request for an injunction, the court noted: "This is a tragic decision, but one that the law compels. The Hills undoubtedly—and justifiably—expected that in exchange for their dutiful payment of premiums, Trustmark would cover their medical expenses in such a desperate situation."[134] Both of these courts, as well as others, seemed anxious to justify their decisions by explaining that, despite their sympathy for the plaintiff, they were obligated to act within the bounds of the law. Ironically, while many of the decisions favoring the plaintiff may have been motivated by sympathy, only those favoring the insurer expressed that sympathy.

Conclusion

The litigation over insurers' denials of coverage of HDC/ABMT for high-risk or metastatic breast cancer is marked by a jumble of fact-specific cases, varying standards of review, and highly divergent outcomes. In the end, the case law really is as inconsistent and difficult to characterize as it appears at first blush. There are some common themes throughout the cases, for example, an emphasis on the policy language and a lack of emphasis on the patient's informed consent, but little can be said about the cases as a whole. Even the *Fox* jury verdict, which generated intense media outrage and frightened the insurance industry into settling many of these cases, failed to generate any trends in the judicial response to HDC/ABMT.

4

Litigation Strategies

We all know here that the law is the most powerful of schools for the imagination. No poet ever interpreted nature as freely as a lawyer interprets the truth.
—Jean Giraudoux

The testimony of those who doubt the least is, not unusually, that very testimony that ought to be most doubted.
—Charles Caleb Colton

The second aspect of our legal analysis is a case study of litigation strategies. At its heart, the litigation reflected dramatically different moral, legal, and scientific views of the world. For patients with metastatic and high-risk breast cancer, high-dose chemotherapy with autologous bone marrow transplantation (HDC/ABMT) represented perhaps their only chance. Clinicians were divided: Breast cancer oncologists and bone marrow transplanters supported the procedure, while academic physicians wanted to wait for the results of clinical trials. For insurers, the procedure represented an unproven treatment that if used could actually adversely affect the patient's quality of life and lifespan.

Given these disparate worldviews, it is not surprising that the attorneys involved in the litigation offered different narratives about how they framed the issue and their litigation strategies. An important consequence of the differing worldviews is that the plaintiffs' narrative can easily be framed in sound-bite terms, while the defense narrative is inherently more complex. To caricature the more complex narrative we elaborate in this chapter, plaintiffs' attorneys framed ABMT as a dying patient's last hope, while defendants talked about the absence of scientific evidence and the need to say no. Not surprisingly, it seems much easier to "sell" the plaintiff's narrative, especially to a jury, than the defense's more complex story. As a result, many of our defense respondents now say that the cases were not winnable. *Fox v. HealthNet* (127 F.3d 196 (1st Cir. 1997)) is usually cited as exhibit A for this position.

Neither the plaintiffs' nor the defense attorneys' interview responses were monolithic. That is, plaintiffs' attorneys adopted different strategies from one another, as did defense attorneys. In part, that is because each trial, arbitration hearing, or settlement negotiation presented a different set of circumstances and tactical decisions that varied across cases. All trial lawyers are not necessarily motivated by common objectives. To be sure, trial attorneys are all motivated by winning and by the money to be made if successful. Yet, one of our plaintiffs' attorneys spoke in terms of a mission, while another used the language of warfare to describe the litigation. Nonetheless, our interviews revealed considerable consistency within each side in the overall strategies and in the narratives they chose to present.

In this chapter, we examine our interview results. We first describe the general legal and nonlegal strategies each side pursued. Then, we analyze the results and the lessons learned. In the final section, we compare and contrast the interview results and the litigation trends described in chapter 3.

Methods

We conducted interviews with leading defense and plaintiffs' attorneys in HDC/ABMT litigation. Together, these respondents have handled hundreds of HDC/ABMT cases, including jury trials, judicial and arbitration hearings, and settlement negotiations. We conducted seven in-person interviews and one by telephone, consisting of four defense and four plaintiffs' attorneys. We identified these respondents by speaking to knowledgeable experts at insurance companies and others familiar with the litigation. During the interviews, we asked respondents to identify other attorneys we should contact. Although our final sample is hardly exhaustive, we believe that the respondents are representative of the broader population and are recognized as leaders in this litigation.

Prior to the interviews, we prepared a semistructured interview protocol. Most of the interviews were conducted by Peter Jacobson, but Jacobson and Wade Aubry conducted the first site interview jointly. The interviews varied considerably in length but generally ran between 60 and 90 minutes. The protocol was designed to elicit discussion about the following specific topics: (1) HDC/ABMT litigation experience; (2) litigation strategies, along with changes in strategies over time; (3) negotiating strategies, along with changes in strategies over time; (4) the respondents' analysis of the reported case law; and (5) lessons learned. During the interviews, we also collected supportive documentary evidence when available. For example, we requested nonconfidential hearing transcripts and legal briefs filed in the cases.

As with any research methodology, the qualitative approach that we took in this analysis has certain inherent limitations. The study, for instance, was not designed to formally test research hypotheses or to be generalizable to the experiences of all HDC/ABMT litigation. Resource constraints limited the number of interviews we could conduct. We believe that we interviewed a sample of very knowledgeable and influential attorneys whose views are likely to be broadly representative of those who have been involved in this litigation. Nonetheless, we recognize that we have no way of assessing whether their views on the issues discussed mirror those of the larger population of attorneys involved in HDC/ABMT litigation.

For the interview results, the primary form of analysis is descriptive, comparing and contrasting information across respondents along several dimensions of interest. To the extent possible, interview notes captured participants' verbatim responses. Based on the interview notes, Jacobson prepared the analysis identifying common themes and differences across respondents; this analysis was reviewed by the other authors for consistency and accuracy. None of our respondents is identified by name because we granted confidentiality to each.

General Strategies

Plaintiffs

Plaintiffs' attorneys agreed on several general strategies they pursued in each case. As an overarching theme, they argued that HDC/ABMT was the patient's only chance for survival. From the opening argument through the closing statement, this theme was central to each case. A typical statement was that "She doesn't deserve to die. This is her only hope." The obvious strategy is simultaneously to create sympathy for the patient and portray the defendant as uncaring, if not greedy, all the while implying that the plaintiff will not die if treated with HDC/ABMT.

A related strategy focused on patient choice. Underlying this approach is the sanctity of the physician–patient relationship. Any attempt by health plans or health insurers to deny HDC/ABMT thus interferes with the treating physician's recommendation, where medical decisions should reside, and the individual patient's right to self-determination.

The third broad strategy was to portray the managed care industry in unfavorable terms (Grinfeld 1999; Larson 1996).[1] Each of the plaintiffs' attorneys characterized the insurer (often a managed care organization [MCO] or a preferred provider organization) as arrogant and tried to demonstrate that arrogance to the judge or jury. According to respondents, the arrogance manifested itself in several ways. Insurers failed to return attorneys' phone calls. More important, insurers failed to communicate directly with the patients to explain why decisions were being made and to answer any questions. In court, the attorneys attempted to demonstrate the arrogance by arguing that the defendant failed to investigate the patient's claim. Take, for example, the following findings of fact from *Adams v. Blue Cross/Blue Shield of Maryland, Inc.*: [2]

> On July 26, Dr. Spitzer [the treating physician] wrote a letter of appeal to Dr. Keefe [the plan's medical director] and Blue Cross, to which neither Dr. Keefe nor anyone from Blue Cross ever responded. On August 22, 1990, Mrs. Whittington's [another plaintiff] attorney wrote to Dr. Keefe, enclosing the phone numbers of nine Maryland oncologists with the suggestion that Dr. Keefe consult them. He did not. Mrs. Whittington never received any formal notification from Blue Cross that her appeal had been denied.

Much more damaging was that, in one remarkable instance, a managed care executive stated during a deposition that his firm went by the Golden Rule: "He who has the gold makes the rules." The jury reacted negatively to this comment. A plaintiffs' attorney interviewed on another project characterized such insensitive remarks as "the gift that keeps on giving" (G. Agrawal, personal communication to P. Jacobson, December 20, 2002).[3]

Defense

In retrospect, it is easy to second-guess defense counsel for not settling cases like *Fox*. Our interviews suggest several reasons why these cases were litigated, which reveal broader defense strategies. First and foremost, respondents indicated that the plans did not believe that HDC/ABMT was in patients' best interests because of the high mortality rates and reduced quality of life. In most cases, the medical director felt strongly that HDC/ABMT was unproven, and that the patient was not an appropriate candidate for experimental treatment. In addition, they felt the weight of the science supported their reliance on the need to wait for clinical trials. For instance, one respondent cited the Eddy (1992) article as demonstrating unknown effectiveness and high risk even for the "right" patients.

Underlying their decisions, defense counsel thought that even if they lost, the cases would be too weak to generate punitive damages. At the worst, the insurer would be required to pay for the treatment (although the attendant litigation costs are not trivial). Defense attorneys also expected that the informed consent documents would demonstrate patients' awareness that the procedure was in fact experimental. Finally, defense counsel believed that the contractual exclusions were sufficiently specific. The procedure's high costs were therefore worth litigating.

A serious strategic problem defendants faced was how to discredit the procedure. Even if the science was not favorable, the procedure could not easily be dismissed as quackery. The problem was that defense attorneys could cross-examine on the scientific validity, but witnesses could easily rely on the Peters and Antman studies or on prevailing clinical practices to refute the defense's claims that the procedure was still experimental. The inability to attack the treatment as mere quackery gave plaintiffs' counsel important openings for attacking the defense case and simultaneously made it difficult to cross-examine the treating physician.

The defense also faced some intangible strategic difficulties, lying in what one defense attorney called the "public mindset" that each individual should have as much care as possible, that nobody really pays for health care, that the chance of life is important no matter what, and that all medical care is good for you. Combined with the anti–managed care sentiment, the public mindset (i.e., the jury pool) would not be favorable to MCOs.[4]

Legal Strategies

Every case involved four separate, but interrelated, legal issues. Across cases, the emphasis on which issue predominated was likely to vary, but in preparing a case for a hearing, attorneys needed to address each issue. There was general agreement among both plaintiffs' and defense counsel that the following—the contract, the standard of care, informed consent, and bad faith—were the major legal issues in play.

The Contract

Each attorney we interviewed said that every case started with the insurance contract. What did the contract promise by way of benefits, what was excluded from coverage, and what did the patient understand about the nature of the contractual agreement? From the plaintiffs' perspective, "Was the person who paid the premiums given fair notice of what would not be paid?" Their attorneys' primary goal was to demonstrate that the contractual language was ambiguous, and that any exclusions could not be enforced unless the language was clear and unambiguous. Since the insurance company drafted the contract, any ambiguity would be resolved against it. The defense argued that the common meaning of the contractual language clearly excluded experimental or investigational procedures. From the defense's perspective, plaintiffs were using the courts to rewrite the contracts when the exclusions were clear.

Yet, according to respondents on both sides, many of the early contracts (i.e., in the late 1980s) were inherently ambiguous.[5] For example, one part of the contract would include bone marrow transplants as a covered benefit, while a separate section would exclude experimental or investigational treatments (as determined by acceptable medical practice).[6] In one section, the bone marrow transplantation benefit might be limited to certain conditions, but chemotherapy would be a covered benefit in another section. Many courts agreed with plaintiffs' challenges that because the sections appeared in different parts of the contract, it was inherently confusing to a patient.

Moreover, plaintiffs' attorneys argued that the definitions of experimental and investigational were often ambiguous and could not be understood by the average patient, particularly in relation to discussions with the treating physician. When asked why the contracts were drafted this way, one respondent referred to statements in a deposition that marketing pressures and fears were responsible. According to this view, the health plan marketers did not want to be viewed as having too many restrictions on care when it marketed the plan to potential subscribers. Two managed care industry attorneys agreed with this analysis.

A related problem, two plaintiffs' attorneys noted, occurred in cases for which the contract language was reasonably specific in excluding HDC/ABMT, but the booklet patients received at enrollment indicated that similar procedures were covered. In conjunction with the ambiguity argument, plaintiffs' attorneys maintained that the insurers created an expectation that HDC/ABMT would be covered. One attorney's closing argument framed the argument this way: "[the plaintiff] looked in his little booklet, looked in the promise and that's what he saw, that bone marrow transplants are a covered benefit. . . . Nowhere in that contract, in this provision here, does it say, 'bone marrow transplants are excluded.'"[7]

Over time, our respondents indicated that insurance contracts came to be more tightly written, making it increasingly difficult to argue ambiguity (Newcomer 1990). In fact, one respondent said that it became so difficult to litigate the newer contracts that he took the matter to the state legislature for legislation to mandate insurance coverage. At least one plaintiffs' attorney argued that payment for HDC/ABMT had been an ongoing controversy before the coverage policy was issued. Therefore, the defendant should have more specifically excluded it from coverage but instead used language that led the patient to believe that the procedure would be covered. At least in the reported decisions, there is no indication that this argument succeeded.

The Standard of Care

At the core of the litigation was whether HDC/ABMT was the appropriate standard of care for patients with metastatic and high-risk breast cancer. To the insurance companies, there was no dispute about the standard of care for HDC/ABMT: it was and remains experimental. Hence, the standard of care for patients with metastatic breast cancer did not include HDC/ABMT (at least outside clinical trials). The plaintiff's job, therefore, was to demonstrate that the procedure's use was widespread among community oncologists. One plaintiff's attorney argued that the defense's best strategy was to show that there was controversy over the science in the medical community. If physicians used a variety of approaches to breast cancer treatment, then there was no standard of care, and the plaintiff should lose her challenge because the procedure should be considered experimental. Defendants wanted the case tried on the lack of proven effectiveness; plaintiffs wanted to try the case based on its widespread use regardless of what the research results indicated.

In many of the cases, plaintiffs' attorneys were able to show widespread use. For example, despite the absence of evidence from phase 3 trials, many community oncologists and transplanters were avid supporters of the procedure. Their testimony carried great weight with the jury and acted to counteract the defense experts. From a judge's perspective, it was difficult to rule that the procedure was experimental when there was strong evidence from community physicians that they were actively using it. At a minimum, it would be justifiable to support a plaintiff's award based on the respectable minority rule (that a respectable number of physicians regard the intervention as the appropriate treatment).

Excerpts from the following trial transcript in 1994 clearly show the dilemma facing the judge and jury in determining the standard of care. The witness, a medical director of a Civilian Health and Medical Program for the Uniformed Services (CHAMPUS) plan, began by stating that HDC/ABMT "does not meet the generally accepted standards of usual medical practice in the general medical community" as defined in the plan's benefit contract.[8] The following colloquy then occurred:

Q: "Ms. X" was a little more straightforward in her affidavit. She stated in paragraph 10 that, "ABMT and PSCR [peripheral stem cell recovery] for breast cancer has gained acceptance among many oncologists." Would you agree with that statement?

A: Yes, sir.[9]

Q: You would also agree that in 1991 the *Journal of Clinical Oncology* conducted a survey wherein 80% of oncologists polled felt that high-dose chemotherapy for the treatment of breast cancer was an alternative that should be offered to women. You would agree with that, wouldn't you?

A: I am not sure, sir.

Q: Are you familiar with the *Journal of Clinical Oncology* study?

A: Yes.

Q: You would agree with me 80% of oncologists felt that it was an alternative that should be offered, is that correct?

A: That is what was reported there, yes, sir.

Q: Do you know some piece of information why that is not accurate?

A: Yes, sir, I do. . . . It would be the consensus conference from Lyon, France, published in last month's *Journal of Clinical Oncology* which states the international consensus of not only the oncologists of America but also the oncologists of the world feel that [HDC/PSCR for] breast cancer should be confined solely to clinical trials.[10]

Q: Now, when we talk about American oncologists, you would agree with me that the *Journal of Clinical Oncology* study . . . polled 465 American oncologists, isn't that right?

A: Yes.

Q: It is 80% of those 465 American oncologists who say that it should be offered as an alternative, isn't that right?

A: Yes.

Q: It is safe to say if 80% of the oncologists polled in America say it should be offered as an alternative, then it is pretty safe to say that it is accepted by American oncologists, isn't that correct?

A: I wouldn't make that assumption.

Q: 80%, that figure speaks for itself, doesn't it?

A: Not in my opinion. [The witness then noted that six of the seven oncologists listed at the end of the article argued that HDC/ABMT was experimental.]

Q: Is it your testimony today that, given the participation of those seven American oncologists at that conference, more weight should be placed upon that than the *Journal of Clinical Oncologists* survey, is that what you are telling the court?

A: Yes, sir.

Q: Isn't it also true that some form of high-dose chemotherapy is available in most every major city and state in the United States, isn't that true?

A: I don't know that to be true.

Q: If you had to take a guess, you would agree it would be a good many?

A: It would be many major cities, yes, sir.

Q: It is available both at many academic institutions and hospitals?

A: That's correct.

Q: It is available from private providers also, isn't that correct?

A: That's true.

Q: It is available inpatient?

A: That's true.

Q: Outpatient?

A: True.

Q: Academicians administer the treatment, isn't that correct?

A: Yes, sir.

Q: Private oncologists administer the treatment. Isn't that right?

A: Yes.

Q: Community-based oncologists administer the treatment, isn't that correct?

A: Yes.

Q: Pretty widespread, isn't it?

A: Yes.

From this exchange, the strategies of both sides can be seen, as can the conundrum facing the court.[11] For plaintiffs' attorneys, if the procedure is widely used, then how can it be considered experimental or investigational? For the defense witness, the mere fact of general use does not define the standard of care. In similar exchanges in other cases, the defense makes a strong case that the science does not support widespread use. Defense counsel attempted to show that what the transplanting physician recommended was unique to the patient, without any agreed-on standards in the community. By contrast, plaintiffs' counsel repeatedly focused on the final set of questions listed to show that the procedure had spread to every corner of clinical practice.

Informed Consent

The contract and standard of care issues can be seen as offensive strategies for each side. Another offensive strategy defense counsel thought would be significant was the insurers' claim that the patient knew about the contractual limitations and, more importantly, was aware that HDC/ABMT was experimental or investigational. Defense counsel used three strategies to put plaintiffs on the defensive regarding informed consent: (1) to show that the patient knowingly signed forms indicating that the procedure was experimental or investigational; (2) to show the discrepancies between what the physician told the patient and the insurance contract; and (3) to show differences between the treatment protocol and the insurance contract.

In deposing a patient, defense attorneys questioned her extensively on exactly what she knew about the procedure (i.e., cure vs. therapy, treatment-related mortality); what her physician had explained about the treatment protocol (i.e., experimental and investigational); and what she knew about the insurance contract. Showing that the patient knew that the procedure was experimental was an important line of defense for insurers. Some of the questions were quite pointed, designed to encourage the patient to reconsider her decision. Defense counsel focused on the forms patients signed to indicate that they were aware that the procedure was experimental and therefore could not claim that the contract was ambiguous. They often cited depositions designed to show that patients had consented to the contractual exclusions.

Defense attorneys also attempted to demonstrate that what physicians told patients indicated that patients were aware that the procedure was experimental. It is not clear that patients actually understood either the contractual limitations or the limitations of HDC/ABMT. For instance, patients in the early 1990s talked in terms of how HDC/ABMT was a cure ("I have a 30% chance of a cure"), when their physicians said that "there is no other therapy that presents the hope of a cure," implying only the hope of HDC/ABMT. More important, one defense attorney argued that informed consent was often vitiated by a physician's simple statement: "You'll die—this might help." After that, it is hard to convince someone that HDC/ABMT might not be good for her.

Plaintiffs' attorneys differed in their concern about informed consent. Although one attorney expressed little concern, he successfully moved to exclude all testimony relevant to the issue. Others noted that it seemed to be an issue in the early litigation but dissipated as time went on, and informed consent seemed to play little role in case dispositions.

For reasons we discussed in the chapter 3 analysis of the case law, informed consent did not play a significant role in the litigation outcomes. Indeed, judges either rejected the link between the signed forms and the contract or ignored the issue altogether. In holding that the contract exclusion was ambiguous, courts tended to dismiss the relevance of the consent forms to whether the contractual language on experimental treatment was ambiguous. This is curious because defendants would seem to have a strong argument that patients knew that HDC/ABMT was experimental once the protocol was explained to them. Perhaps the problem was that the contract language rarely explicitly excluded bone marrow transplants for breast cancer. Arguably, then, patients were not informed when they signed the contract.

Bad Faith

For both sides, the issue of bad faith was key to their legal strategies. Plaintiffs' attorneys wanted to demonstrate that the insurer not only inappropriately denied the treatment, but also did so in bad faith. The defense argued that there was a legitimate dispute about the coverage, and that the insurer acted reasonably and in good faith. The stakes for avoiding bad faith were high. The reason lies in the level of damages to be awarded and hence the recovery of attorney's fees. Absent bad faith, even if the insurer lost, its damages were limited to the amount of the procedure. For plaintiffs, a finding of bad faith could result in punitive damages (i.e., the $77 million punitive damages award in *Fox v. HealthNet*) and a high payday for the attorneys.

Thus, plaintiffs' attorneys attempted to show that the insurer wrongly denied coverage, interpreted the contract provisions inconsistently, or failed to investigate thoroughly the patient's case. In short, the plaintiffs' strategy was to demonstrate that the insurer was unfair to the patient and should be punished. A key part of this strategy was to show that the insurer did not adequately investigate the appropriateness of the treatment for the individual patient, and that the plan medical director never examined the patient.

Plaintiffs' attorneys began by probing the contract language, focusing on the exclusions and definitions of experimental therapy. From there, they relied on the treating physician's recommendation for HDC/ABMT to show that the insurer's denial was unreasonable or failed to follow the appropriate process. In California, this was somewhat easier than in other states because the California courts presume that the treating physician's recommendation should be followed.[12]

Perhaps the easiest way to show bad faith was to show that the insurer was inconsistent. Plaintiffs' attorneys did so in two very effective ways. In some instances, the insurer covered HDC/ABMT for some patients but not for the plaintiff. In *Fox,* for instance, it was widely reported that HealthNet covered one of its employees (over some internal objections) and at least one other subscriber. During the trial, this inconsistency became a cudgel not only for liability but also, most importantly, may account for the large punitive damage award.[13] In others, the attorneys were able to show that different treatments with characteristics similar to HDC/ABMT were covered.

For instance, a plaintiff's attorney argued in one trial that the defendant itself

pays for the same treatment for other solid tumor cancers which have not advanced any further in the scientific literature than has the treatment of breast cancer. Indeed, [the defendant] pays for HDC/ABMT treatment of multiple myeloma, germ cell carcinoma, testicular cancer and acute myelogenous myeloma in adults. The peer review studies regarding this treatment as applied to these cancers is [*sic*] no more conclusive than are the studies regarding breast cancer. The *only* difference is that these cancers appear with far less frequency than does breast cancer. . . . The *only* apparent, though not justifiable, basis for the disparity is expense.[14] [emphasis in original]

Another plaintiffs' attorney estimated the prevalence of testicular cancer at 1 in 7000 men compared to a breast cancer prevalence of 1 in 8 women. In a brief submitted to the court, this attorney also argued that "the 'cure' rates, safety, efficacy, peer review studies and acceptance in the medical community of such treatment for testicular cancer is essentially identical to that of breast cancer."

In another set of cases, the treating physician (at an academic institution) initially recommended HDC/ABMT only to be overruled by the medical director after the insurer put pressure on the institution. Although perfectly understandable to those familiar with utilization review practices, it exposed the insurer to a bad faith claim. Plaintiffs' attorneys argued forcefully that the insurer put undue pressure on the treating physician to abandon what he or she thought was in the patients' best interests.

For defendants, the question was how to insulate themselves from bad faith claims in cases that did not concern the Employee Retirement Income Security Act (ERISA). Under ERISA, the plaintiff can only collect the amount of the benefit denied; punitive damages are not allowed. *Fox* exposed the industry's vulnerability to punitive damages in non-ERISA claims. In most of the cases, defendants were able to avoid bad faith damages by showing that their actions were reasonable under the circumstances and thus in good faith. Even community oncologists testifying for plaintiffs would admit that reasonable physicians could differ on HDC/ABMT, making it difficult to show bad faith.

To insulate itself further from bad faith damages, at least one major insurer responded by developing an external grievance process for any patient denied care based on the experimental/investigational exclusion. After the denial, the case would be reviewed by three experts, with majority rule determining the plan's response. This strategy did not fully inoculate plans from bad faith damages as at least one hearing following external review resulted in a punitive damage award (Larson 1996). Nonetheless, the strategy seems to have largely reduced such exposure. Although we were unable to obtain data tracking the results, one respondent indicated that plans continued to deny treatment after *Fox*.

Expert Witnesses

Expert witnesses played a crucial role in the litigation once the contractual issues were decided. Each side faced strategic and tactical challenges regarding which witnesses to call, how to avoid devastating cross-examination, and how to shape the standard of care determination. The use of expert witnesses is integrally connected to the role of the science discussed below.

The plaintiffs' attorneys' strategy regarding expert witnesses seems straightforward. They relied on the treating physician to make the case that standard chemotherapy offered no hope, and that HDC/ABMT was best for this particular patient. The plaintiffs' strongest witness was usually the treating oncologist. In fact, one plaintiff's attorney preferred the treating physician over an outside expert.

For one thing, the respondent noted that jurors were not always receptive to experts. For another, use of the treating physician allowed the attorney to frame the case as "the physician was just trying to help the patient." Other plaintiffs' attorneys, however, relied on experts in part because they could not always rely on local physicians to testify in areas dominated by one managed care plan.[15]

Aside from the judiciary's traditional deference to the treating physician, another reason for relying on the treating physician was defense counsel's dilemma in how to cross-examine. As one defense attorney noted, even when confronted, the treating physician could simply respond by saying "I did it to help the patient." To be sure, the defense could cross-examine on the literature and the procedure's toxicity and danger and suggest that the treating physician was raising false hopes. None of this seemed to influence judges and jurors. The defense strategy, therefore, was to get the treating physician on and off the witness stand quickly.

Plaintiffs had another advantage. By all accounts, its expert witnesses, especially community oncologists, were enthusiasts of the procedure and willing to testify about it.[16] At least in one important trial, the defense's expert was at best equivocal. On direct examination, he testified that the procedure was not proven scientifically but said during cross-examination that he favored it for this patient. Thus, the treating physician managed to come down on both sides of the issue.

> I signed two declarations. Each side used one of those declarations. The two were consistent. For [the insurer], I listed the conditions that should govern coverage and concluded that HDC should not be covered for metastatic breast cancer. For [the patient], I listed the factors that she understood and indicated that she wanted the treatment, after I had explained it, and that I thought she should have it. (Glaspy 2002)

This may have seemed consistent to the physician, but it was effectively exploited by the plaintiff's counsel as inherently contradictory. The jury awarded a substantial verdict to the patient.[17]

The primary witness for the defense was usually the plan's medical director, who relied on the literature to show that the procedure was experimental.[18] A problem with relying on the medical director was that he or she rarely saw the patient, a fact that was not well received by either judges or juries. According to one defense counsel who did not participate in any of the litigation, medical directors gave the impression of not caring and being unsympathetic to the patient. As a result, the plans appeared to be excessively bureaucratic, interested only in saving money, and having no empathy for the patient's feelings.

Defendants had trouble convincing outside experts to testify. Even when they identified outside experts prepared to testify on the state of the available literature, they were often undermined on cross-examination with the question: "Dr. 'X,' how many breast cancer patients do you see on a daily basis?"

Equally important, several respondents (two plaintiffs' attorneys and a defense attorney) suggested that defense counsel missed numerous opportunities to challenge plaintiffs' witnesses on the science or to show the potential harm from HDC/ABMT. The defense attorney commented that "no one would take on the aura of Peters and Antman."[19]

Settlement Negotiations

Our respondents varied considerably in describing their settlement negotiation experiences. One common element is that settlement negotiations were easier once defendants sensed that plaintiffs' attorneys were learning how to litigate the cases successfully.

For the most part, our respondents suggested that settlement negotiations can be divided into two time periods: pre-*Fox* and post-*Fox*. Before *Fox*, plaintiffs' attorneys said settlement negotiations were very difficult. Insurers did not return calls and were arrogantly unwilling to negotiate. After *Fox*, the environment changed dramatically as insurers were increasingly unwilling to "bet the company" against one large punitive damages award.[20] One defense attorney indicated that his client settled nothing before *Fox* and covered everything after the verdict to avoid going before a jury. However, two defense counsel indicated that their settlement policies did not change post-*Fox*, and that they continued to maintain an aggressive stance regarding the lack of scientific evidence favoring HDC/ABMT.

Insurers were not initially interested when first approached to place patients in randomized clinical trials (RCTs), pilot projects for nonrandomized trials, or special programs normally not covered. After *Fox*, insurers expressed increased willingness to place patients in trials since offering clinical trials could help avoid punitive damage claims. By then, the costs of standard therapy and HDC/ABMT were roughly equivalent. Nevertheless, a defense attorney said that settlement negotiations were actually harder after *Fox* because the price of settlement escalated. If so, this helps explain why litigation continued for several years after *Fox*.

Nonlegal Strategies

The Science

In many ways, the science seems to have been a distraction to both sides. Neither dealt effectively with the results of studies of patients with high-risk breast cancer as they might apply to plaintiffs with metastatic breast cancer. Plaintiffs' attorneys were especially cautious with the science, trying both to ignore the fact that HDC/ABMT had, at least initially, a high mortality rate and to "muddy" the issue.

Our interviews revealed several strategies plaintiffs' attorneys used to defuse the science. First, one respondent argued that HDC/ABMT was simply an extension of procedures that had been used for many years. A defense attorney lamented that community oncologists and transplanters would say that "I've been doing this for 25 years, so it can't be experimental." Patients with breast cancer had been given bone marrow transplants beginning in 1977, with the procedure becoming more widely available by the end of the 1980s (Weiss 2001). Instead of being seen as a radical new development, he argued that this was part of how science evolved. Since bone marrow transplants had been used for many years to treat breast cancer patients, the addition of HDC should not transform the procedure into an experimental or investigational category. Another respondent built on this to argue that all medicine is experimental and constantly evolving.[21]

A second strategy was to highlight the defendant's inconsistencies in coverage decisions. As noted, this was a particularly critical factor in *Fox v. HealthNet,* which was an important reason for the large punitive damage award. A related strategy built on the inconsistencies by attempting to show that the insurers did not follow the same criteria across diseases. If, plaintiffs argued, insurers did not pay for HDC/ABMT because the results were unproven, then why did they cover other procedures equally lacking evidence of success? For example, one attorney created a chart showing seven or eight different treatments. None of the treatments had been proven effective through phase 3 trials, yet the only one not covered was HDC/ABMT. Insurers countered that not every treatment requires a phase 3 trial to show effectiveness, but HDC/ABMT was one of those that did.[22]

A third strategy was to argue that the peer-reviewed literature questioning the value of HDC/ABMT was outdated. Because of the length of time it takes to go through the peer review process, plaintiffs' attorneys argued that the data were too old to be reliable, that the procedure had evolved since the studies were conducted. Speaking of a plan's medical director, one attorney said that he "relied on medical practices that were 8 years old."[23]

Finally, the scientific evidence was hardly monolithic. For all of the questions about the procedure's effectiveness, especially given the treatment-related mortality figures in the early stages, plaintiffs' attorneys were able to cite the Peters and Antman studies as a counterweight. With the Peters and Antman studies, plaintiffs' attorneys were able to undermine through cross-examination the insurers' claims of experimental or investigational treatment. While it is tempting to dismiss the Peters and Antman research as drawing conclusions unsupported by the data (from the beginning, and certainly in retrospect), these studies provided considerable support to plaintiffs' witnesses. Defense experts were repeatedly forced to explain why Peters and Antman should not be accepted as demonstrating the procedure's efficacy. Doing so was easier once the National Cancer Institute trials began, but data showing declining treatment-related mortality over time further complicated the defense strategy.

In addition, plaintiffs' attorneys were able to solicit letters of support in 1992 from some very prestigious academic institutions, including physicians at Scripps Clinic, the University of Michigan Medical Center, Stanford, and the University of California at Los Angeles, among others. This support reinforced the finding of the 1990 American Medical Association survey that the safety and effectiveness of ABMT was "established or promising" (AMA Diagnostic and Therapeutic Assessment 1990).

For defense attorneys, the science should have been the strength of their cases. At first glance, it seems reasonable to expect that the lack of scientific evidence favoring HDC/ABMT (especially the absence of phase 3 clinical trial results) would doom a plaintiff's case. Curiously, the defense attorneys provided a key reason why that rarely happened. Each of the defense attorneys noted that HDC/ABMT is not equivalent to laetrile. In other words, the physicians recommending and using the procedure were not "quacks" and were not experimenting with "quackery," even if there was little evidence supporting the procedure's superiority over standard chemotherapy. This enabled plaintiffs' attorneys to introduce testimony from community oncologists and transplanters with reasonable certainty that judges would allow them to testify.

Another reason was the difficulty of defense cross-examination given the Peters and Antman studies. When questioned about the scientific evidence, plaintiffs' experts could always rely on Peters and Antman. As questionable as the application and conclusions of their work may be scientifically, it had a powerful influence in the courtroom, in part because of their pedigrees and reputations.[24]

A final problem defense counsel faced was the difficulty of proving a negative—that HDC/ABMT was ineffective. In the few jury trials, defense observers noted that jurors' eyes tended to glaze over when complex scientific evidence was introduced.

For defendants, the problem was less the science than the willingness of experts to testify against community oncologists. Defense counsel used two basic strategies, with only partial success.

First, defendants relied on academic physicians to question HDC/ABMT's scientific validity absent RCTs. When willing to testify, they provided credibility for and bolstered the insurers' claims that the procedure was still experimental. The problem was that many were unwilling to testify, even if they opposed widespread use (Rose 2002). Academic experts agreed to review cases informally for defendants, participate in technology assessments, and perhaps write a letter, but often would not testify.

A second strategy was to show the jury how complex the scientific reality was and the need for RCTs. The purpose was to discredit the plaintiff's contention that HDC/ABMT was the appropriate standard of care. Because it was often difficult to recruit academics willing to testify that the procedure was experimental, defendants were left with "the supervisors rather than the doers." Thus, the defense was usually relegated to relying on the plan's medical director to convince the judge or jury that the procedure was experimental or investigational.

In considering the appropriateness of these strategies, it is important to understand that lawyers and the law tend to think anecdotally as opposed to looking at population-based statistics. As a result, the attorneys' personal experiences dominated their approach. Three of the four plaintiffs' attorneys recounted specific instances when one of his or her clients survived after HDC/ABMT. To say that they were disdainful of the science is not correct, although they were certainly skeptical of the insurers' arguments given their individual experiences. But, they were unapologetic about using the courts to obtain the treatment. One respondent said that "No clients died on the treatment. I got a higher quality of life for at least 6 months, even with a relapse." In contrast, one plaintiff's attorney watched each of five clients die or see their condition worsen as a result of the treatment and refused to take any new cases.

In sum, because of the trial process and the importance of expert witnesses, plaintiffs had an advantage. It was easier for plaintiffs' attorneys to obtain expert testimony from the transplant community in favor of the procedure. Ironically, defendants were unable to take advantage of the stronger argument on the science. The defense witnesses were simply less effective. Even when highly respected academics such as David Eddy testified, judges and juries usually deferred to the treating physician. In one memorable case, the court detailed Dr. Eddy's exhaustive statistical analyses and concluded as follows:

Indeed, Blue Cross' primary expert, Dr. Eddy, is not a practicing physician but is an expert in biostatistics. However, scientific data only provides statistical results from research. After reviewing the relevant scientific data, the practicing medical commu-nity must make an overall value judgment about whether a treatment is accepted, that is, has a sufficiently acceptable risk–benefit ratio to justify offering, or indeed recom-mending, the treatment as an option. According to the contract, Blue Cross must defer to that practical medical judgment if a consensus among Maryland oncologists agrees that the treatment is accepted medical practice. Thus, the Court accords little weight to the opinion of the Blue Cross experts.[25]

Costs

The cost of HDC/ABMT relative to standard treatment was an important considera-tion in the early trials. As the cost differential narrowed (along with the mortality dif-ferences), cost naturally became less of an issue. Most of our respondents tried to avoid the issue. One took it off the table entirely by arranging for reduced cost treat-ment before going to court. The others argued that ultimately the costs of standard chemotherapy, with its follow-up clinical expenses, were not that much different from the HDC/ABMT regimen.

At least in one case, the defendant argued that it lacked the assets to pay for all who might be in the HDC/ABMT pool. The plaintiff's attorney was able to introduce an actuarial study showing that the money was instead going to executive bonuses, which apparently angered the jury. The defense witnesses were not prepared for this line of cross-examination. Another attorney was able to show that the amount of money in the transplant pool was several million dollars higher than the defendant asserted. One plaintiff's attorney recognized the importance of costs but tried to turn it to his advantage. He argued that the insurer was saving $200,000 to remove the patient's best hope.

A defense attorney raised an interesting cost issue in passing. In commenting on testimony from community oncologists, the respondent noted that they, along with community hospitals, had a financial incentive to encourage HDC/ABMT's wide-spread adoption. Although the respondent cross-examined the witnesses on this point, it was not a significant line of attack.

Sympathy and Emotion

Somewhat surprisingly, our respondents differed on the role sympathy and emotion played during the litigation. Each admitted that emotion was a factor (along with gen-erating sympathy for the dying patient), yet there was no agreement on how much it factored into decisions or how to handle it. Indeed, two defense attorneys distinctly downplayed sympathy as a major factor, and most respondents did not differentiate between how judges and jurors reacted. While recognizing that judges and jurors would identify with the patient's dire condition, they both felt that judges focused on the reasonableness of the treatment option and how the plan handled the case rather than responding emotionally to the patient's illness. One defense counsel suggested that judicial sympathy might play a role in hearings for an injunction against denying the procedure. The least-damaging mistake to make would be to err on the side of cov-erage and issue the injunction. Otherwise, the patient's last chance is removed.

Sympathy undoubtedly played a role in the bad faith damage award in *Fox v. HealthNet*. In reading various transcripts, it is hard to avoid a lingering sense that emotion and sympathy were subordinate to purely legal issues in any of these cases. From the plaintiff's opening statement, through witness examination, to the closing argument, the patient's suffering and lack of alternatives were front and center. At various points in one closing argument, the plaintiff's attorney made the following statements: "This was [her] best chance to live a better quality of life, to possibly extend her life, and with the outside chance of a cure. But there's no guarantees, and no guarantees with any medical procedure. . . . [The defendant] did not cause [the patient's] cancer, but they abandoned the [family] when she was fighting for her life" (*Fox v. HealthNet*, no. 219692, Superior Court of California, 1993).

Perhaps that is why a defense attorney stated: "Once opening arguments begin in an emotional case, the defendant is in trouble. If you lose the pre-trial motions, it is better to settle" (interview by P Jacobson). Another put it this way: "Juries are interested in hope, not science"[26] (interview by P Jacobson).

The defense also had to be wary about aggressive cross-examination. Using smart trial tactics, plaintiffs' attorneys often called the patient as the first witness. Defense counsel had to be careful not to arouse sympathy for the dying patient.[27] As one plaintiffs' attorney put it, "she did not deserve to die" was a difficult hurdle for the defense to overcome (interview by P Jacobson).

In contrast, managed care was largely viewed unsympathetically by the public and certainly by participants in the litigation. In choosing between a dying patient and a bureaucratic enterprise, it is not surprising that the sympathies lay entirely with patients. As noted, plaintiffs' attorneys complained that plans were arrogant and dismissive of the patients. Some defense counsel agreed. One said that cases were brought because patients got a bureaucratic runaround instead of an organization trying to work with the patient to get the best care. Better customer relations might have mitigated the urge to sue and the jurors' response to the cases. In this view, plans might have averted litigation by reaching out to patients and their physicians to share information and decision making.[28]

A related problem was the process that insurers used to decide coverage requests. Aside from the inconsistencies in the *Fox* case, numerous respondents discussed the health plans' lack of attention to individual patients.[29] Not only patients, but also judges and jurors wanted to see that cases were handled individually. Jurors expected a deeper analysis of the individual case than insurers were providing. In those instances when the insurer lacked consistent processes for making individual clinical decisions, jurors punished them. From the insurers' point of view, however, individual decisions that were not "standardized" in some way to conform to their medical policy raised the risk of liability from inconsistent decision making. To insurers, this was a double-edged sword: They might be "damned if they do, damned if they don't."

Quality of Life

Respondents discussed patients' quality of life in virtually every interview, but quality of life seemed not to play much of a role in the litigation. Our interviews revealed two very different worldviews about the patients, at least in the early 1990s. Repeatedly, plaintiffs' attorneys framed the issue as their clients having no other hope and as individual choice or preference. Insurers and their attorneys looked at the same phenomenon and said, in the words of a defense attorney, "Why would women go through this? They have 2 years to live and [the procedure presents] the possibility of dying right away" (interview by P Jacobson). Insurers did not view HDC/ABMT as lifesaving or improving the patient's quality of life. Rather, they viewed it as a painful, highly toxic, and life-threatening intervention, as "technology in search of an application" (interview by P Jacobson).

Without exception, defense counsel maintained that HDC/ABMT more often than not reduced the patient's quality of life. According to defense counsel, women did not really understand the nature of the procedure and its potential (to insurers, likely) mortality consequences. Defense attorney respondents raised the issue in two contexts: to question patients about higher mortality rates from HDC/ABMT and to understand patients' motivations for undergoing what insurers believed was a brutal and fruitless procedure. One defense counsel said his clients had trouble following the shifting explanations for why patients wanted the treatment, ranging from curative to quality-of-life improvements.[30]

With one exception, plaintiffs' attorneys disagreed with the insurers' quality-of-life assertions, citing specific instances when the patients lived longer or are still living. It is important to note, however, that the attorneys were vague on which breast cancer stage the survivors had reached when treatment began (although one acknowledged that his surviving clients were stage II nonmetastatic). The plaintiffs' lawyer who disagreed represented five women in the early 1990s, won each of the cases, and then watched each of them die, probably sooner than they would have with conventional chemotherapy and certainly in far more painful circumstances. After that, she refused to take additional cases because all of her clients died painfully and "used up their time" with substantially reduced quality of life.

Analysis of the Interviews

Naturally, the defense and plaintiffs' attorneys offer very different narratives to explain their strategies. Where the narratives overlap is on the issue of bad faith. All along, the driving concern for plaintiffs' counsel was to show bad faith, while defense counsel tried to portray the industry as acting reasonably and in good faith. Plaintiffs' attorneys cannot make much money if the remedy is just to provide care, but that would be a result that the defense seemed resigned to accept. Strategically, therefore, the cases were largely struggles over whether the industry acted in good faith or unreasonably denied appropriate care.

Strategies

These cases are not all about emotion and sympathy; trial tactics and strategy matter, in both large and small ways. For instance, the first jury trial was a defense verdict because the plaintiff's treating physician did not testify. The *Fox* jury awarded punitive damages in part because of the plaintiff's successful procedural tactics (i.e., in excluding informed consent testimony) and in part because of statements defense witnesses made about the Golden Rule.

Our interviews suggest some changes over time in the respective strategies. Three factors account for most of the changes: (1) the verdict in *Fox v. HealthNet;* (2) the rising anti–managed care sentiment that reached a pinnacle in the mid-1990s; and (3) declining treatment-related mortality rates.

It is hard to disentangle the effects of *Fox* and the attendant rise in anti–managed care sentiment. It may be that the attendant publicity surrounding *Fox* contributed to the managed care backlash.[31] *Fox* captured everyone's attention and has dominated the breast cancer litigation environment ever since. There is no evidence that *Fox* altered juror attitudes, but the decision and attendant publicity certainly reinforced the rising anti–managed care sentiment. A defense attorney familiar with all four jury trials commented that juror attitudes changed between 1992 and 1994 as jurors became increasingly distrustful of managed care industry arguments and increasingly favorable to the treating physicians.

The decline in treatment-related mortality rates added to the defense's difficulties. Defendants lost the opportunity to show that HDC/ABMT was more harmful than standard therapy, a key line of argument. Disputes over safety and effectiveness (i.e., that the plan is protecting patients) lost force when there were no differences in mortality. On the contrary, if there were no differences in mortality, the arguments for patient choice gained momentum. Once the mortality from standard treatment and HDC/ABMT were equivalent (as were the costs), the plaintiffs' patient choice arguments became increasingly powerful.

According to defense counsel, the industry's biggest response to *Fox* was to establish an external grievance process for any denials based on the experimental or investigational exclusion. We discuss this under lessons learned.

At the same time, some strategies did not change. As a general observation, it seems clear that the defense's failure to introduce evidence from a treating physician or at least from someone who saw the patient undermined their position. A problem, which did not appear to be corrected over time, was that the insurers relied almost exclusively on the medical director to make the coverage decisions, without any effort to examine the patient or have outside physicians/experts involved from the beginning.

One other point on changing strategies is worth noting. Like any other area, plaintiffs' attorneys learned from the early cases. In this area, most respondents commented on how much more sophisticated plaintiffs' attorneys were after the first round of the litigation. For example, in the second round of hearings and trials, plaintiffs' counsel effectively introduced evidence showing that insurers cover a range of diseases (such as HDC/ABMT for testicular cancer) that are no less experimental than HDC/ABMT for patients with high-risk and metastatic breast cancer. One plaintiff's attorney successfully focused on finding stronger and more motivated experts after losing an early trial. In the early trial, this attorney also underestimated the informed consent issue. In subsequent proceedings, the attorney tried to defuse it right from the start by saying: "She knew, but the alternative was certain death, so she willingly accepted the risks" (interview by P. Jacobson).

As a footnote to this discussion, the *Fox* case settled for an undisclosed amount (estimated by a knowledgeable source unconnected with our interviews to be in the range of $5 million to $10 million). Given the mythic status the *Fox* case has achieved and its subsequent dominance of the legal debate, an interesting strategic question is whether the industry would have been better off had the defendant chosen to fight the verdict rather than settle. Our interviews revealed no consensus, although most seemed to support the settlement. Those supporting the settlement noted the costs of continuing litigation, the need to post a large bond, and the potential that the verdict might stand. Most important, they argued that the public relations damage had already been done, and that a reduced award or a reversal would get very little media attention.

Standard of Care

For our defense counsel respondents, probably the most frustrating aspect of the litigation was the judiciary's willingness to consider HDC/ABMT as the legal standard of care. Although the published opinions vary considerably, and also display each judge's struggle to weigh the reality of diffusion in the oncology community with the limited scientific validity, defense counsel uniformly rejected the idea that unproven procedures could ever constitute the clinical standard of care. One problem for the defense was that, objectively, many clinicians were using the procedure. At a minimum, a court could easily decide that a respectable minority of physicians considered HDC/ABMT to be the standard of care even if the physician community was split on its use.

This is not to suggest that it is easy to determine whether HDC/ABMT constitutes the legal standard of care under these circumstances. In many ways, this case study reflects the difficulty of even defining a legal standard of care. In most instances, physicians think of a spectrum of care, while the law focuses on a standard of care as a single metric of a complex process (Jacobson and Rosenquist 1996; Morreim 2001).[32] At best, our interviews revealed an ambiguity regarding when and whether there was any consensus about the procedure. As noted in our analysis of the reported cases, courts have disagreed with each other about the extent to which the procedure is generally accepted.[33] For instance, one court rejected the following (*inter alia*) as establishing the standard of care:

a. Letters from 22 universities and cancer centers, dating 1988–90, stating that HDC-ABMT for the treatment of breast cancer [was] not experimental and were generally accepted by the medical community.
b. Letters from 34 universities and cancer centers in 1992 stating the same.
c. A letter from the AMA encouraging third-party payors to be flexible I applying the "investigational" exclusion (Brown 1998).
d. Seventeen abstracts from peer-reviewed medical literature stating that HDC-ABMT [is] generally accepted in the medical community.[34]

Yet other courts have relied on fundamentally similar evidence to rule that the procedure was in fact the standard of care in the community. What stands out is the courts' deference to the treating physician, in this instance at least, at the expense of scientific proof of the procedure's efficacy. In any event, there is no rigorous or accepted methodology for determining the legal standard of care.[35]

In an odd way, perhaps both sides were correct: The procedure was indeed widespread, but it lacked scientific justification and was experimental.[36] If so, the legal question is to ascertain when the "widespread disagreement among qualified medical experts over whether the treatment or procedure at issue has crossed the line from being an experimental procedure to become an acceptable medical practice."[37] This dilemma was eloquently captured by the Seventh Circuit Court of Appeals in an HDC/ABMT case:

> The pace of medical science is ever-quickening; yesterday's esoteric experiment is today's miraculous cure. . . . That is noteworthy because at issue here is the point where a treatment which has been experimental in the past crosses the line into general acceptance—the point at which the medical value of a treatment is no longer generally disputed. Perhaps no such line exists; we are probably dealing more with a zone of perceived effectiveness than a precise dividing line. What is evident, though, and foremost in our minds as we consider this case, is the incompetence of courts to decide when exactly that line or zone has been traversed. Such decisions are judgment calls for medical scientists and health-care professionals, not judges . . . which is why our standard of review in these cases is highly deferential. To repeat, our narrow duty is to monitor those charged with knowing and deciding these matters for decisions that are patently wrong.[38]

The policy question is to determine the proper forum for deciding the issue, which we address in the "Lessons" section.

Courts are reluctant to overrule medical standards of care as determined by physician testimony. In this situation, however, a strong argument can be made that courts should have overridden physician custom given the lack of evidence suggesting HDC/ABMT's effectiveness. The scientific basis for the procedure's validity was so thin that courts could have disregarded its widespread use without fear of setting a precedent that could undermine the traditional deference to the medical community. Had the courts, for instance, adopted a standard based on what a reasonable MCO would have decided as opposed to a reasonable physician, the result may have been entirely different (Bovbjerg 1975; Jacobson 2002, pp. 1989–1993).[39] Taking this approach could have had the salutary effect of compelling a more productive dialogue between physicians and plans, along with accelerating the clinical trials' process.

One question is how the standard of care could have been set to encourage RCTs. Arguably, a standard of care favoring patients would provide an incentive for plans to participate in and fund RCTs but might discourage patients from agreeing to participate in them. On the other hand, a standard of care favoring insurers would diminish the urgency of participating in RCTs. It is difficult to see a middle ground once the issue is framed around the appropriate standard of care. That suggests the need to develop a more robust contractual relationship.

The Contract

Aside from less-than-precise contractual language, insurers faced a serious challenge in seeking to exclude last-chance experimental therapies. Despite winning a fair number of the reported cases, insurers seemed to be at a constant disadvantage in developing adequate trial tactics to defend their contracts and certainly in appealing to juries. This dilemma was nicely captured as follows:

> The case law shows that the investigational exclusion is an effective and appropriate barrier to payment for zany treatments, such as coffee enemas and tomato therapies. For this reason alone, it is worth maintaining. However, for potentially life-saving treatments, the case law suggests a trend that may render standard medical coverage language insufficient to protect against claims for investigational treatments. Even the finest of investigational exclusions and decision-making processes will face an uphill battle in court in life-threatening cases where the plan is characterized as asking the court for a death sentence for the subscriber. (Ader 1995, p. 5)[40]

In support of the insurers' position, defense counsel argued that it is hard to craft a contract with sufficient confidence to exclude emerging technologies that judges and plaintiffs' attorneys cannot circumvent. Perhaps so, but two plaintiffs' attorneys noted that it became more difficult to win their cases after the plans redrafted and tightened the contract. Several respondents (on both sides) also observed that the contracts generally did not specify a standard of care beyond "safe and effective."

There is an ongoing debate among insurers and scholars regarding whether and how to write contract exclusions that are sufficiently comprehensive and unambiguous (Morreim 2001). The responses from our interviews mirrored the range of options being discussed. One defense attorney suggested that using a laundry list of exclusions would avoid ambiguity. This respondent also talked extensively about the need for a consistent process, such as a well-functioning external grievance mechanism.

Lessons Learned

Finding the Right Forum

The two sides differed dramatically over the proper forum for resolving these types of cases. Plaintiffs' attorneys argued strenuously that this is an issue traditionally decided in the courts, and that "there was no other way to get their attention." Defense attorneys equally strenuously argued that courts were exactly the wrong forum. To defense counsel, there is an inherent judicial bias in favor of the treating physician. Defense counsel strongly maintained that the legal process is incapable of evaluating the scientific dispute, and that judges and juries have no real basis for making these decisions. Arguing the absence of proof of effectiveness can never be as persuasive as testimony from a physician who is actually using the procedure.

As an alternative, respondents agreed that RCTs would be the best way to sort out these disputes. They disagreed on who should pay. Most defense respondents rejected the need to have the insurers pay for the trials. One respondent characterized this as a tax on health plans. Defense counsel objected that this would reduce funds available for clinical treatment. Instead, the respondents viewed the process as a societal responsibility to be funded through the National Cancer Institute or similar governmental agency.

One respondent argued in favor of a science court, although he had rejected this approach in the past. The use of science courts has been debated among legal scholars and judges for many years but may be ripe for reconsideration because of the success that special drug courts have had. The reason why the respondent's opinion has changed is interesting. In response to my concern that it is difficult to find unbiased experts, the respondent argued that the current dynamic rewards "medical zealots" who seek to market their ideas for academic fame and future grants. These entrepreneurs are more likely to be careful and constrained before other scientists and academic peers, to maintain their credibility, than they are in a judicial forum. The respondent's argument is that the science court would impose some bounds and norms because if witnesses go beyond the bounds, they may lose funding and related academic privileges. At a minimum, the science court is able to recognize where the biases lie, through full disclosure, and adjust accordingly.[41]

An alternative to a science court would be to require the judge to obtain the views of an independent panel of scientists. As with the science court, the problem would be to find knowledgeable scientists who had not already taken a position on the issue. This would at least give judges the benefit of the best possible science without being encumbered by presenting it through the adversarial process. To avoid potential bias, the panel would only be asked to determine whether the proposed treatment is likely to be better than the standard available therapy and whether the panel recommends this treatment for the patient. The goal would be to provide the litigants with the best possible science. In one respondent's view, the panel will not be asked whether the treatment is experimental or investigational (but it would be hard to assemble an expert panel that would not consider experimental status). While not perfect, the respondent argued that this would be a better process for deciding scientific disputes than leaving it to a judge and jury. The respondent added that he was not impugning the judicial system's fairness. Instead, "the question is what are you asking the courts to be fair about? You can't resolve scientific questions through the adversarial system" (interview by Jacobson).[42]

Science versus Law

Nowhere are the contrasting worldviews between plaintiffs' and defense counsel more apparent than when they describe what they learned from their involvement. Each of the plaintiffs' attorneys said that the legal system performed as it should and each was reluctant to recommend changes. According to one dramatic response: "It was the science that failed, not the law" (interview by Jacobson). Each of the defense attorneys concluded that the legal system failed miserably and was an inappropriate forum for resolving these difficult issues. As one defense attorney put it: "I continue to believe that I save more lives than [the plaintiffs' attorneys] by preventing the unsupported and rapid diffusion of technology." Pointedly, this respondent added: "It is clear in hindsight that defense litigators knew more about the long-term toxicity than treating physicians." Another added that "the courtroom is not a good scientific laboratory."

All of the respondents were critical of the scientific process. A common sentiment was that science failed because the treatment diffused too quickly, before it was tested in RCTs. It became a panacea for patients without much hope and gained unstoppable momentum until being discredited in the later 1990s. Thus, all agreed that we need better strategies to fund and complete RCTs for new technologies and treatments.

External Review

Not surprisingly, defense counsel offered a range of alternative suggestions for resolving similar future scientific and technological controversies. One defense attorney is an avid proponent of external review. Most of the time, he argued, the plan will be vindicated, and the enrollee obtains an independent and impartial review of his or her dispute. Despite some contentions that this is a costly burden, the respondent argued that external review was both quick and cheap (at least relative to litigation). The primary benefit is that the focus is on getting the best scientific answer: providing the best treatment for the individual patient. The process can adapt to changes in the state of the science. "People want treatment, not a lawsuit" (interview by Jacobson). Side benefits will be to reduce the probability of litigation and inoculate plans against punitive damages if litigation occurs, and patients who do not prevail may still feel that the process was fair.

According to proponents, the external review process makes it easier to defend the cases in court, especially on bad faith. Not only does external review present an additional hurdle, but also it makes it difficult for plaintiffs' attorneys to argue that the defendant acted in bad faith.[43] Therefore, the litigation would often settle for covering the cost of the procedure with no additional damages. From the industry's perspective, this had the added benefit of discouraging plaintiffs' attorneys from pursing the cases aggressively.

Not all defense respondents agreed with external review as the solution. One objected because care will usually be provided, while another said it would reduce some pressure but was not the ultimate solution. When afforded the opportunity to request external review, plaintiffs' attorneys reportedly rejected it in favor of going to court. Plaintiffs' attorneys seemed generally indifferent about it.

Technology Assessment

Very few of our respondents focused on the broader issue of technology assessment. Only one defense attorney explicitly mentioned a satisfactory technology assessment process as a solution to the HDC/ABMT controversy. In contrast, one plaintiffs' attorney was dismissive of the technology assessment process as applied to HDC/ABMT, calling it "eyewash." Another plaintiffs' attorney noted that the plan needs to make clear in the contract how the technology assessment process will be handled for new technologies.

Cost Containment

Some respondents noted that we need to have a public discussion about cost containment. Before controversial cases like HDC/ABMT can be resolved, the stigma of cost containment needs to be resolved. Defense attorneys were especially likely to raise the concern that patients believe they should have unlimited access to care without concern for overall health care costs.

Postscript

Defense counsel strongly maintained that these cases were not winnable, although none anticipated the sizable punitive damages awarded in *Fox v. HealthNet*. In their view, it was ultimately too hard for judges and jurors to look at the patient and say no, especially when Americans generally do not view limits on health care very favorably.

Plaintiffs' counsel strongly maintained that courts did their job. More than one noted being "proud to be a part of it."

In this sense, their narratives are disconnected. Paradoxically, the narratives may actually be reconcilable. After blaming the science, a plaintiff's attorney concluded the interview by saying that the saga should not be viewed as good versus evil: we were "all sold a bill of goods" (interview by Jacobson).

In the end, this is a classic example of the judicial focus on individuals vs. the insurers' concern for patient populations. The courts have struggled unsuccessfully to resolve the inherent tensions between these competing policy objectives. It is no wonder, then, that our respondents reflected this struggle in the HDC-ABMT litigation saga.

Comparisons between the Cases and the Interviews

We conclude with a few observations about the similarities and differences between our review of the published cases and our interview results. Simply put, the differences far outweigh the similarities. This is largely because many of the cases involve summary judgment motions under ERISA preemption, which means that few appellate courts reviewed trial transcripts. Without reviewing transcripts of the appellate arguments, it is hard to know what was actually argued in the cases. In fact, our attorney respondents mostly discussed strategy in preparing for trial rather than for appellate arguments, although only four jury trials were actually held. Presumably, their approach was fundamentally different in jury trials than in arguments for summary judgment.

Perhaps the most interesting comparison between the interviews and cases is the disparity between anticipated results and case outcomes. Defense attorneys repeatedly said that these cases were not winnable. Yet, our case analysis shows that defendants won a majority of the cases before both juries and judges, even after the breathtaking award in *Fox v. HealthNet*. Since the jury trials in which plaintiffs won were subsequently settled, we have no way of knowing how those verdicts would have fared in the appellate process.

Not all of the legal strategies attorneys considered in preparing for trial were discussed in the written judicial opinions. A single case usually emphasized one over the others. The contract language came up in almost every case, with some exclusively reviewing the language of the contract. The plaintiffs pushed the ambiguity of the contract, at times going so far that the courts accused them of trying to create an ambiguity where none existed. Similarly, the widespread use of HDC/ABMT was an important point in the cases, as suggested by the interviews, although it was definitely less of a factor than the contracts. Informed consent was raised in a few of the cases but was not likely to persuade the judge that the treatment was experimental. Plaintiffs' attorneys were able to spin the informed consent as merely a formality of a big research hospital.

Indeed, three of the articulated strategies revealed in our plaintiffs' attorney interviews—the treatment was the plaintiff's only chance, preservation of the doctor–patient relationship, and unfavorable portrayal of the managed care industry—are not obvious from reading the cases. A few of the cases make note of the fact that the treatment is the patient's last chance, but the opinions do not talk explicitly about who should make medical decisions or about the evils of the insurance industry (although there is some implicit suggestion of that in several of the cases, for example, the *Adams* case).

Perhaps the most significant difference was over the claim of bad faith denial of insurance coverage. The concept of bad faith comes up only very rarely in the cases; a search of Westlaw for the words "bad faith" in an ABMT case yielded very few results. Elements of bad faith do show up in the cases (e.g., emphasizing that the insurer relied on outdated data to refuse treatment or that the insurer refused to consider certain studies demonstrating the HDC/ABMT was effective), but they are not labeled as bad faith. In contrast, our respondents maintained that bad faith was central to the trial strategy.

The interviews referred many times to the scientific studies by Peters and Antman, but those studies are actually referenced very little in the cases. It is unclear whether the evidence offered by the plaintiffs was based on or incorporated Peters's and Antman's studies, but the courts did not focus on Peters and Antman. Obviously, there is no way to know whether the studies simply were not introduced by the plaintiffs or whether the courts found the other materials adequate or more accessible. Their absence is not surprising in a summary judgment hearing.

A curious difference is that the cases do not discuss the fact that insurers covered other unproven treatments (so why not ABMT?), even though the interviews suggested that stressing this inconsistency was an important strategy. One would think that this would be an important plaintiffs' argument regarding why the defendants' contract interpretation is arbitrary and capricious.

Cost almost never comes up in the cases except to note that the procedure was very expensive, and that the patient could not afford it on her own. None of the cases discussed the difference in cost between HDC and standard-dose chemotherapy. A few of the cases discussed the larger issue of health care costs in general, but mostly only in passing.

Quality-of-life issues played almost no role in the litigation. The facts that the treatment was grueling, leaving patients debilitated for months; that it did not improve quality of life; and that, in the beginning, may have had a higher mortality rate were not discussed at all. Although courts acknowledged that there was a question regarding whether the treatment would be successful, they did not recognize that there are varying degrees of success or that success may not mean a full recovery.

A disturbing similarity concerns how the science was treated. Some cases, such as *Pirozzi,* delved deeply (if not convincingly) into the science, but most courts and most of our respondents simply glossed over it. For many courts, almost anything counted as science, and as we have seen, the courts often disregarded expert academic testimony. No studies or individual experts appear repeatedly in the opinions. In fact, the opinions can best be characterized as failing to inquire into the procedure's scientific validity, a factor that surely favored plaintiffs. The reality that "everyone is doing it" is an underlying theme in the cases and, while not always explicit in the opinions, is another factor favoring plaintiffs.

All told, there were very few thoughtful opinions that grappled with the complex issues presented. Two of them, *Pirozzi* and *Bossmeyer,* reached different conclusions, making it difficult for subsequent courts to identify a seminal opinion for guidance. Perhaps the most dispiriting cases were decided in 2002. Despite 14 years of litigation and strong scientific evidence that the procedure is not effective, the cases mention two opinions (ignoring the rest) and somehow manage to find in favor of plaintiffs.

Finally, it is difficult to capture how important sympathy for the dying patient was in the opinions. Occasionally, a judge dealt with sympathy forthrightly (and not always in favor of the patient), but most often the issue was never directly mentioned. It is, however, somewhat difficult to believe that plaintiffs won as many cases as they did without sympathy playing at least some role.

5

Entrepreneurial Oncology

What's the subject of life—to get rich? All of those fellows out there getting rich could be dancing around the real subject of life.
—Paul A. Volcker

Wise are those who learn that the bottom line doesn't always have to be their top priority.
—William A. Ward

People are usually much more moved by economics than by morals.
—Norah Phillips

In the early 1990s, it became clear to many that the high-dose chemotherapy with autologous bone marrow transplantation (HDC/ABMT) procedure for breast cancer would diffuse rapidly into clinical practice. Increasing utilization might be slowed but not stopped by health insurers and health plans. Physicians claiming that the procedure represented standard of care, desperate patients persuaded that it was their best hope for cure, highly visible litigation in the courts, and media coverage of the drama associated with denials of coverage ensured that HDC/ABMT was well under way to becoming the treatment of choice for patients with metastatic and high-risk breast cancer. In this chapter, we examine national HDC/ABMT utilization data for the treatment of breast cancer. Then, in the context of the business of oncology, we analyze the effort of one for-profit corporation, Response Oncology, to provide the HDC/ABMT treatment in community settings. We also consider the provision of the procedure by not-for-profit oncology providers.

National Utilization Data

One of the most difficult problems in grappling with the introduction of new medical procedures is determining how many are being performed in a given period of time. There is no uniform terminology for describing the procedure and thus no clear basis for counting. Voluntary reporting is often driven by the specialists providing a procedure and typically reflects scientific and clinical interest in the extent of use. It is subject to self-interest behavior by providers, both for reporting and for withholding data. Mandatory reporting is best when tied to payment requirements and claims processing for a procedure by health insurers. The fragmentation of the U.S. health insurance system and the controversy surrounding coverage of new procedures militate against the establishment of effective reporting systems. Finally, data systems independent of providers and payers typically have limitations.

All these issues come into play in efforts to determine a "true count" of the number of HDC/ABMT procedures performed to treat breast cancer. Data are available from a voluntary registry and an independent database; there are no payment-based data. Data are presented for 1989 through 2002. These are broken into two periods: data for 1989–1992 are retrospective; those for 1993–2002 are available from both the voluntary registry and the independent database.

Data Sources

Two sources of data describe the U.S. experience with HDC/ABMT for breast cancer: the Autologous Blood and Marrow Transplant Registry (ABMTR) and the Nationwide Inpatient Sample (NIS) of the Healthcare Cost and Utilization Project (HCUP) database (Steiner et al. 2002). The ABMTR is a voluntary organization of more than 200 institutions that perform allogeneic and autologous transplants in North and South America.[1] These institutions provide information on all patients who receive a transplant at their center, including women with breast cancer. The ABMTR began collecting data from these centers in 1993; it also collected data retrospectively on women treated from 1989 until 1992, and it collects follow-up data for several years after transplantation as the Center for International Blood and Marrow Transplant Research.[2] Registry data indicate only the total number of women receiving a BMT at reporting centers and the specific cancer for which treatment is provided.

The second source of aggregate data, the HCUP database, is a federal-state-industry partnership sponsored by the Agency for Healthcare Research and Quality (AHRQ). The HCUP database, which is independent of both providers and payers, provides national estimates of inpatient discharges from acute care community hospitals in the United States. The database contains 7 million discharges from about 1000 hospitals located in 22 states, approximating a 20% stratified sample of U.S. acute care hospitals (AHRQ 2004). HCUP NIS data are available only from 1993 onward; they are not available for the 1989–1992 period. These data include women identified as having any diagnosis or history of breast cancer (*International Classification of Diseases, Ninth Revision, Clinical Modification* [*ICD-9-CM*] diagnosis codes V103, 1740–1749) and receiving high-dose chemotherapy (*ICD-9-CM* procedure codes 4101 and 4104).[3] The age, in-hospital death, diagnoses, primary payer, charges, and length of stay were abstracted for all selected observations. Payers are categorized as Medicare, Medicaid, private commercial payers, health maintenance organizations (HMOs), and other (including the uninsured).

Advantages of using NIS data over the ABMTR include the availability of data on inpatient mortality, length of stay, total hospital charges, and the source of the payment for the inpatient hospital care. This additional information allows for further analyses and provides a better understanding of the personal burden that patients and their families endured over the many months of treatment. It also provides some insight into the considerable financial burden on payers.

High-Dose Chemotherapy with Autologous Bone Marrow Transplantation Breast Cancer Procedures

The ABMTR data provide us the basis for an upper estimate of breast cancer patients receiving HDC/ABMT. Among centers that report their transplants to ABMTR, 18,223 women with breast cancer received the HDC/ABMT procedure in the United States in the 1993–2002 period (table 5.1); another 2559 women were treated in the earlier 1989–1992 period. A total of 20,782 transplants were reported for 1989–2002 by this count.[4] Submission of data to the ABMTR by cancer centers is voluntary, however, so transplants performed at nonparticipating centers are not included. The ABMTR estimates that it collects information on 50%–60% of all autologous transplants. If the 20,782 reported transplants for the years 1989–2002 represents 60% of the total, it is possible that 34,787 (or nearly 35,000) received the procedure for breast cancer treatment; if the reported cases represent 50% of the total, as many as 41,564 (or over 40,000) women received the procedure.

The NIS HCUP data provide the basis for a lower estimate of HDC/ABMT recipients. Using the NIS, we obtained data on the number of women in U.S. community hospitals with breast cancer, the number of women receiving HDC, and the number of women with breast cancer receiving HDC. For those identified with a diagnosis of breast cancer and receiving the HDC procedure, we calculated the median length of stay, median charges, the number of in-hospital deaths, percentage in-hospital deaths, median age, and distribution of primary payer.

From 1993 to 2002, according to NIS data, 20,817 women with breast cancer as a primary or secondary diagnosis in the United States underwent the HDC procedure on an inpatient basis (table 5.1). The number nearly doubled from 2132 to 3930 in the 5-year period from 1993 to 1997. Cases coded with a less-definitive diagnosis (chemotherapy, metastatic cancer, and anemia) may also include some breast cancers as well, so the total identified in the national data set for 1997 may be higher and may exceed 4000 (table 5.2).[5]

The most conservative lower estimate of HDC/ABMT breast cancer recipients for 1989–2002, then, is based on NIS data for 1993–2002 of 20,817 plus the ABMTR figure of 2559 women for 1989–1992, or 23,376. In any event, we can safely say that 23,000 approximates a lower estimate and 35,000–40,000 an upper estimate of the number of women who received HDC/ABMT for breast cancer in the years from 1989 to 2002. In this same period, perhaps 1000 women entered high-priority randomized clinical trials sponsored by the National Cancer Institute (NCI) (AHRQ 2004; Stadtmauer et al. 2002).

The discrepancies between the two data sources cannot be resolved. Coding problems may account for some of the difference. Moreover, NIS data do not capture discharges performed in active military hospitals, Veterans Health Administration hospitals, or facilities of the Indian Health Service, although the last two were unlikely to have performed these procedures. In addition, the NIS inpatient database

Table 5.1 Women with breast cancer and high-dose chemotherapy, 1993–2002[a]

	1993	1994	1995	1996	1997	1998	1999	2000	2001	2002
Number of women with any diagnosis of breast cancer[b]	510,095	520,001	539,400	545,423	560,685	560,188	556,403	580,069	618,031	623,137
Total number of women receiving HDC[c]	4,225	3,863	5,243	5,629	6,424	4,850	4,511	2,456	3,163	2,197
Total number of women with breast cancer and HDC	2,132	2,421	3,073	3,312	3,930	2,769	2,033	466	563	118
Data from the Autologous Blood and Marrow Transplant Registry	1,459	1,963	2,466	2,978	3,333	3,478	1,876	567	231	83

[a] Sources: Nationwide Inpatient Sample (NIS), Release 6, 1997, Healthcare Cost and Utilization Project, Agency for Healthcare Research and Quality; Autologous Blood and Marrow Transplant Registry.

[b] Defined as primary or secondary diagnosis *ICD-9* code 1740-1749, 1759

[c] Defined as primary or secondary procedure *ICD-9* code 4101, 4104.

Table 5.2 Women receiving high-dose chemotherapy for all purposes, by frequency of diagnosis, 1997

Diagnosis[a]	Number	Percentage
Breast cancer	3894	60.6
Non-Hodgkin's lymphoma	632	9.8
Multiple myeloma	347	5.4
Leukemia	294	4.6
Solid tumors[a]	292	4.6
Hodgkin's lymphoma	189	3.0
Chemotherapy[b]	306	4.7
Metastatic cancer[c]	140	2.2
Anemia and diseases of white blood cells	73	1.1
Other noncancerous conditions	257	4.0
Total	6424	100

Source: Nationwide Inpatient Sample (NIS), Release 6, 1997; Healthcare Cost and Utilization Project (HCUP), Agency for Healthcare Research and Quality.

[a] Diagnoses grouped using the Clinical Classification Software.
[b] Cancer of the ovary, brain, bone, bronchus, testis.
[c] No other diagnostic category possible.

would not capture HDC/ABMT procedures performed on an outpatient basis, but the likely distribution between inpatient and outpatient settings is not known. An examination of an outpatient database of the NIS (only available for six states currently: Colorado, Connecticut, Maryland, New Jersey, New York, and Wisconsin) did not find any cases of HDC being performed in outpatient settings in the state of New York (AHRQ 2004). New York State may not be representative in this regard given its history of high regulation of providers. Moreover, Response Oncology, which we examine in a separate section, only had three centers in one of these six states, Colorado; the absence of patient data on Response centers elsewhere in the country would result in an undercount of outpatient procedures. The only other national data set that could be used is the National Hospital Discharge Survey. Unfortunately, the survey cannot provide useful national estimates as it is based on small survey numbers (U.S. Department of Health and Human Services 1991).

In 1993, women treated for breast cancer represented 50% of all women receiving HDC for any reason; that proportion rose to 60% in 1994 and hovered there through 1997. By 2001, however, the percentage of women receiving HDC for an indication of breast cancer had dropped to slightly less than 18% of all women receiving HDC for any reason (figure 5.1). We address this decline in chapters 8 and 9. All indications for HDC in 1997 are shown in table 5.2.

Treatment-related mortality associated with the procedure in the early 1990s was more than 10% (Peters et al. 1986). The death rate decreased from 3.7% in 1993 to 1.1% in 2001, and no deaths were reported in 2002 according to NIS data. Overall, 490 in-hospital deaths occurred from 1993 to 2001 (table 5.3). The NIS data are likely to underestimate treatment-related mortality, however, as they are based on hospital discharge data, and additional treatment-related deaths may have occurred after discharge. The ABMTR reported treatment-related mortality of 5% in 1995,

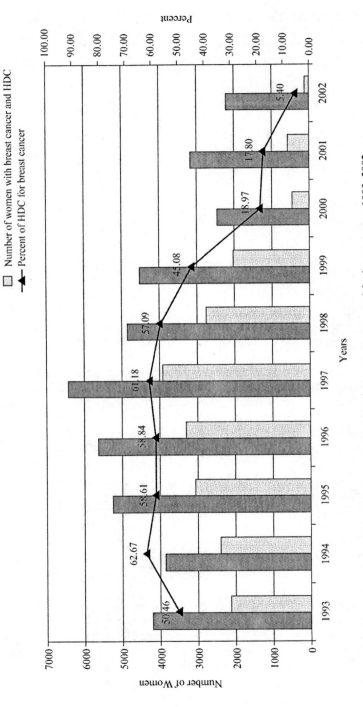

Figure 5.1. Women receiving high-dose chemotherapy (HDC) for all purposes and for breast cancer, 1993–2002.

Table 5.3 In-hospital mortality, median age, median length of stay, and median total charges for women with breast cancer who undergo high-dose chemotherapy

	1993	1994	1995	1996	1997	1998	1999	2000	2001	2002
In-hospital mortality (%)	3.7	3.6	2.0	2.9	1.9	1.8	1.3	1.2	1.1	0
Number of deaths	78	85	60	96	73	48	25	5	20	0
Median age	44	45	45	45	47	47	47	45	46	52
	(39–49)[a]	(38–50)	(39–50)	(39–51)	(41–52)	(41–52)	(41–53)	(39–52)	(40–53)	(47–57)
Median length of stay (days)	24	23	20	20	20	20	19	20	21	21
	(20–31)	(19–28)	(18–25)	(17–24)	(17–23)	(17–24)	(16–21)	(17–21)	(20–26)	(20–26)
Median charges ($)	103,924	103,540	87,062	86,415	82,881	78,468	71,760	90,029	107,412	
	(78,593–145,535)	(78,546–147,906)	(63,182–120,869)	(56,451–119,757)	(57,451–112,718)	(57,080–101,000)	(51,551–94,329)	(61,881–109,961)	(75,898–145,805)	

Source: Nationwide Inpatient Sample (NIS), Release 6, 1997, Healthcare Cost and Utilization Project (HCUP), Agency for Healthcare Research and Quality.

[a] Figures in parentheses indicate 95% confidence intervals.

which is also likely to be an underestimate for a number of reasons: Missing data account for 4% of the total; a healthier population is typically represented in a voluntary registry; and only 100-day mortality is reported (Vahdat et al. 1998). To date, clinical trials have reported treatment-related mortality varying between 0% and 7.4% (Stadtmauer et al. 2000). The largest U.S. trial, sponsored by the NCI and conducted in the United States, reported 7.4% treatment-related mortality (Peters et al. 2001). The data from the clinical trials is probably the most reliable figure for treatment-related mortality because of better data collection in clinical trials. However, women willing to enter clinical trials and be randomized may not represent all women with breast cancer who sought HDC.

The ABMTR data show 1998 as the peak year of utilization of HDC/ABMT for breast cancer, followed by a dramatic decline in 1999. NIS data show 1997 as the peak year, followed by marked declines in 1998 and a dramatic fall-off in utilization in 1999. This discrepancy cannot be resolved. We can only speculate on factors that might have influenced a slowing or decline before the May 1999 American Society of Clinical Oncology (ASCO) meeting. A shift from inpatient to outpatient provision of treatment was occurring but cannot be documented, which might account for the NIS showing an earlier peak year. A technology assessment by ECRI, which had findings that were made public in February 1995, concluded that HDC/ABMT provided no benefit and involved harm (ECRI 1995) (see also chapter 7). The ECRI 1996 patient brochure may also have influenced some prospective patients to avoid the procedure. In addition, Hortobagyi in 1997 analyzed patient selection bias as a source for overestimation of the benefits of the procedure. A Dutch pilot study published in 1998 showed no benefit (Rodenhuis et al. 1998). Response Oncology encountered market competition in 1998, as discussed in the section on Response Oncology. Whether these factors contributed to a waning of enthusiasm for HDC/ABMT among patients and physicians before the May 1999 ASCO meeting is unknown.

Data about payers for HDC in women with breast cancer are shown in table 5.4. Private commercial insurers were the most frequent payers; they included the Blue Cross Blue Shield Preferred Provider Organizations and other fee-for-service insurers. Medicare and Medicaid were primary in only 8% of cases. However, median total charges were highest in the Medicare population, as was length of stay. Median total charges were lowest for Medicaid patients and those in the other category, which includes a significant proportion of uninsured.

The total national hospital charges for the years from 1993 to 2001 based on the median total hospital charges for each year reached nearly $1.7 billion. (Charges do not represent costs and are not payments, which are generally lower, whether paid by insurers or patients.) Total per treatment charges have declined steadily from 1993 through 1999, then have increased. The median length of stay declined early in this period but has remained constant at 19–20 days since 1995. Median total charges also declined from $103,924 in 1993 to $82,881 in 1997, but by 2000 had increased again to $90,029 (table 5.3). High-end charges for HDC/ABMT were often very high: Some outlier patient cases had total hospital charges as high as $800,000. By comparison, the charges for standard chemotherapy for breast cancer typically vary

Table 5.4 Primary payer, median length of stay, and median total charges for women with breast cancer receiving high-dose chemotherapy, 1997[a]

	Percentage	Median length of stay (days)	Median total charges ($)
Medicare	1.2	24	98,241
Medicaid	6.8	20	75,980
PPO/FFS[b]	53.9	20	85,801
HMO	23.4	19	83,731
Other	10.9	20	82,881

Source: Nationwide Inpatient Sample (NIS), Release 6, 1997, Healthcare Cost and Utilization Project, Agency for Healthcare Research and Quality.

[a] Missing data, 3.8%.

[b] PPO stands for preferred provider organization; FFS means fee for service.

between $15,000 and $40,000. Although HDC/ABMT charges represent only a small proportion of total health care spending in the United States, HDC/ABMT was one of the five most expensive procedures in the United States in the mid-1990s (Hurd and Peters 1995). Moreover, high-cost procedures applied to a large patient population represent a major challenge to all purchasers and providers of health insurance.

The NIS data have important limits. They include only hospital charges and not physician fees. The NIS data do not record the additional charges for treating adverse events that occur more frequently with HDC/ABMT compared to standard chemotherapy, especially as many deaths are related to the development of new hematologic malignancies such as leukemia (Imrie et al. 2002). These charge data do not include the indirect costs to the patient and her family as time lost from work and the need for additional supportive care. Finally, the intangible cost of lost time at the end of a woman's life due to premature death secondary to treatment toxicity should not be overlooked.

The analysis demonstrates that the procedure was widely utilized throughout the United States during the 1990s. Payers were primarily private fee-for-service insurers and HMOs. Widespread use has been attributed to many factors: resistance by women to be randomized; reluctance of physicians to randomize to a treatment that many believed to be beneficial; financial incentives to provide HDC/ABMT; patient litigation against insurance companies for coverage; federal and state mandates; and decisions by insurers to cover the treatment. We examined the legal issues in previous chapters. We turn now to the commercial exploitation of the procedure.

Two important changes in HDC/ABMT utilization occurred in the mid-1990s (table 5.5). Hudis and Munster (1999), using data from the ABMTR, showed that the preponderant use of the procedure shifted from metastatic breast cancer to high-risk breast cancer (adjuvant/neoadjuvant); the proportion of women receiving the procedure for metastatic disease went from 88% in 1989–1990 to 49% by 1995. These data also show a marked shift in type of transplant: The proportions went from 80% BMTs and 14% peripheral blood stem cell (PBSC) transplants in 1989–1990 to 10%

Table 5.5 Trends in autotransplants for breast cancer reported to the ABMTR, 1989–1995

Variable	1989–1990	1991–1992	1993–1994	1995
Ave. no. patients transplanted/yr	310	920	1400	1700
Age (years)				
Median	42	44	45	45
Range	23–66	22–72	24–66	22–71
Disease stage at transplant (%)				
Adjuvant/neoadjuvant	12	30	35	49
Metastatic	88	70	65	50
Other	<1	<1	1	1
Graft type (%)				
BM	80	52	24	10
PBSC	14	20	49	72
BM+PBSC	6	28	27	18
100-day mortality	18	8	5	5

Source: CA Hudis and PN Münster. High-dose therapy for breast cancer. *Seminars in Oncology* 1999; 26(1):35–47. © 1999. Reprinted with permission. Data from Autologous Blood and Marrow Transplant Registry, http://www.ibmtr.org.

Abbreviations: ABMTR, Autologous Blood and Marrow Transplant Registry; BM, bone marrow; PBSC, peripheral blood stem cell.

and 72%, respectively, by 1995, with recipients of both types increasing from 6% to 18% in this period. These data reflect both the expanding nature of the patient population and the changing technology of the procedure. A 2005 update of these data from the ABMTR registration database for 239 teams in North and South America for the years 1996–1997 and 1998–1999 showed patients with metastatic cancer accounted for 55% of patients and 50%, respectively; and peripheral blood transplants accounted for 87% and 95%, respectively, while bone marrow alone fell to 5% and 2% for the two periods in question, respectively, and bone marrow plus peripheral blood declined to 8% and 3%, respectively.

The Entrepreneurs

The HDC/ABMT procedure was both expensive and profitable. Charges were initially quoted by some providers as $150,000 for hospital services only, independent of physician services. These fell over time to approximately $80,000, still substantial. True costs were not readily known but included the cost of drugs, hospitalization, and nursing care. Profit came from the substantial differential between revenues and costs. Revenues were substantially higher for HDC/ABMT than for other oncological services and costs less so. Providers faced the prospect of doing well by doing good. They could provide leading-edge medical care to otherwise hopeless patients and make money in the process.

Both for-profit and not-for-profit providers responded to the demand for HDC/ABMT, often encouraging it. We examine Response Oncology, the most prominent for-profit entity. First, we place it in the context of oncology practice management.

Oncology Practice Management

The 1980s and 1990s saw the emergence of for-profit oncology service providers. Some were physician practice management firms, but one involved specialized cancer treatment centers providing complex cancer therapies. Mighion et al. (1999) identified the factors driving this development as a large, fragmented oncology market; the growth of managed care; a shift toward risk sharing and capitation; the emergence of oncologists as gatekeepers; technology and capital requirements; and the demand for practice management services. Oncology services provided by these firms included contract negotiation with managed care companies, pricing, planning, information system support, and marketing. Mighion et al. focused on American Oncology Resources, Inc. (AOR); Physician Reliance Network, Inc. (PRN); Salick Health Care; and Response Oncology, Inc.

Salick Health Care, the oldest of these firms, pioneered the development of the market for outpatient cancer treatment in a site located between the academic medical center or the specialized cancer center and the oncologist's office practice. Bernard Salick, a nephrologist, had developed a small chain of for-profit dialysis centers to serve Medicare-financed patients with end-stage renal disease. As a result of his daughter's treatment for bone cancer (osteogenic sarcoma), Salick concluded that he could provide cancer care more efficiently and with greater attention to patient needs than could academic medical centers (Paris 1986; Salick 2002, 2003). He founded Salick Health Care in 1983 (Mighion et al. 1999). The firm's cancer centers were located mainly in California and Florida, but also in Kansas, Pennsylvania, and New York.

What was innovative about Salick Health Care?[6] According to its founder, physician fees were "sacrosanct and went [solely] to the physician" (Salick 2003). All the other companies (AOR, PRN, Response Oncology) derived some of their revenues from physician fees. Second, Salick outpatient centers were open 24 hours a day, 7 days a week, for both diagnostic and therapeutic services (Rebello 1987). "We were always open and provided every possible service that could be done in the outpatient setting" (Salick 2003). Third, the firm was affiliated with academic medical centers. "That assured us of top quality physicians" (Salick 2003). Fourth, Salick provided benefits to third-party payers. We were the first-ever organization to establish capitated management of cancer. We had an arrangement with a Florida HMO that had 100,000 members. We used their historical data, we calculated the percent of patients who would get cancer and what type of cancer. If they had 100,000 members, we might calculate 500 or 5,000 cancer patients. We then calculated what it would cost treat these patients. We then charged them a premium. We relied on careful examination of good databases. In order to provide treatment this way, we needed practice guidelines and outcome measurements" (Salick 2003; see also Olmos 1994a, p. D1, and 1994b, p. D3).

Salick turned to Robert Gale for help in developing guidelines for BMT. Gale, with Ed Park of RAND, prepared guidelines for three leukemias (acute myelogenous leukemia, chronic myelogenous leukemia, and acute lymphoblastic leukemia) and breast cancer. The purpose was to help Salick develop predictive models for capitating cancer care (Salick 2002). Since Salick did not employ physicians, he could not require their use by oncologists. Since Salick Health Care was not an insurer, it could not make reimbursement contingent on their use. Salick never entered the BMT market, so the guidelines were not used.

The breast cancer guideline was not published until 2000 (Gale et al. 2000). It argued that, for women with local/regional breast cancer, "autotransplants" were appropriate for those with 10 or more cancer-involved lymph nodes; uncertain in women with 4–9 cancer-involved nodes; and inappropriate for those with 3 or fewer cancer-involved nodes. For women with metastatic breast cancer, autotransplants were appropriate when metastases involved "favorable" sites (skin, lymph node, pleura) and a complete or partial response to chemotherapy; uncertain in women with metastases to "unfavorable" sites (lung, liver, or central nervous system) and a complete response to chemotherapy or those with bone metastases and a complete or partial response or stable disease after chemotherapy; and inappropriate in other settings. By the time the guideline was published, however, the fate of HDC/ABMT had largely been decided for both local/regional and metastatic breast cancer (as we discuss in chapter 8).

The AOR firm, based in Houston, provided comprehensive management services to its oncology affiliates (Mighion et al. 1999). In 1997, there were 311 physicians in 16 states affiliated with AOR. Its strategy was to build integrated networks of oncologists who were leaders in their regions. The integration of medical and radiation oncology and the development of comprehensive cancer centers characterized AOR. Its management services included practice operations, billing, facility development, marketing, managed care contracting, information systems management, and clinical research development. It had a scientific advisory board for the development of treatment guidelines and the review of clinical trial results. It also had created a site management organization for the conduct of industry-sponsored clinical research. Total revenues in 1997 were $322 million, up nearly 60% from the prior year.

Based in Dallas, PRN was incorporated in 1993 by the reorganization of Texas Oncology, P.A. (Mighion et al. 1999). At the end of 1997, there were 326 oncologists in 12 states affiliated with PRN. It provided practice management services and facilities, equipment, ancillary services and personnel to Texas Oncology. It emphasized the development of comprehensive cancer centers. PRN Research, a wholly owned subsidiary, contracted with pharmaceutical companies for research studies, which included clinical trial protocols for standard chemotherapy, BMT, and gene therapy. Its total revenues in 1997 were $317 million, up one third from the prior year. It derived substantially more revenue from Medicare and Medicaid than did AOR. In mid-1997, it was announced that AOR and PRN had agreed to a merger. This was accomplished successfully by mid-1998, with the resulting firm now known as U.S. Oncology.

Response Technologies/Response Oncology

Response Technologies, Inc., founded in 1989, was the most prominent entrepreneurial advocate for treating breast cancer with HDC/ABMT. Its IMPACT centers (so named for Implementing Advanced Cancer Treatment) were dedicated outpatient facilities at which affiliated community oncologists could provide chemotherapy as an extension of their office practices. Trained nursing and technical staff, specialized technology, and an electronic medical data system, along with comprehensive support, were the hallmarks of these Response-owned centers.[7]

Response was the successor to Biotherapeutics, a firm founded in 1984 in a Memphis suburb by Dr. Robert K. Oldham. Oldham, an oncologist, had been at the NCI on two different occasions, leaving initially in 1975 to establish the cancer program at Vanderbilt University and returning in 1980. He left the NCI again in 1984 to found Biotherapeutics, where he developed immunological treatments, monoclonal antibodies, and adaptive immunotherapy, which were marketed to cancer patients (Raeburn 1988). Although the Food and Drug Administration (FDA) classified these treatments as Investigational New Drugs (INDs), Oldham avoided FDA regulation because none of his drugs were sold in interstate commerce. Using the corporate recipe, they were compounded and sold through 17 local Biotherapeutics laboratories, mainly in Tennessee, Florida, and California. Insurers were reluctant to cover these experimental treatments. As one analyst wrote: "The company ... came to discover that the non-reimbursable nature of experimental treatment did not make for a viable business" (Banchik 1991).

Dr. William H. West joined Biotherapeutics in 1985 and became chief executive officer in 1989. He first sought to reorganize as financial difficulties increased, then bought the company, renamed it Response Technologies (it would be renamed again as Response Oncology), and changed the management, line of business, capital structure, and ownership. Biotherapeutics was an unprofitable venture, losing $30 million in 1989. According to West, "the relative benefit" of the laboratory services provided to cancer patients "was not real," "third party reimbursement was not satisfactory," and it had "an excessive overhead structure" (West 1992, p. 21). What, then, did Response inherit from Biotherapeutics? "A stock symbol," said Robert Birch, who ran clinical trials for the firm. "Biotherapeutics was dead. It was a laboratory research organization. We took it over in June [1989] and reduced it from 220 employees to five. We [also] inherited relations with physicians and a clinical trials units, a research group" (Birch 2004).

West, like Oldham, was an oncologist. He had been at the NCI from 1975 through 1979, first as research associate in the immunodiagnosis laboratory involved in biological response research, then as a clinical associate in the medical oncology branch dealing with dose response and chemotherapy in lung cancer treatment (West 1992). He left the NCI in 1979 to become staff oncologist at Baptist Memorial Hospital in Memphis and concurrently founded and maintained West Laboratories to continue research begun in Bethesda. His firm was absorbed into Biotherapeutics when he joined that organization in 1985.

Response Technologies began with the intention of delivering advanced cancer treatments as newer, more complex chemotherapies became available. As it evolved, however, it became exclusively identified with HDC with PBSC rescue for breast cancer on an outpatient basis. Therapeutic advances were linked to treatment setting and business strategy. Birch recounted:

> The first center was opened in Memphis in 1989. Bone marrow transplantation (BMT) was the standard therapy. We looked at peripheral blood stem cell (PBSC) rescue.

Some work was being done at Nebraska. But there was a sense that stems cells would wear out, they would not restore the white cells. Some work was being done using both BMT and PBSC together. But there was no data to support the superiority of bone marrow. No one knew how to quantitate the number of cells needed for effective transplant. The thinking was that 108 cells were needed and one hoped for engraftment. But some patients engrafted fast with PBSC, some slowly. . . . We looked at two ways to evaluate product [i.e., the number of cells needed for engraftment]. Colony forming units (CFUs) could be measured using a functional assay for growth. Cells were grown in an incubator for 2 weeks. The other way was CD34+ +, where surface antigens appear early and then disappear. Flow cytometry could be done within 24 hours and give a measure of the number of cells. . . . The fundamental question was what made good PBSC and how could you measure this. No one knew how to evaluate this. We did correlation analysis between CFUs and CD34+ +. The second question was how many cells do you need. Response was trying to get a quantitative measure of stems cells and a sufficient cohort of patients. The issue was whether it was feasible to provide high-dose chemotherapy with PBSC. If so, then the question was how to provide support. (Birch 2004)

Response's methodology was to provide treatment and support through its IMPACT centers. (In addition to HDC/PBSC, it also provided home infusion intravenous therapy for those patients of its affiliated oncologists who were not being treated in centers.) Birch elaborated: "Initially, we sent patients to the hospital very quickly for reinfusion. We took a very conservative approach. Over time it became clear that this was not necessary. What was needed was a dedicated staff that understood the procedure and was trained to respond to side effects. So we had protocols, standard orders, and guidelines" (Birch 2004).

According to an analyst's report in 1991, 5 centers were operational at the end of fiscal 1991, 7 more were planned for fiscal 1992, and 6 to 8 centers for each year thereafter (Banchik 1991). Response met these plans by the end of 1997 with 52 centers; the number would increase to 60 centers before declining demand in 1998–1999 took its toll. (A list of centers is found as table 5.6.) Centers were located in leased space, typically 2800 square feet in area, and included an apheresis suite, a six-bed treatment area, a pharmacy, and a specimen preparation area. The initial investment of $600,000 covered leasehold improvements; equipment; start-up expenses; and working capital. Centers typically became profitable in the third month of operation and realized positive cash flow in the fourth month. The typical center was expected to produce $2.0 million in revenues in its second year. Of this amount, $1.5 million would be generated from treatment for only four new patients per month at $30,000 per patient. Treatment revenues were from pharmacy (53%) and laboratory (47%) charges. The Memphis center, which opened in 1989, was expected to gross $3.6 million in fiscal year 1992.

Response Technologies marketed itself to community oncologists, who found it attractive because it represented leading-edge technology. It also allowed them to treat their patients in the community rather than sending them long distances to a tertiary cancer center and losing them to that center's physicians. The incentives to oncologists to participate were described in the following way: "Most oncologists in community-based private practice, as opposed to academically-based practice, do

Table 5.6 Response Technologies/Response Oncology: IMPACT centers, cooperative agreements, and physician practice management affiliations

Location of	Affiliation	Date	No. of centers	Cumulative no. of centers
IMPACT Center				
Memphis, TN		11/01/89	1	1
Tampa, FL		04/09/90	1	2
Hollywood, FL	Cancer Treatment Holdings (relinquished interests in 1994*)	05/1990	1	3
Columbia, MO		08/08/90	1	4
Nashville, TN		04/01/91	1	5
Miami, FL	01/03/96 RO develops physician's group with 9 doctors	05/1991	1	6
	at Baptist Hospital*, receives FAHCT accreditation	10/12/98		
Macon, GA		07/1991	1	7
Kansas City, KS		09/1991	1	8
Savannah, GA		12/05/91	1	9
Atlanta, GA	07/1994 transitions to a cooperative agreement with DeKalb Medical Center	12/05/91	1	10
Hampton, VA		12/05/91	1	11
Asheville, NC		12/05/91	1	12
Greenville, SC		02/19/92	1	13
Houston, TX		02/19/92	1	14
St. Louis, MO	09/28/95 transitions to a cooperative agreement with St. John's Mercy Medical Center	04/28/92	1	15
Dayton, OH		07/22/92	1	16
Clearwater, FL		09/15/92	1	17
Knoxville, TN	04/16/96 RO develops physician group (with Knoxville Hematology Oncology Associates)*	09/22/92	1	18
Columbia, SC		11/25/92	1	19
Colorado Springs, CO		11/25/92	1	20
Albuquerque, NM		12/08/92	1	21
St. Paul, MN		12/08/92	1	22
Philadelphia, PA		02/02/93	1	23
El Paso, TX		04/24/93	1	24
Ft. Wayne, IN		05/10/93	1	25
Norfolk, VA		10/05/93	1	26
Long Beach, CA		10/05/93	1	27
Grand Rapids, MI		12/1993	1	28
Worcester, MA	The Medical Center of Central Massachusetts	02/23/94	1	29
Blue Bell, PA	U.S. Healthcare—provider contract	05/10/94	0	29
Elgin, IL	Hines & Associates, Inc.—provider contract	06/08/94	0	29
Port Jefferson, NY	North Shore Hematology Oncology Associates	08/04/94	1	30
Indiana	PARTNERS Health Plans of Indiana—provider contract	08/10/94	0	30

(*continued*)

Table 5.6 (*continued*)

Location of	Affiliation	Date	No. of centers	Cumulative no. of centers
New Orleans, LA	Touro Infirmary	09/07/94	1	31
Munster, IN	Munster Medical Research Foundation	10/25/94	1	32
Richmond, VA		10/26/94	1	33
Burlington, VT	The Medical Center Hospital of Vermont	11/03/94	1	34
Johnson City, TN		02/21/95	1	35
Scranton, PA	Mercy Hospital	02/22/94	1	36
Glendale, CA	Glendale Memorial Hospital and Health Center (affiliate of UniHealth)	05/08/95	1	37
National	USA HealthNet— national contract	06/29/95	0	37
Northridge, CA	Northridge Hospital Medical Center	07/05/95	1	38
El Monte, CA	ProHealth, Inc.— provider contract	07/06/95	0	38
Mobile, AL	Providence Hospital	07/11/95	1	39
National	HealthNet, Inc.— national contract	07/12/95	0	39
National	American Postal Workers Union Health Plan (APWU)—national contract	07/13/95	0	39
Bayonne, NJ	Bayonne Hospital	09/11/95	1	40
Albany, GA	Phoebe-Putney Memorial Hospital	12/29/95	1	41
Oceanside, CA	Tri-City Medical Center	12/29/95	1	42
Miami, FL	Baptist Hospital, Oncology Hematology Group of Southern Florida—practice management affiliation	01/03/96	0	42
South Florida	South Florida Oncology Disease Management, GP— provider network	02/05/96	0	42
Washington, DC	Medlantic Healthcare Group (Washington Hospital Center)	02/07/96	1	43
Mt. Diablo, CA	Mt. Diablo Health Care District	02/08/96	1	44
Knoxville, TN	Knoxville Hematology Oncology Associates—practice management affiliation. Terminated 02/12/99*	04/16/96	0	44
St. Petersburg, FL	J. Paonessa, MD, PA—practice management affiliation (16 physicians)	06/20/96	0	44
Ft. Lauderdale, FL	Rymer, Zaravinos, & Faig, MD, PA—practice management affiliation (20 physicians)	07/08/96	0	44
Memphis, TN	West Clinic, PC—definitive agreement for a practice management affiliation	07/16/96	0	44

Table 5.6 (*continued*)

Location of	Affiliation	Date	No. of centers	Cumulative no. of centers
Tamarac, FL	Rosenberg & Kalman, MD, PA—practice management affiliation (22 physicians)	09/03/96	0	44
Port S. Lucie, FL	Hematology Oncology Associates of the Treasure Coast—practice management affiliations	10/09/96 Center established in 1997	1	45
West Boca Raton, FL	The Center for Hematology Oncology, PA—practice management affiliation	10/09/96 Center established in 1997	1	46
Miami Beach, FL	Lawrence A. Snetman, MD—practice management affiliation (31 physicians)	10/09/96	0	46
Florida	CIGNA Healthcare of Florida—provider contract	10/18/96	0	46
Knoxville, TN	Drs. Harf, Antonucci, McCormack & Kerns general partnership—practice management affiliation	12/02/96	0	46
Tamarac, FL	Weinreb, Weisberg & Weiss, PA—practice management affiliation (38 physicians)	12/09/96	0	46
Jackson, MS		1997	1	47
Billings, MT	Jointly owned with 2 community hospitals	1997	1	48
Little Rock, AK		1997	1	49
Corpus Christi, TX		1997	1	50
Houma, LA		1997	1	51
Miami, FL (added physicians)	Lessner & Troner, MD, PA—practice management affiliation (added physicians)	12/22/97	0	51
Lafayette, LA		End of 1997	1	52
Bangor, ME		04/16/98	1	53
Tacoma, WA	Multi Care Health System	04/16/98	1	54
Harrisburg, PA		04/16/98	1	55
Greely, CO	Northern Colorado Medical Center	04/16/98	1	56
National	Aetna U.S. Healthcare—10/08/98 national provider contract	0	56	
St. Joseph, MO		10/20/98	1	57
Youngstown, OH	Case Western Reserve	10/20/98	1	58
St. Petersburg, FL		10/20/98	1	59
Colorado Springs, CO		10/20/98	1	60
Knoxville, TN	Hematology Oncology Associates—terminated contract	02/12/99	0	60
National	Intracorp (largest U.S. case management company)—national contract	04/08/99	0	60

(*continued*)

Table 5.6 (*continued*)

Location of	Affiliation	Date	No. of centers	Cumulative no. of centers
Southeast Florida	Southeast Florida Hematology Oncology Group, P.A.—terminated contract	05/07/99	0	60
Nationwide	RO closes 6 IMPACT Centers and announces plans to close an additional 4 over the next quarter	08/04/99	−6	54
Nationwide	RO terminates 2 more PPM contracts	11/15/99	0	54
Pensacola, FL		11/15/99	1	55
New York, NY	Beth Israel Medical Center— administrative services agreement	11/15/99	0	55
Nationwide	RO closes 6 IMPACT centers (for a total of 12 in 1999)	11/15/99	−6	49
Nationwide	RO terminates more PPMs	1999	0	49
Nationwide	RO closes 8 IMPACT centers	08/11/00	−8	41
Nationwide	RO reports having a total of 37 IMPACT Centers (21 wholly owned, 13 managed programs, and 3 centers owned and operated in a joint venture with a hospital	09/30/00		37
Nationwide	RO announces closing of 14 under-performing IMPACT centers during December and the first quarter of 2001	12/00		23

[a] Information found below in chronology.
Abbreviations: RO, Response Oncology; FAHCT, Foundation for the Accreditation of Hematopoietic Cell Therapy.

not have the time to stay abreast of the science in cancer care; nonetheless, they want to provide their patients with every opportunity for remission" (Banchik 1991, p. 3).

The company recognized that the procedure was usually not reimbursable by insurance companies as it remained experimental. Consequently, they billed for "the component parts," mainly the laboratory studies and the intravenous drugs. FDA-approved drugs were typically reimbursable costs of treatment and thus eligible for reimbursement by insurers. Company collection of charges for drugs ran about 90%–95%; that for laboratory services was at 60% due to the complexity of one protocol.

The target population of patients—the national market—was estimated at 40,000 patients per year. This estimate included patients with breast cancer, ovarian cancer, and lymphoma and leukemia and patients under 65 years of age and responsive to chemotherapy. It was estimated that if HDC proved effective against lung cancer, the target population would double. Overall, the national market for HDC was estimated at $1.2 billion according to an analyst, who though that it could "double or triple over the next 5 years" (Banchik 1991, p. 3). In 1991, it was projected that 18–20 centers in place by April 1993 would give Response the physician base to capture 5% of the market, or $60 million in revenue. The analyst recommended "aggressive accumulation" of Response stock: The company was expected to become profitable in fiscal 1992; revenue and earnings per share (EPS) were expected to grow at annual rates of 69% and 123%, respectively, through fiscal 1996; the company was "a relatively new player in segments of the industry that are commanding EPS multiples of 28×–50× current fiscal year estimates" (Banchik 1991, p. 10). The analyst's recommendation was "STRONG BUY for long-term growth" (p. 1) and "aggressive accumulation of this stock" (p. 10).

Where Oldham had ignored the U.S. government by marketing cancer drugs not yet approved by the FDA, West took a much more sophisticated approach. He sought close identification, not confrontation, with the FDA. An internal Response Technologies document written in 1991 or 1992 (Response Technologies n.d., pp. 4, 6, 32) outlined the firm's approach to "the delivery of complex cancer therapy" in the outpatient setting: All patients received treatment "in the context of a clinical trial"; HDC regimens followed literature-based standards; all clinical protocols were "registered with the FDA"; treatment programs were modular to ensure maximum benefit and avoid unnecessary therapy; and recovery from HDC was supported by PBSC products and bone marrow growth factors.[8] (Response Technologies n.d., pp. 3–4). Response Technologies provided HDC/ABMT according to 12 different protocols, which basically meant tailoring protocols to individual patients. All chemotherapy drugs were FDA approved, but doses ranged from 3 to 50 times those of standard chemotherapy. These dosages fell outside the FDA-approved range for single agents, but Response registered all its protocols with the FDA as Investigational New Drugs. This was not required but may have provided some marketing advantage.

At the time the internal report was written, over 300 patients had been treated by HDC with PBSC support, and mortality of 4% had been achieved by "refined [patient] eligibility criteria" (Response Technologies n.d., p. 4). It was anticipated that over 500 patients would be treated within the Response "network" in 1992. All preparative chemotherapy, stem cell preparation, HDC, and reinfusion of stem cells were done in the outpatient setting. Two of three Response-affiliated oncologists were participants in the NCI Community Cooperative Oncology Program or another NCI-sponsored cooperative group. Patients with severe myelosuppression were hospitalized in affiliated hospitals, all of which were tertiary referral centers that met the ABMT guidelines of ASCO or the American Society of Hematology (p. 4).

Response achieved major cost savings by providing treatment in the outpatient setting; using PBSC rescue rather than the more expensive, more invasive ABMT; using PBSC and growth factor to stimulate recovery; and engaging in "rational patient selection" based on the IMPACT database and the clinical trials experience that guided treatment decisions (Response n.d., p. 4).

Several aspects of the Response strategy are noteworthy. First, although treatment was provided in the context of clinical trials, no one was randomized to standard therapy. The use of 12 treatment protocols tailored to individual patients meant that no experimental controls existed, and the value of the experience depended on the quality of the data acquired from the individual centers by the centralized data system. Birch explained the absence of randomization as follows:

> It's very difficult to randomize. The same barriers to randomization that appeared in the universities appeared here also. They were multiplied here. Also, we didn't know who to randomize. The barriers included: it took a lot of time to randomize; physicians wanted to differentiate themselves from others in the community by HDC. Patients

came and wanted HDC. If patients are referred to you for HDC, it is very difficult to randomize them. (Birch 2004)

Second, registration with the FDA for the use of approved drugs outside approved dosage ranges was unusual. Although the FDA drug approvals specify indications for use within given dosages, the oncology community routinely ignores these limits. Physicians are free to use approved drugs as they see fit. Response was not required to register these protocols. Why did it do so? "Every protocol has to be reviewed by an IRB [institutional review board]," Birch (2004) said. "One IRB asked whether we had an IND [Investigational New Drug application]. We did not. We were using all approved drugs but in higher than approved doses. West called FDA and said, 'We are using standard drugs. Do we need an IND?' 'No,' they said, 'but we would like you to submit one.' They had no data on HDC" (Birch 2004). Response provided data to the FDA. Third, Response took advantage of the developments related to PBSC and growth factors, which facilitated more rapid reconstitution of bone marrow. Thus, it positioned itself competitively with respect to academic oncology practices, which were initially engaged mainly in HDC with ABMT.

Fourth, in designing protocols based on ASCO and ASH guidelines, which were quite elementary in 1991, Response said to community oncologists that it would translate the latest advances in cancer research into working clinical practices for them. It doing so, it also provided specialized facilities that the community oncologist could use without giving up his or her patients to a tertiary academic center. "We thought we should be a translational arm," Birch said. "The universities should push the envelope: graft versus host disease, new drugs, that was the province of the universities" (Birch 2004).

Finally, Response also positioned itself with insurers in two ways. It sold them information about HDC for cancer treatment, especially breast cancer treatment, recognizing that a market for such information existed among smaller health insurers who could not support their own technology assessment effort. It also presented itself as more cost conscious than academic centers: PBSC was less expensive than ABMT, and the outpatient setting was less expensive than a major teaching hospital.

Response Technologies/Response Oncology did not intend to enter the physician practice management market. It owned treatment centers, not physicians. But in the late 1990s, AOR and PRN, pursuing the model of physicians-as-employees, began buying up oncology practices. As they did so, Response found some of its previously affiliated oncologists barred from treating their patients in its IMPACT centers. Hence, Response entered into a number of physician practice management arrangements in the mid-1990s. (A Dow Jones news service article about the creation of U.S. Oncology commented that the implications of this development for Response Technologies, a substantially smaller firm, was that the larger firm provided different, but more comprehensive services, although some competitive overlap existed.)

The data shown in figure 5.2 indicate that Response was profitable in 1992–1993, just a few years after it began and during a time when it was rapidly adding new centers, that it was briefly unprofitable in 1993–1994, and it continued making money until it hit the competition from AOR and PRN in 1998.

Response had its supporters. Three Georgia "former university oncologists with transplant specialization," in a March 29, 1993, letter to the *Wall Street Journal*,

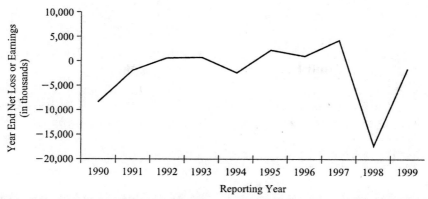

Figure 5.2. Response Technologies/Response Oncology finances for fiscal years 1990–1999.

remarking on a Karen Antman prediction that PBSCs would replace BMTs, said, "They already have" (Leff et al. 1993, p. A13). In concert with Response Technologies, community oncologists had been providing this treatment in outpatient settings for several years, and costs had fallen to $60,000 to $100,000 compared to bone marrow averages of $125,000 to $180,000. Their experience with 25 patients had resulted in "no procedure-related mortality, minimal morbidity and an average hospital stay of only 14 days." "We are witnessing a dramatic improvement in our ability to cost-effectively lengthen the lives of and possibly cure an increasing number of women with this dread disease" (Leff et al. 1993, p. A13).

Response also had its critics. The Sunday, September 26, 1993, broadcast of *60 Minutes* included a segment asking, "Is Bone Marrow Transplant Really the Answer to Curing Breast Cancer?" (Kroft 1993). Among the interviewees, Steve Kroft, the narrator, asked Dr. William West, chief executive officer of Response Technologies, "How much training do they get?" referring to physicians who practiced in Response centers. West hemmed and hawed: "They spend considerable time reading the protocols and the background information . . . [and] the reference literature." Kroft asked again, "How much training do they get?" West replied, "Oh, they've had a lifetime of training." Kroft pressed, "No, but from you, how much training do they get?" West responded, "Well, there's an ongoing interchange of ideas and experience, but the idea that they should come and go through a 2-month period of on-site training is not efficient." Finally, this from Kroft: "How much training do they get? How much time do they spend here with you learning how to do this procedure?" West answered, "I would say that the average physician is here 1 day?" Croft, incredulous, said "It sounds inconceivable to me that you can take an oncologist from Tampa or Miami or anywhere where you've got one of these centers, bring them to Memphis for 1 day, give them a list of doses and drugs . . . [and] send him back to begin doing this procedure."

The camera cut to Dr. Bruce Cheson of the NCI. "You can't learn it in a couple of days, and spending a day or two off in another city somewhere learning how to do it, and then going back and setting up 'Transplants-R-Us' is not the way to manage patients" (Kroft 1993). Kroft summarized this exchange: "Dr. Cheson says it takes years of specialized training to learn how to deal with the dangerous side effects that frequently accompany bone marrow transplants."

Not-for-Profit Entrepreneurs

Not-for-profit cancer centers, whether independent or university affiliated, discovered the financial attractiveness of cancer treatments in the 1990s. There was sometimes direct competition between for-profit and not-for-profit cancer providers. In 1996, Salick Health Care announced its plans to team with St. Vincent's Hospital as an entrée into the lucrative New York City market. This jarred four New York City cancer centers: Memorial Sloan-Kettering, Mt. Sinai Cancer Center, Columbia-Presbyterian, and the Albert Einstein Cancer Center (Lagnado 1996b). Salick's proposed entry was challenged by Memorial Sloan-Kettering, which requested that the New York State health commissioner delay approval and provide Sloan-Kettering the opportunity to review the financial documents behind the proposal (Lagnado 1996c).

While this competition for a share of the New York market was occurring, Memorial Sloan-Kettering signed "a sweeping contract" with Empire Blue Cross and Blue Shield (Lagnado 1996a). Months of secret negotiations, according to the report, had resulted in a contract that would increase the flow of new cancer patients to the center in return for cutting its rates as much as 30%. The episode underlined the general conflict between managed care and the providers of cancer care, against a background of competition among those providers. It makes the point quite clear that oncology is a very big business. In the 1990s, HDC/ABMT was a very profitable segment of that business.

Unfortunately, one cannot search Dow Jones archives for financial information about not-for-profit medical centers. Anecdotes indicate that BMT was very lucrative for those centers providing HDC/ABMT, that transplanters were very highly paid, and that railing against for-profit providers by academic and not-for-profit entities often disguised financial self-interest. Dr. Roy Jones, in a 1994 Denver newspaper, would concede that the BMT program was a "cash cow" for the University of Colorado. "We make a lot of money," he was quoted as saying. "And it causes some problems for us." But, the account continued, Jones added that his personal income did not depend on the success of the BMT center. The center's profits did finance other "worthwhile CU medical programs" (Dexheimer 1994, p. 2). Craig Henderson, who had been instrumental in persuading the Blue Cross Blue Shield Association to organize a demonstration to support randomized clinical trials, recounted a visit from the hospital administrator of the Dana-Farber Cancer Institute. Reimbursement under the demonstration was approximately $60,000 per patient. The administrator complained to him that the demonstration reimbursement rate was substantially lower than that received from insurers being billed directly.

The economic dimension of HDC/ABMT is largely hidden from public view. A great deal of information is available about publicly traded companies such as Response Oncology. But the economic data behind the provision of a specific medical service by non-profit institutions, whether academic medical centers or community hospitals, is not readily available. In this chapter, we have suggested only the economic side of HDC/ABMT. But, in an interview on September 1, 2004, Dr. Susan Love emphasized money as a driver of HDC/ABMT's widespread use. In her view, it was similar either to other medical interventions adopted before adequate evaluation, or to interventions not adopted if "an economic advantage to the physician" was absent. "We tried to get women to understand science, randomized clinical trials, evidence-based medicine," Love maintained, but "encountered a lot of opposition. . . . Doctors and hospitals were making a lot of money; these were the drivers. . . . It's a huge market: blood products, hospitalizations." Response Oncology was "a clear sign that a lot of money is to be made." The other piece, the belief women held that it was their only chance, was "wishful thinking." The therapy was not that good. "But hope drives belief and that drives behavior." Physicians say, 'Well, the patient asked for it.' However, "you can't underestimate the economic pull; BMT meant more money for the oncologists and the hospitals. . . . It is one of the dirty secrets of medicine: no one is greedy; no one is in it for the money. It's subtle, not conscious" (Love 2004).

6

Government Mandates

If you like laws and sausages, you should never watch either one being made.
—Otto Von Bismarck

The greater the ignorance, the greater the dogmatism.
—Sir William Osler

Any law that takes hold of a man's daily life cannot prevail in a community,
unless the vast majority of the community are actively in favor of it. The laws that
are the most operative are the laws that protect life.
—Henry Ward Beecher

Widespread clinical use of high-dose chemotherapy with autologous bone marrow
transplantation (HDC/ABMT) was partly driven in the mid-1990s by administrative
and legislative mandates that required health plans to cover the procedure for breast
cancer. In this chapter, we examine a mandate in 1994 from the federal Office of
Personnel Management (OPM) that required all health plans participating in the
Federal Employees Health Benefits Program (FEHBP) to provide HDC/ABMT for
breast cancer as a covered benefit. We also examine the enactment in 1995 by the
Minnesota legislature of a mandate that all plans in the state cover the procedure. We
introduce these cases with a discussion of the context.

Antecedents

Innumerable health and medical proposals were debated in 1993 and 1994 in relation to the health care reform initiative of President and Mrs. Clinton. Breast cancer
medical research, mammography, and clinical trials were discussed in this larger
context. When the Clinton health plan failed in the fall of 1994, many specific initiatives also fell by the wayside. Some breast cancer initiatives survived.

Against a background of successfully promoting increased Congressional appropriations for breast cancer research in 1992 (see chapter 2), the NBCC first discussed
HDC/ABMT at a board meeting in Los Angeles on January 9, 1993. The board
debated vigorously whether HDC/ABMT should be provided only within clinical
trials or whether it should be available without regard to trials. In either case, board
members thought that insurers should pay. Kay Dickersin of Arm-in-Arm, Susan
Love of the University of California at Los Angeles, and Sharon Green of Y-ME

argued that the procedure should not be supported outside randomized clinical trials. Dickersin (2004) recalls: "We [the board] had a huge argument. We [she, Love, Green] said 'the evidence is not in' " (Dickersin 2004). Love (2004) concurs: "The key to the response of NBCC was Kay Dickersin and me arguing very strongly for science-based, evidence-based medicine. Many women wanted access to it [ABMT] at the time. We tried to get women to understand science, randomized clinical trials, evidence-based medicine" (Love 2004). Both credit Green for voicing a concern for resources. If insurance coverage was provided for the procedure outside trials, then it would cost a good deal of money. "If you start allowing coverage on bone marrow transplant outside of clinical trials, it will cost hundreds or thousands of dollars," the minutes record someone (TD) saying (NBCC 1993, p. 4). Answers to effectiveness would not be obtained.

Belle Shayer, of Breast Cancer Action of San Francisco, countered by arguing that women had the right to obtain the kind of treatment that would help them, and NBCC did not have the right to say yes or no. "I was for giving a woman the right to choose what she wished to do and having the insurers pay for it. Not everyone wanted HDC. But those who wanted it should be able to get it. I had friends who were very involved in fighting insurers. This was also the view of Breast Cancer Action at the time" (Shayer 2004). Importantly, NBCC would not endorse unrestricted access to the procedure. The experience of Ricki Dienst tells the story of a women who wanted to take advantage of potentially beneficial treatments.

Ricki Dienst was one of the Breast Cancer Action members Shayer had in mind. Dienst had described her battle with breast cancer in the organization's newsletters. Diagnosed in 1986 with a 3-cm tumor and 24 positive lymph nodes, she was treated by surgery and aggressive chemotherapy but had a recurrence in November 1989 (Dienst 1993a). After failed hormonal treatments, a computed tomographic liver scan revealed metastases. Dienst had previously had uncontaminated bone marrow collected and frozen. So, after a 1-year battle with her insurance company for coverage, she wrote in 1993, "I entered Alta Bates Hospital in October 1991 for high-dose chemotherapy and autologous bone marrow transplantation. I was there for 5 weeks. Now, 18 months later, I am treatment free (except for tamoxifen) and have no evidence of cancer. My scans are clear and my CA 15–2 tumor marker is 17—well within normal range. So far, so good. I am optimistic and grateful" (Dienst 1993a, p. 1). Dienst later described what she had learned for others interested in HDC/ABMT (Dienst 1993b). But, in "One Woman's Dying Wish," she reported a recurrence, recounted the resistance she met at Genentech to enter the trial of Herceptin, a monoclonal antibody, and made a plea for Food and Drug Administration (FDA) compassionate use access to experimental drugs (Dienst 1995). Such testimonials exerted a strong influence on advocates.

Other NBCC board members endorsed freedom of choice but condemned centers that lacked experience and were providing the treatment for financial reasons. Betsy Lambert remembers "a very hot debate, very emotionally charged" (Lambert 2004). "There were two sides," she remembers. "One side said the science was not there. We all had anecdotal contacts with people, families and friends, who were involved. It was a mixed bag." The minutes suggest that the "heated discussion" resulted in a tabled motion. The HDC/ABMT issue would later be rolled into a policy statement dealing with "health care reform/payment for clinical trials," endorsing the view that insurers should pay for treatments offered in the context of publicly funded randomized clinical trials. Importantly, NBCC did not endorse providing the procedure outside randomized trials.

Although NBCC may have been divided about what to do about HDC/ABMT, advocates for the procedure were not. In this context, William Peters's June 1993 article in the *Journal of Clinical Oncology* made the case for HDC/ABMT for high-risk patients (Peters et al. 1993). His data, which showed dramatic differences in actuarial probability of relapse or event-free survival between the experimental treatment and historical controls, were sufficient to make the case for many oncologists that HDC was superior (see chapter 1, figure 1.2). In October of that year, he presented a different type of data to support his case and in a markedly different venue.

At a Capitol Hill luncheon on October 14, the Duke physician introduced a busload of women to interested members of Congress and their staff. These women, who had traveled from Durham, North Carolina, had all received HDC/ABMT (*Cancer Letter* 1993). They had come to Congress to argue that the Clinton health care reform should include reimbursement for patients enrolled in clinical trials, and that initially expensive innovative treatments became less so over time. Peters reported, for example, that the price of BMT at Duke had fallen from about $140,000 to about $65,000 as it had begun to be performed on an outpatient basis. It was now "roughly the price of a Lexus automobile," he was reported as saying. "As you look at a woman across the table from you, ask yourself, 'Is the price of this woman's life worth the price of a car?'" (Cancer Letter 1993, p. 4). Individual patients testified to the effectiveness of the treatment. Dramatically, Peters said, "I could give you a lot of statistics about the effectiveness of this treatment protocol. But I think it would be easier to do this with a simple demonstration. 'Would the women who received the transplants please stand up!'" (Cancer Letter 1993, p. 4). More than 70 women stood up.

Senator Tom Harkin (D, Iowa) also spoke. As chair of a Senate appropriations subcommittee, he had increased funding for breast cancer research in response to the NBCC. At the luncheon, he urged the patients to lobby for a surcharge on health insurance premiums that would finance biomedical research and for making mammograms available to all women without a copayment.

The following week, on October 18, 1993, President Clinton, who would later lose his mother to breast cancer, met with representatives of the National Breast Cancer Coalition (NBCC), from whom he received a petition containing 2.6 million signatures, the number of women in the United States estimated to have breast cancer, diagnosed or undiagnosed (Slatella 1993, News p. 17; Goldstein 1993, p. A1). At the meeting, after which Clinton signed the National Mammography Day proclamation, the president said that Donna Shalala, secretary of Health and Human Services, who herself had lost her three paternal aunts to breast cancer, would begin drafting a "national action plan" for preventing, diagnosing, and treating breast cancer (Clinton 1993, p. 1762). While the meeting was being held, breast cancer advocates were marching on the national mall chanting, "one in eight, we can't wait," a slogan derived from the statistic that breast cancer affects one in eight women during their lifetime (Goldstein 1993, p. A1). A few days later, on October 27, a special commission on breast cancer from the President's Cancer Panel, initiated 14 months earlier by President George H. W. Bush, reported that federal agencies need to spend at least $500 million a year on breast cancer to make substantial progress against this killer disease (Presidential panel, 1993, p. A25; Slatella 1993, News, p.17). This report reinforced the continuing demands for more money for breast cancer research. All this occurred as Clinton was submitting his plan for health care reform (Devoy 1993, p. A1).

Sooner rather than later, these developments would focus attention on the OPM and its FEHBP, which under federal law covered approximately 5 million federal government employees, retirees, and their families. Arlene Gilbert Groch, a New Jersey attorney, had drawn a bead on the FEHBP exclusion of HDC/ABMT coverage for breast cancer for women federal government employees. In mid-December 1992, she had written a memorandum to the NBCC board entitled, "Political Action to Compel the Federal Government to Mandate Insurers of Federal Employees Cease Excluding Bone Marrow Transplants for Women with Breast Cancer while Covering the Same Treatment for Men with Testicular Cancer" (Groch 1992). At that time, Groch represented Sherry and Tom Flatley, who had prevailed the prior week in federal district court in New Jersey, in an action to compel Blue Cross of New Jersey to pay for HDC/ABMT for stage IV breast cancer for Ms. Flatley. She expressed the hope that Sherry "is the last woman who has to fight her insurer while fighting cancer" (p. 2). FEHBP plans had previously covered bone marrow transplantation "without limitation as to the illness for which [it] was needed" (p. 1). In 1991, after several court cases declared that HDC/ABMT was not experimental, "The Blues and similar national insurers changed their contracts to cover BMTs for specified illnesses (including testicular cancer), and to *exclude* BMTs for any unspecified illnesses (including breast cancer)" (Groch 1992, p. 1). Making the case for political action, she wrote the following:

> In March 1993, OPM will be negotiating its 1994 contracts with Blue Cross and 300 other insurance companies for coverage of the 5+ million people. The results of those negotiations will directly affect those millions, and will indirectly affect all other insureds. OPM reports directly to the President, rather than to any Cabinet Officer. Significant public pressure on Congress and the White House during this window of opportunity can result in an agreement that OPM will require all insurers to cover BMTs and other "medically necessary" treatment for women with breast cancer. (p. 2)

Groch had received assurances from the two New Jersey Senators, Bill Bradley and Frank Lautenberg, and from Representative Bill Hughes that they supported OPM or legislative change to provide such coverage for women with breast cancer who were federal employees (Groch 1992). She would miss the "window of opportunity," but only by 1 year.

Groch would litigate a number of HDC/ABMT cases, including at least three in Colorado. In addition, she continued her political activity. In early February 1993, she wrote a widely circulated nine-page "MEMORANDUM" to "INDIVIDUALS CONCERNED ABOUT BREAST CANCER," indicating that the issue was "ACCESS TO HDC/BMT/APCR, AN ACCEPTED MEDICAL TREATMENT FOR

ADVANCED BREAST CANCER, AND WOMEN'S RIGHT TO CHOOSE AMONG TREATMENT OPTIONS [emphasis in original]" (Groch 1993). The HDC/ABMT procedure, she wrote, "is a treatment which provides the best hope of long term remission and/or cure for women with advanced breast cancer" (p. 1). But although insurers would pay for this procedure for patients with other diseases, including testicular cancer, "many, including all national insurers of federal employees, refuse to pay for it for women with breast cancer." In the memorandum, Groch quoted Dr. Roy Jones of the University of Colorado as indicating that HDC/ABMT "appears to be the only long term option providing any significant likelihood of long-term remission and control" of breast cancer. She went on to criticize the Blue Cross and Blue Shield Association (BCBSA) and other national companies that provided health insurance to federal government employees for consistently rejecting payment for HDC/AMBT for breast cancer.

Groch attacked the BCBSA demonstration project (described in the next chapter), which supported the National Cancer Institute (NCI) randomized clinical trials of HDC/ABMT. The BCBSA, she argued, had never required a randomized study of HDC/ABMT treatment for "any disease other than breast cancer" (p. 4). The insurers' support of these trials appeared to stem more from fiscal concerns than the impact of the treatment on patients. In any event, the BCBSA only agreed to fund the NCI study after courts had rejected claims that it was "experimental" or "investigational." Indeed, after deciding to support the NCI trials, Blue Cross plans had redrafted their OPM contracts. Quoting from the Blue Cross FEP Plan, Groch's memorandum said that these terms had been defined as applying to a treatment that was "the subject of on-going phase 1, 2, or 3 clinical trials or under study to determine its maximum tolerated dose, its toxicity, its safety, its efficacy, or its efficacy as compared with the standard means of treatment or diagnosis" (p. 5). Thus, Groch argued, the Blues had "created the basis for exclusion of treatment by funding the study" (p. 5).

The Blues had done this, even though an NCI public information pamphlet described HDC/ABMT for breast cancer as "state of the art." Groch's concluding "WHAT YOU CAN DO" focused on influencing the contract negotiations for the OPM 1994 contracts for the FEHBP (Federal Employees Health Benefit Program). Members of Congress and the Clinton administration needed to hear from other parties than the national health insurers.

What were the issues associated with HDC/ABMT? The general issue was what the OPM FEHBP health plans should cover. Up to this time, the OPM had deferred to the plans' exclusion of coverage of experimental or investigational treatments and most excluded coverage for HDC/ABMT for breast cancer. If HDC/ABMT was to be covered for breast cancer, as advocates were urging, what restrictions should apply? Should coverage be restricted to patients participating in phase 3 randomized clinical trials, available to women participating in any trial, or available without regard to trial participation? The BCBSA demonstration project covered women participating in NCI-sponsored high-priority randomized trials. Finally, should HDC/ABMT be available only in major cancer centers or in community cancer centers as well?

Each year, usually in March, the OPM issues a "call for proposed benefit and rate changes" to the health plans participating in the FEHBP. Plans respond, negotiations follow, and new contracts are usually completed during August for the coming calendar year. The 1994 language in contracts between the OPM and health insurers indicates clearly the FEHBP policy before Congress intervened. We cite below from contracts with the Blue Cross and Blue Shield Service Benefit Plan, the Kaiser Foundation Health Plan of the Mid-Atlantic States, Inc., and the Government Employees Hospital Association, Inc., Benefit Plan, which use similar, if not identical, language (OPM FEHBP 1994a, 1994b, 1994c, 1995a, 1995b, 1995c). Contracts typically include definitions of "experimental or investigational drug, device and medical treatment or procedure" (OPM FEHBP 1994a, p. 10). These definitions applied to a drug or medical device not yet approved for marketing by the FDA; or if "reliable evidence" showed that a drug, device, or medical treatment or procedure was under study in an ongoing phase 1, 2, or 3 clinical trial to determine toxicity, safety, or efficacy; or if reliable evidence showed that "prevailing opinion among experts" held that further studies or trials were necessary to make such determinations (OPM FEHBP 1994a p 10). Reliable evidence, in turn, meant "published reports and articles in the authoritative medical and scientific literature"; the protocols used to study the treatment in question; or the written informed consent used by a treating facility or one engaged in studying a treatment (OPM FEHBP 1994a, p. 10).

The reason for the definitions was clear. Under "General Exclusions," investigational or experimental treatments were described as benefits "not provided for services and supplies." These general contract exclusions were explicit in "Organ/Tissue Transplants and Donor Expenses." In the Blue Cross and Blue Shield contract, allogeneic bone marrow transplants were covered for a number of itemized diseases, mainly hematological malignancies. ABMTs were covered specifically for acute lymphocytic or nonlymphocytic leukemia; advanced Hodgkin's lymphoma; advanced non-Hodgkin's lymphoma; advanced neuroblastoma; and testicular, mediastinal, retroperitoneal, and ovarian germ cell tumors (OPM FEHBP 1994a, p. 23). Under "What Is Not Covered," the language read: "Allogeneic and autologous bone marrow and stem cell transplants for breast cancer are not covered" (OPM FEHBP 1994a, p. 23).

As the following discussion in this chapter suggests, the issues would be parsed with political skill but with little attention to the larger policy issue of access versus evaluation. A few skeptics argued that HDC/ABMT should be provided only within the context of randomized clinical trials. More well represented advocates argued that the procedure should be available in any clinical trial, randomized or not, but only if provided in academic or reputable cancer centers. OPM would resolve these issues in a way that generated some surprise and substantial confusion.

On October 29, 1993, Representative Patricia Schroeder and 52 other members of Congress wrote the OPM to urge that the agency cover HDC/ABMT for breast cancer (Schroeder et al. 1993). The letter cited data from Duke University terming HDC/ABMT "eight times more effective than conventional dose chemotherapy," (U.S. House, p. 146) but urging that its use be confined to major academic centers. Cost alone should not determine coverage for the treatment, the letter said, but waiting for clinical trials to be completed appeared to be "a delaying tactic." A second letter of June 1994 signed by the directors of five major cancer treatment centers, including Roy Jones and Bill Peters, increased pressure on the OPM to modify its policy (Jones et al. 1994).

Curtis Smith, then associate director of the OPM for retirement and insurance, would recall several years in which he took "painful calls" from Congressional offices, preachers, and other individuals regarding women federal employees who were being denied coverage for HDC/ABMT (Smith 2004). But, this was "case work," in bureaucratic language, involving individual employees. It was not organized lobbying to influence policy. That would come later.

Congressional Hearing, August 11, 1994

Representative Patricia Schroeder enlisted early as an enthusiastic supporter of more funds for breast cancer research. Educated at the University of Minnesota and Harvard Law School, Schroeder was elected as a Democrat to the House of Representatives from the First Congressional District of Colorado in 1972, where she served 12 terms before retiring in 1996. During her years in the House she served on the Judiciary Committee, the Post Office and Civil Service Committee, and the Armed Services Committee and chaired the House Select Committee on Children, Youth, and Families in 1991–1993. She also cochaired the Congressional Caucus on Women's Issues for 10 years and carried the unofficial title of Dean of Congressional Women. She unsuccessfully sought her party's nomination for president in 1988.

Mandating coverage for HDC/ABMT for breast cancer patients through the FEHBP was Schroeder's cause within Congress. The House Committee on Post Office and Civil Service served this cause well as it exercised jurisdiction over the OPM. Her colleague-in-arms in this endeavor was Representative Eleanor Holmes Norton, the nonvoting member of the House of Representatives from the District of Columbia, who chaired the Subcommittee on Compensation and Employee Benefits.

Cynthia Pearson, of the National Women's Health Network, recalls learning in the summer of 1994 that Norton's subcommittee would try to have the OPM declare the HDC/ABMT procedure effective for treating breast cancer. In disbelief, she visited the staff of Representative Norton, arguing that there was no evidence of effectiveness. Although not persuasive, she made it clear that not all women viewed the procedure in the same way and did persuade the staff to invite Craig Henderson as a witness (Pearson 2004).

At 10:00 A.M., August 11, 1994, Representative Norton called to order a hearing on FEHBP coverage of HDC/ABMT treatment for breast cancer. The hearing was a vehicle for advocacy, not one for finding of fact. Testimony overwhelmingly supported making HDC/ABMT available to breast cancer patients immediately, as did statements for the record from a number of members of the House. Witnesses included four breast cancer survivors who had undergone the treatment, two federal agency representatives, three BMT specialists, and two lawyers and an officer of a patient support organization. Norton turned to Schroeder for an opening statement, which set the tone for the entire hearing. Schroeder said:

> I represent a lot of Federal employees, and we came upon horror show after horror show of family members of Federal employees or their doctors clearly telling them bone marrow was the way to go, and then they find out that the only thing OPM could let them do is get into this clinical trial where they do a coin flip, which means half the

people won't get bone marrow transplant. . . . And you are going to hear from Dr. Roy Jones, who's an expert in this area . . . [and] has shown that a five-year relapse-free survival for high-risk breast cancer treated with the bone marrow treatment is 35 percent better than any other result reported in the medical literature by any research using conventional treatment. That's amazing. And yet OPM continues to insist upon having a gold standard for this that they have not required for testicular cancer or the others where they do permit payment. Why is the standard higher on breast cancer? Madam Chair, you put that in your opening statement, and I—I think that is a real question to ask OPM when they come up. (U.S. House 1994, p. 5)

Although Schroeder supported clinical trials, "insurance payment should be available to patients who participate in other NCI approved treatment programs," she said in her prepared statement, and the OPM "should require carriers to pay for coverage under these circumstances" (U.S. House 1994, p. 6). Schroeder saw HDC/ABMT as both a women's issue and a Colorado issue, especially as a number of her constituents had been denied coverage. In addition, Dr. Roy Jones, a University of Colorado constituent, was a vocal advocate of insurers paying for patient care in clinical trials.

Curtis J. Smith represented the OPM and Dr. Bruce Cheson the NCI. Together, they set out the administration's position. Smith, the associate director of the OPM for retirement and insurance, agreed that FEHBP "needs to provide reasonable access to medically necessary treatments that have been demonstrated to be effective" (U.S. House 1994, p. 34). All plans provided for treatment of cancer, including breast cancer. "However," he added, "not all methods of treatment are covered under all plans, which is the issue we have before us today." He continued:

Simply stated, the reason ABMT is not generally covered for treating certain conditions, such as breast cancer, is that in such cases, this treatment is not proven to be more effective than conventional treatments, while we know it carries a much higher risk. For this reason, OPM has not required carriers to cover the procedure, to carry the coverage. Also, to aid in determining whether ABMT therapy for breast cancer is efficacious, OPM has arranged to allow FEHBP plans to participate in an outside non-FEHBP demonstration project sponsored by the Blue Cross and Blue Shield Association and the National Cancer Institute involving clinical trials in order to establish if both the trials are good and safe. This issue is of serious concern to us at OPM, to FEHBP carriers, and certainly to our employees and their families. We will continue to actively monitor and review current published studies in the medical literature and to correspond with NCI and our FEHB's medical directors to update our knowledge of the HDC autologous bone marrow transplant for breast cancer while we await the results of the ongoing clinical trials. We will not hesitate to modify FEHBP coverage requirements as soon as reliable clinical evidence indicates ABMT is as effective and worth the greater risk. We expressly advised our carriers in 1994 that once the clinical evidence establishes the efficacy and safety of ABMT for breast cancer, we would expect all plans to provide coverage, including changing coverage provisions in midyear. (U.S. House 1994, p. 34)

In his written statement, Smith noted that the majority of FEHBP plans excluded coverage of HDC/ABMT for breast cancer at that time. He also said "there is as yet no consensus in the medical community" that the procedure was more effective than standard therapy. The OPM had maintained close contact with the NCI, and "they emphatically advise that AMBT therapy for breast cancer should not be performed outside of the clinical trial setting" (U.S. House 1994, p. 35). Importantly, he acknowledged that the OPM lacked the medical expertise to make independent determinations. It based its policy on two things: the absence of scientific evidence supporting claims that HDC/ABMT was more effective than conventional therapy and its dependence on the NCI to make that determination.

Cheson, who headed the medicine section of the NCI's Clinical Investigations Branch, Division of Cancer Treatment, testified that ABMT had been used for over a decade for patients with "leukemias and other disorders" and more recently with solid tumors, including breast cancer. Results at "high-caliber institutions supported by the NCI," such as Duke, the Dana-Farber Cancer Institute, the University of Colorado, and M. D. Anderson in Houston, were "encouraging" for women with metastatic or high-risk breast cancer. Even so, such results "must be viewed with care." They had been compared to treatments that were no longer considered optimal, and studies had been conducted in highly selected women "who are otherwise in good health." Therefore, he said, "We are faced with one of the most important and certainly one of the most controversial and unanswered questions in cancer therapy: Is autologous bone marrow transplantation better than current standard therapy in comparable breast cancer patients?" (U.S. House 1994, p. 38). Cheson expressed concern that treatment was "being increasingly delivered by inexperienced physicians outside of clinical trials," which jeopardized patient safety and reduced the likelihood of benefit. The intended target of this indirect reference was Response Technologies, as Cheson had criticized Dr. William West on precisely this point the preceding September on *60 Minutes* (Kroft 1993; see chapter 5).

Cheson, noting that NCI-sponsored clinical trials were addressing "these important issues," laid down the following policy marker:

> For breast cancer patients, more data are needed to definitively establish the role of ABMT as standard therapy. Although it is not within the mandate of the NCI to determine coverage policy, we believe it is scientifically and clinically responsible for formal scientific evaluation to precede the routine use of such a toxic and expensive therapy in clinical practice. We believe routine use in clinical practice should occur only after scientific evaluation establishes its value. In the case of ABMT, this has not yet definitively occurred. (U.S. House 1994, p. 39)

In the questions and answers that followed the testimony of Smith and Cheson, Norton would deftly undermine the OPM policy by sundering its reliance on the NCI (U.S. House 1994). Norton, who still taught a course at Georgetown Law School, began by expressing "great respect for the way in which scientific evidence must be accrued, . . . for the kind of research it takes to prove anything, whether it is a matter in law or a matter of scientific evidence" (U.S. House 1994, p. 42). Her first question to Cheson was whether Sloan (Memorial Sloan Kettering Cancer Institute) had participated in NCI trials. Yes, he answered. "How would you characterize Sloan's reputation?" she asked. "It was one of the finest cancer centers in the country," he responded. Norton then asked: "You wouldn't consider it malpractice for Sloan to recommend a treatment similar to the one under discussion here for a patient who comes to Sloan?" It would "depend on the patient," but the NCI position was that "the therapy would be appropriate if conducted in the clinical trial setting."

"Well," Norton bored in, "if an institution like Sloan ordered the treatment outside of a clinical trial setting, would you believe that Sloan was doing something inappropriate?" (U.S. House 1994, p. 43). Not necessarily, Cheson replied, as they had a number of clinical trials "for patients with this particular condition." "So while you recommend that the treatment be administered only in clinical trials, I take it that is controlled studies?" the representative asked. Not necessarily, Cheson said. Developmental (nonrandomized phase 1 and phase 2) studies were also ongoing. "So," Norton queried, "while the NCI recommends that this treatment be administered in clinical trials, you are not prepared to say it is inappropriate for it to be recommended outside of clinical trials?" Cheson replied:

> It would depend on the setting in which it is being conducted. If it is conducted at an institution which is experienced in the conduct of clinical trials and has some form of quality assurance, institutional review, et cetera, that is fine. But what I am saying is that there are now a large number of small hospitals that are undertaking this procedure, which is being performed by individuals who lack the experience and expertise to do this safely and from which no useful information will be gained to improve this field and to improve on therapy. (U.S. House 1994, p. 43)

Norton solicitously agreed that not any Podunk hospital should do HDC/ABMT. But, she said, "We have testimony from an attorney, Robert Carter, that suggests that many of the country's top medical institutions refuse to participate in NCI trials because they believe that HDC/ABMT treatment is far superior to conventional treatment and that the continued use of randomized trials is, at least in this situation, unethical." Was Cheson proposing that conventional treatment was superior to HDC/ABMT? "It remains to be demonstrated," he replied. Was there a point at which knowledge of a treatment was sufficient that randomized trials were unethical? Yes. "What is that point? What is that standard?" Norton asked. Cheson suggested that the experimental treatment be "at least as good as and not significantly more toxic" than conventional treatment.

Relentlessly, the chairwoman pursued: "We are faced with the fact . . . that a substantial number of court cases have specifically rejected the argument that this treatment for breast cancer is experimental." Cheson responded, "We [speaking for NCI] do not like to use the word 'experimental' or the word 'investigational' because they are vague. They mean different things to different people. We prefer to base determinations on whether it is appropriate for a particular patient and whether, based on the appropriateness, it should be considered standard treatment." In short, Cheson did not defend randomized trials against other clinical trials if done at a reputable institution. He also did not defend the need for population-based data that such trials generated but deferred to a standard of appropriateness for an individual patient.

Smith interjected himself at that point, and he and Norton continued the colloquy. In his prepared statement, he had stated that the OPM, beginning in contract negotiations for 1993, had required plans to state exclusions "in plain language in the plan's benefit brochure to avoid any enrollee confusion and potential for litigation" (U.S. House 1994, p. 36). In the question period, Smith acknowledged that the majority of FEHBP plans did exclude HDC/ABMT coverage for breast cancer at that time. He also indicated, "Out of the NCI trial arrangement, very few people cover it. There are a number of HMOs [health maintenance organizations] throughout the country on the fee-for-service side. None of the open fee-for-service nationwide plans cover it outside—some of those larger plans do participate in the NCI clinical trials. But, no, there is not very much coverage. You are right about that" (p. 49). He added later, "We have looked particularly to NCI to tell us when this particular therapy crosses over and becomes standard medical practice, and it has not done that" (p. 54).

In the continued give and take of questions and answers, Norton wrung this concession from Smith: "I had agreed earlier that we owe you a look at whether or not we should expand the definition of clinical trial in which we pay. And NCI's recommendation will be important. We look to them for the medical and scientific basis for what we should do but welcome their advice on the reimbursement as well" (U.S. House 1994, p. 58). Cheson had affirmed the value of providing the treatment not only in randomized studies, but also in developmental studies if done at reputable cancer institutions. Consequently, Smith was no longer in a position to defend the OPM's policy to limit coverage to participants in randomized trials.[1] Norton greeted the OPM's willingness to review its policy appreciatively, asking how long it might need. "That is a hard question for me to answer just on the spot," Smith said. "Does a couple of months sound reasonable?" "A couple of months is reasonable," Norton replied.

Three oncologists followed the OPM and NCI witnesses. Dr. Craig Henderson, then chief of oncology at the University of California at San Francisco, led off and raised a note of caution. Describing the FDA's review of drugs, he defended "the long-standing tradition . . . of restricting the right of a physician to prescribe a drug or for a patient to have access to a drug until these [phase 1, phase 2, and phase 3] studies are completed" (U.S. House 1994, p. 67). For HDC/ABMT, which did not require FDA approval, the most important question had not been answered: "Are the high doses of chemotherapy and bone marrow transplant as good as or better than conventional therapy?" He asked how the conflict was to be resolved, "between the humanistic desire to comfort the seriously ill and the scientific need to find out which treatments really work." "I am convinced," he answered, "it is not by abandoning rigorous assessment of new treatments" (U.S. House 1994, p. 70). His was a lengthy, thoughtful statement, but in that setting not persuasive.

Dr. Roy Jones, a protégé of William Peters, and a University of Colorado constituent of Schroeder's, followed. First, somewhat derisively, he agreed "with the NCI staff, OPM and Dr. Henderson that coin flip trials are required to definitively prove the superiority of these treatments" (U.S. House 1994, p. 78). "But," he added, "available evidence from 8–10 years of research is clear. These [HDC/ABMT] programs are very effective." Five-year tumor-free survival for metastatic breast cancer patients was 15–20 times greater than the results of conventional therapy when "given at three of America's most prestigious cancer hospitals." For high-risk patients, 5-year relapse-free survival was 35% better than anyone reporting results with conventional treatment. He attacked the OPM policy that recommended coverage approval only for participation in coin-flip trials. This meant the patient and her doctor could not select HDC/ABMT treatment if they wished. He wished to expand coverage beyond randomized trials.

Second, Jones also sought to restrict the provision of the procedure. "Until this technology is optimized for cost-effectiveness, its administration should be restricted to research centers with proven research productivity. Otherwise, half-way technology is given to patients at the price of reduced benefit and increased cost" (U.S. House 1994, p. 79). He suggested that "new high-technology treatments for cancer should be reimbursed if they are approved by the NCI, its cooperative groups, or its designated cancer centers." Behind the abstract language, Jones was attacking the challenge to academic cancer centers raised by Response Technologies, which had opened several IMPACT (Implementing Advanced Cancer Treatment) centers in Colorado (Jones et al. 1994).[2]

The final oncologist to testify was Dr. Richard Champlin from the M. D. Anderson Cancer Center, speaking as president of the American Society for Blood and Marrow Transplantation. He endorsed HDC/ABMT as "probably the most promising treatment that has been published in the last decade in the field of breast cancer" (U.S. House 1994, p. 86). It fell between experimental and standard therapy. But insurers should not be allowed to deny coverage for it. In his concluding statement he said: "So I want this committee to give instructions to your own insurance carrier to indeed cover this service; perhaps this and other treatments do require further evaluation, but are clearly a benefit to patients and clearly should be covered in the scheme of health care" (U.S. House 1994, p. 87).

The skepticism of Smith, Cheson, and Henderson had little effect on the subcommittee as it pursued its advocacy agenda. The day after the hearing, Schroeder and Norton wrote James B. King, the OPM director, to underscore the breach between the OPM policy and the views of the NCI—as they interpreted those views:

> During yesterday's hearing . . . Dr. Bruce Cheson testified that NCI does not support OPM's decision to limit insurance coverage for autologous bone marrow transplantation for breast cancer patients to patients in "randomized" clinical trials only.
>
> Dr. Cheson's testimony contradicts earlier testimony by Curtis Smith, who said, "We maintain close contact with the National Cancer Institute and they emphatically advise that ABMT therapy for breast cancer should not be performed outside of the clinical trial setting."
>
> The key point brought out in the hearing is that there are different kinds of clinical trials approved by NCI. OPM reimburses only the randomized or coinflip trials, while NCI advocates reimbursement for *all* NCI approved trials, including non-coinflip trials.
>
> The NCI-approved non-coinflip trials, conducted at centers like Duke University and the University of Colorado, have shown extremely promising results. According to Dr. Roy Jones . . . the 5-year relapse-free survival for high-risk primary breast cancer treated with ABMT is 35 percent better than any result reported in the medical literature by any research group using any conventional treatment. (Schroeder and Norton 1994)

On August 16, Representative Norton sent King another letter "to confirm that OPM is, in fact, considering expanding its current insurance coverage to include patients in all [emphasis in original] NCI approved clinical trials of a promising new breast cancer treatment—HDC/ABMT" (Norton 1994). The issue for her turned on coverage for all trials:

> In an important development from the hearing last Thursday. . . . OPM Associate Director Curtis committed that OPM would reconsider within 2 months—that is, by October 11, 1994—its policy of limiting coverage to an extremely small number of "randomized" clinical trials only. Particularly in light of NCI testimony that there was

no reason that patients should not be treated through NCI-approved facilities, such as Georgetown University Hospital and Sloan Kettering, the Subcommittee would anticipate that OPM would require coverage of appropriate breast cancer patients. (Norton 1994)

Norton had selectively interpreted Cheson's testimony to make the point she wished to make and simply ignored his other arguments. Her letter continued: "[I]n light of the testimony of federal employees whose lives have apparently been saved by this therapy but whose applications for reimbursement were denied by their insurance carriers, it would have been remarkable and cruel if OPM had adhered to its original position of refusing to consider expanding access to this life-saving treatment until randomized trials were completed" (Norton 1994). When an experimental treatment is shown to have "higher success rates" than conventional chemotherapy, she wrote, "it would seem the height of callousness to impose bureaucratic obstacles that effectively deny women the chance to participate in approved programs that might well save their lives."

Norton's letter struck at the Achilles' heel of efforts to evaluate HDC/ABMT in randomized clinical trials. She had differentiated between randomized and earlier stage clinical trials and argued that both should be covered. If the OPM policy changed accordingly, it would sanction the provision of therapy outside of multisite phase 3 randomized clinical trials as long as patients were enrolled in single-site phase 2 studies. This expansion of coverage was precisely what believers such as Roy Jones hoped for: If a woman approached them for access to therapy and refused to participate in a randomized trial, they could easily enroll her in a nonrandomized, no-control phase 2 study that examined some technical question related to improving the HDC/ABMT procedure (e.g., a study of techniques to ensure that bone marrow was purged of occult cancerous cells that might otherwise increase the risks of reinfusion). Academic researchers were quite adept at such maneuvers. The only problem was that the OPM could not adopt a policy that restricted for-profit providers, such as Response Technologies, from doing the same as the academic centers were doing. Policy determinations are often a blunt instrument.

The OPM took less than 6 weeks to review its policy. On September 20, James King, OPM director, held a press conference to indicate the 1995 "open season" highlights, including the policy change pertaining to HDC/ABMT. The accompanying press release read: "Effective immediately, OPM will now require coverage by all plans (HMO and fee-for-service) of high-dose chemotherapy with autologous bone marrow transplantation (HDC/ABMT) in the treatment of breast cancer, multiple myeloma, and epithelial ovarian cancer, in addition to the other conditions for which each plan currently provides coverage" (OPM 1994d, pp. 1–2). King was quoted in the press release as saying: "With the addition of this coverage under the FEHBP, the choice of appropriate treatment options will be back with the patient, doctor and insurance plan. It simply was time to move the decision from the hearing room to the hospital room" (OPM 1994d, p. 2). (King would convey this information a week later to Rep. Norton [King, U.S. House, pp. 60–64].) In a same-day letter to participating plans, the OPM wrote that it was "mandating immediate coverage of HDC/ABMT for all diagnoses for which it is considered standard treatment and, in addition, specifically for breast cancer, multiple myeloma, and epithelial ovarian cancer" (Harris 1994, p. 1).[3] Plans not then covering the procedure, the letter indicated, were allowed to limit coverage to nonrandomized clinical trials if such trials were available in a service area. According to the *Washington Post* story covering the press conference: "At a time when efforts to reform the nation's health system and cut its costs have all but collapsed on Capitol Hill, the Federal Employees Health Benefits Program will expand benefits and cut average premiums for the 1995 benefit year" (Rich and Brown 1994).

Schroeder described the OPM policy change as "a victory for women who ha[d] been denied treatment that is routinely provided for other forms of cancer. . . . This decision will save lives" (Brinkley 1994). Looking back, Schroeder explained the OPM's action in terms of various factors that came together in the mid-1990s:

There was a lot of research going on in Denver, and federal employees in the area (57,000 in Colorado at the time) who had breast cancer were very frustrated that they could not be reimbursed for the treatment. No one in my family had breast cancer, but it seemed like Denver was having an epidemic. Rocky Flats was a nuclear facility and Denver was down wind, plus the higher altitude meant higher fall out. No one knew why the incidence seemed higher, but it did. There was no question this [HDC/ABMT procedure] was experimental, but the issue was what constituted "experimental." This was when breast cancer awareness was really surging. There was such anger that the mammograms were crap in many instances, we discovered only one mammography clinic in Denver met federal standards, more anger that the federal government had totally ignored research into any women's health issues, and panic that there were no treatments that had been vetted drove the train. Therefore, many women didn't catch the cancer in the early stages and were ready to try anything. At that time it looked like this had more promise that we know it has now. Since the trials hadn't been done, no one had any final conclusions. I'm not so sure it was seen as a "miracle cure" but as the only other alternative known at the time. The only thing women could do was get in experimental programs where only half would get the treatment and you couldn't control which half you were in. I felt since the federal government had not done any research on breast cancer (one study using men), according to the Government Accounting Office, they could reimburse women desperate to try something that appeared to have a greater chance of survival. Once NIH [National Institutes of Health] and NCI finally started the research, it seemed harsh that the only way you could get treatment was to get in the study. The research should have been done long ago and if breast cancer impacted men, it would have been done. (Schroeder 2002)

What led to the OPM decision? Ron Winslow, in the *Wall Street Journal* (1994), analyzed the "tremendous political press to abandon its policy of supporting the treatment only within randomized clinical trials." In addition to the letter from Congress in October 1993 and that from the cancer centers in June 1994, "staffers for the committee, which oversees the OPM, were disturbed by a Cable News Network story about a federal worker who was denied coverage" before the August hearing, Winslow wrote. In addition, many women's advocacy groups had listed access to the treatment as "an important goal for health care reform."

Winslow's last point deserves elaboration. In the hearing, Cancer Care, Inc., was the only advocacy group to testify but took "no position on access to or reimbursement for HDC/AMBT" (U.S. House 1994, p. 133). Instead, Kim Calder testified, "Our relevant position is based squarely on our firm belief that people with cancer should have access to state-of-the-art anti-cancer therapy as recommended by cancer specialists and that they have the right to expect their insurer to provide for such coverage" (U.S. House 1994, p. 133). In short, patients should have what their physicians recommend and insurers should pay. In this instance, this was a distinction without a difference.

Where were the national patient advocacy organizations? The National Alliance of Breast Cancer Organizations did not testify. Amy Langer recalls writing a letter but not being invited to testify (personal communication, April 29, 2004). The NBCC also did not testify. Fran Visco said flatly, "We weren't invited. We didn't know about it" (personal communication to R. A. Rettig, September 2, 2004). The subcommittee staff undoubtedly knew in advance that neither organization would endorse the provision of the HDC/ABMT procedure outside randomized clinical trials.

Arlene Gilbert Groch, the New Jersey lawyer who had litigated several cases, also testified. She had it right from the start. The OPM was vulnerable to political pressure from Congress and was not protected by a cabinet-level department. A single-day hearing by a House oversight subcommittee that lacked authority to write legislation, chaired by a nonvoting member of the House, had led an administrative agency to reverse an explicit policy within 6 weeks. That reversal reflected the strength of feminism and the inadvertent undermining of the OPM by the NCI.

On the other hand, some observers suggested that the OPM action could have been anticipated. A managed care newsletter published an account in September 1994 that said: "Plans have known for some time that OPM this fall likely would begin requiring them to cover ABMT/HDC for federal workers with breast cancer" (Darby 1994). "Earlier this year," it continued, "OPM told carriers that contract with FEHBP that it was considering requiring them to cover ABMT/HDC. 'It's not as if this is a big, complete surprise for them,' the OPM official notes. 'They were well aware of this.'"

What were the consequences of the OPM decision? FEHBP participating plans were caught off guard by the requirement of immediate coverage and by extending coverage to ovarian cancer and myeloma (Darby 1994). An upward but mild impact on premiums was expected. It was also expected that plans providing coverage for federal government employees would find it hard to deny coverage for others. Defense in litigation was unlikely to be affected, as one lawyer surmised, because "the 'experimental' nature of the procedure is no longer the key issue in court" (Darby 1994, p. 10). Rather, the issue was exclusionary language used in insurance contracts. One view, however, was that such clauses had been "torpedoed" (DeMott 1994).

More broadly, the decision meant that 300 health plans participating in FEHBP were suddenly required to cover HDC/ABMT for breast cancer for federal employees and their beneficiaries. The indirect effects virtually extended coverage to all by reason of the difficulty in sustaining discriminatory coverage between federal and nonfederal workers. A domino effect was anticipated with employers, "purchasing groups and state legislatures" following with demands similar to the OPM decision (DeMott 1994, p. 2). The financial impact was estimated at $120 million (DeMott 1994). The BCBSA filed a compliance statement the day after the OPM announcement, seeking to minimize the effects of the policy change by limiting coverage to women who agreed to enter nonrandomized trials. It listed three criteria for coverage: the institution was a member of a cancer cooperative group; it was an NCI-designated cancer center; or it received a special grant for a particular trial (DeMott 1994).

The NCI was embarrassed. Cheson was quoted in the *Wall Street Journal* saying that a portion of his testimony was misinterpreted to mean "that everybody who wants this procedure should get it whether they're on a clinical trial or not" (Winslow 1994). For NCI and the high-priority clinical trials of HDC/ABMT, the decision would compound the already significant challenges of enrolling women in its randomized trials, which were at least two years from completion (DeMott 1994). The agency worried that coverage mandates "could undercut incentives for women to enter those trials," which were necessary to determine treatment effectiveness. Michael Friedman, head of NCI's Cancer Treatment Evaluation Program, termed the OPM decision "unfortunate." NCI could no longer avoid demands from patients that they be provided treatment under a nonrandomized phase 2 protocol.

Karen Ignagni, the president and chief executive officer of the Group Health Association of America (GHAA), the trade association for health plans, managed care organizations, and HMOs, voiced "serious concerns" about the decision and "the inappropriate manner in which it has been implemented" (Ignagni 1994, p. 1). She expressed concern about the "detrimental impact on medical research . . . and [on] the ongoing need to evaluate new technologies and experimental treatments." Mark Jordan, senior counsel for Kaiser Permanente, would do the same a few weeks later. Kaiser physicians, he wrote, "firmly believe, based on the available scientific data, that ABMT/HDC has not been demonstrated to be a scientifically proven procedure for the treatment of solid tumors such as breast or ovarian cancer" (Jordan 1994, p. 1). In light of the probable interpretation by individuals and courts that the procedure was no longer experimental, he asked that the OPM formally acknowledge that its decision was "not based upon the scientific merits of the procedure," that it was made "regardless of its experimental nature," that premiums charged by plans did not include coverage for ABMT/HDC, and that "its decision was not a determination that the procedure is no longer experimental" (Jordan 1994, p. 2).

The confusion created by the OPM decision was not reduced by an exchange between the GHAA and the agency. The GHAA general counsel, Alphonse O'Neill-White, asked how clinical trial was to be defined and by whom (O'Neill-White 1994). Ed Flynn, who had succeeded Curtis Smith as OPM Associate Director for Retirement and Insurance, responded that the agency had "no special definition for 'clinical trial'" (Flynn 1995, p. 1). "Any FEHB plan," he wrote, "that chose to limit its coverage to services performed in a clinical trial setting was free to choose those trials it wished its members to participate in, *provided coverage was not limited to only randomized clinical trials* [italics added]."

The OPM found itself explaining its action well into calendar year 1995. The OPM assistant director for insurance programs, Lucretia F. Myers, wrote Dr. Clifton Gaus, then administrator of the Agency for Health Care Policy and Research, to provide "more background information" on the decision to require all FEHBP plans to cover HDC/ABMT for breast cancer (Myers 1995, p. 1). Obviously responding to some criticism, Myers asserted, "we believe we made the right decision." She wrote: "Although there is lack of unanimity in the medical community [about HDC/ABMT for breast cancer], there is much more agreement that health insurance coverage should be available for the associated patient care costs despite the ongoing clinical research." The OPM acted, she wrote, "not as medical authorities or regulators of the insurance industry, but as purchasers of health insurance coverage in the market-place." It would be the political marketplace, however, not the economic or medical science markets, that drove this major policy shift.

The 1995 contract for the Blue Cross and Blue Shield Service Benefit Plan reflected the changes. In addition to the previous covered conditions for ABMT, new language stated that it was now covered for

> 1) breast cancer; 2) multiple myeloma; and 3) epithelial ovarian cancer; only when per-formed as part of a clinical trial that meets the requirements noted in the Limitations below and is conducted at a Cancer Research Facility. In the event no non-randomized clinical trials meeting the requirements set forth below are available at Cancer Research Facilities for a member eligible for such trials, the Plan will make arrange-ments for the transplant to be provide at another Plan-designated transplant facility. (OPM 1995a, p. 15)

The language further indicated that for ABMT procedures covered only through clinical trials, prior approval by the plan was required; the trial "must be approved and funded by the National Cancer Institute at the Cancer Research Facility where the pro-cedure is to be delivered"; and the patient must be "properly and lawfully registered" in the trial (OPM 1995a, p. 15). Similar language was included in other contracts.

State Government Mandates

Efforts to mandate health insurer and health plan coverage for HDC/ABMT for breast cancer were not restricted to the federal government, but were also being enacted by state governments. A few state actions preceded the OPM mandate; a number followed it. In table 6.1, we list the states with legislatures that have adopted statutes that require health plans operating within their borders to cover HDC/ABMT for breast cancer. We examine one state mandate, Minnesota, next.

Of the states that mandate HDC/ABMT, we chose Minnesota for three reasons. First, the mandate occurred at a time when legislators would have a clear picture of the

Table 6.1 State government statutes regarding HDC/ABMT for breast cancer

Florida (Fla. Stat. Ann. § 627.4236; enacted in 1992; West 1996)
New Hampshire (N.H. Rev. Stat. Ann. § 415:18-c; enacted in 1992; 1998)
Massachusetts (Mass. Gen. Laws ch. 175, § 47R; enacted in 1996 to replace a 1993 emergency act; 1996)
Virginia (Va. Code Ann. § 38.2-3418.1:1; enacted in 1994; Michie 1999)
New Jersey (N.J. Stat. Ann. §§ 17:48-6k, 26:2J-4.8; both enacted in 1995; West 1996)
Tennessee (Tenn. Code. Ann. § 56-7-2504; enacted in 1995) (1994 & Supp. 1999)
Minnesota (Minn. Stat. Ann. § 62A.309; enacted in 1995; West 1996)
Missouri (Mo. Ann. Stat. § 376.1200; enacted in 1995; West 2002)
Georgia (Ga. Code Ann. § 33-29-3.3; enacted in 1995; 1996)
Kentucky (Ky. Rev. Stat. Ann. § 304.38-1936; enacted in 1996)
Montana [Mont. Code Ann. § 33-22-1521 (1998)] (enacted in 1985; not specific to breast cancer)

scientific controversy, which allowed us to examine the role that science played in the legislative debate. Second, the state's extensive managed care market penetration allowed the industry to speak with a unified voice, which provided us an opportunity to assess the industry's strategy by interviewing a relatively small number of participants. Third, we had extensive contacts in Minnesota, which facilitated the interviewing process.

Minnesota

On March 29, 1995, Representative Dee Long introduced legislation in the Minnesota House of Representative that would require health plans in the state to cover HDC/ABMT for breast cancer. Her cosponsor, House Speaker Irv Anderson, conveyed the "powerful blessing" attached to the proposed mandate by the House leadership (Grow 1995). A *Minneapolis Star Tribune* reporter surmised that the bill came "late in a [legislative] session, perhaps too late to pass this time around" (Grow 1995). The bill was referred to the House Committee on Health and Human Services, an identical proposal was introduced in the Senate, and both House and Senate committees would approve the bill 8 days later.[4] After perfunctory floor debate, conducted under suspension of the rules to allow immediate consideration, the proposed mandate was adopted. On June 1, 1995, Governor Arne Carlson signed the mandate into law.

The straightforward language of House File No. 1742, which became the statute, stated:

> Every health plan must provide to each covered person who is a resident of Minnesota coverage for the treatment of breast cancer by high-dose chemotherapy with autologous bone marrow transplantation and for expenses arising from the treatment. The treatment shall not be considered experimental or investigational. Coverage shall not be subject to any greater coinsurance or copayment or deductible than that applicable to any other coverage the health plan provides. (Minnesota 1995, p. 1)

The basic story is deceptively simple: Sympathetic patients with few if any realistic treatment options and little hope for cure were arrayed against an evil, avaricious managed care industry. The story also reveals the limited ability of the political system to cope with complex issues of clinical science. As with most narratives, there is an element of truth to this simple portrayal, but the interview nuances reveal a much more interesting story.

The not-so-behind-the-scenes advocate for the mandate was a Minneapolis attorney, Mike Hatch, who had "regularly gone to court to win the life-saving treatment for his clients" (Grow 1995). Hatch was repeatedly accused of using the HDC/ABMT issue as a platform for seeking political office and of using the media to portray opponents as antiwomen.[5] (He would run for governor, partly on the basis of his advocacy for the procedure, but without success. More recently, he was elected state attorney general.) A "handful of people battling breast cancer" met in his office the morning of the day that Representative Long introduced the proposed mandate. These included Corrine Zweber and her husband, Mark, who were suing Blue Cross Blue Shield of Minnesota for denial of coverage for the procedure. "We've had a [Blue Cross] policy for seven years," she said. "It's got a $2000 deductible, but we said, 'We need the health insurance for that catastrophic situation.' In the 7 years we've had the policy, we never made a claim, but then when we did have the overwhelming need, what happened? They fought us" (Grow 1995). Ruth Erickson, 42, another breast cancer patient, had also been denied coverage for HDC/ABMT by the Minnesota Comprehensive Health Administration, which is administered by Blue Cross Blue Shield of Minnesota.

Litigation preceding the legislative debate had garnered considerable media attention, which usually portrayed the "nasty" insurance industry denying women an opportunity for lifesaving treatment. In the late 1980s, the University of Minnesota and the Mayo Clinic, both major transplant centers, had experimented with HDC/ABMT. Insurers initially denied coverage for the procedure for breast cancer because it was considered experimental and investigational. At that point, the insurers and the two medical institutions agreed to participate in clinical trials (a timetable of 5–7 years was anticipated). Insurers covered the procedure for those enrolled in the trials but refused to pay for off-trial use.

One woman, denied participation in the randomized clinical trial, became the "poster patient" in the legislative debate. Phyllis Anderson, wife of the speaker of the House, had been diagnosed with high-risk (stage II) breast cancer, but her insurer had determined that she was ineligible for the clinical trial and denied her coverage.[6] In a court trial that received considerable media attention, she had sued the insurer and won. As a teacher and wife of an elected representative, she was an ideal candidate for the media, and her case stimulated substantial television coverage. She maintained that "I'd be dead" without the HDC/ABMT procedure and argued that it should be made available to all who could benefit. Her advocacy generated sufficient political momentum that the mandate became virtually unstoppable.

Not surprisingly, once the proposal got to the floor of the legislature, there was little formal opposition. Republicans viewed opposition as a losing proposition. Several legislators who thought the mandate unwise nevertheless regarded opposition to it as political suicide. A vote against the mandate would be interpreted as a vote for the unpopular insurance industry. The Republican governor, Arne Carlson, signed the legislation without voicing an opinion on it. Likewise, his insurance commissioner took no position on the mandate, even though the state insurance department did not require health plans to cover HDC/ABMT as there was no evidence of its effectiveness.

Three factors provide the political context for the mandate. First, Minnesota is a leading state in enacting health benefit coverage mandates, most of which are general, covering, for example, mental health services. The HDC/ABMT procedure, then, was only one of many mandates, albeit the only procedure-specific one. Second, large managed care organizations (MCOs) dominate the Minnesota health care market, and the managed care backlash was beginning to take hold in 1995, making it difficult for the industry to oppose the legislation effectively. Third, the Minnesota political environment then was relatively liberal. Although the governor was a Republican, Democrats dominated both houses.

The Legislative Debate

Crucial to the outcome of most policy debates is how the issues are framed. It might be reassuring to characterize the legislative debate as science versus a woman's choice, which would at least suggest an important role for evidence in the proceedings.

Instead, as in the OPM hearings, the debate was framed as a woman's issue, primarily as a patient's right to choose among various treatments recommended by her physician versus the evil, greedy insurance industry. This characterization put the insurance industry on the defensive from the outset. As one respondent noted, the debate "was positioned as—these women will die. There is no other alternative" (Minnesota 2004). Another characterized the story as "emotion overrode the science" (Minnesota 2004).

The debate was an entirely Minnesota debate—no national experts were directly involved or testified before the legislative committees. Insurers noted, however, that nationally prominent physicians arguing the procedure's potential benefits had led to the mandate. One respondent, for example, called Peters's studies "a shameful display. What failed was that scientists with national reputations in research behaved in unethical ways that gave lie to science to enhance their own remuneration and careers and institutions that turned a blind eye. Human individuals failed, not the science" (Minnesota 2004). The debate was also framed as access to physician-recommended treatment versus cost increases, in which access clearly dominated. The cost of the procedure would become more salient in a later effort to repeal the mandate.

The actual debate was short and dominated by proponents, who used two basic approaches. They first argued that the patient should have the choice of treatments, conventional or HDC/ABMT. Given their view that there was no hope without it, and as patients were likely to die anyway, it would be "mean" to disallow coverage of the treatment, even unethical. As one legislator put it, "Images of women were the debate" (Minnesota 2004). Legislators were more interested in "looking out for the little guy" (as one mandate opponent stated) rather than waiting for the results of the clinical trials. Equally important, mandate proponents consistently attacked the industry as "greedy and self-interested," caring only about money. As some respondents noted, "Insurers sounded evil." Patients were viewed as double victims—first by the disease and then by unsympathetic insurance companies.

In addition, four respected community oncologists testified that they were using the procedure and presented anecdotal evidence of success. "I save lives and use HDC/ABMT every day," said one (Minnesota 2004).These anecdotes played a powerful role in the debate as the legislature was apparently uninterested in broader population-based statistics. William Sage observed (1996) that the courtroom is "the bastion of the identified life" (p. 208). The legislative forum also qualifies. Anecdotal testimony by reputable physicians, including transplanters, made it "hard for legislators to be against doing something" and lent credence to HDC/ABMT as an acceptable procedure. Our respondents generally praised the community oncologists' testimony. Even a legislator opposed to the mandate indicated that "they did not have much of a financial incentive and were taking the patients' interests into consideration" (Minnesota 2004). [7]

The few academic and research physicians who testified against the mandate argued that it was inappropriate given the state of the science. They were unified in arguing that clinical trials were needed, and that the mandate would destroy the ability to conduct the trials. One respondent added that the academics made poor witnesses: "They were arrogant and gave the impression that anyone who disagreed with them is less ethical." The Minnesota Medical Association took no formal position on the mandate. Both the Mayo Clinic and the university were on record saying that clinical trials were needed to determine the procedure's efficacy, and that both were willing to participate in such trials. According to a legislator who tried to marshal the scientific evidence against the mandate, researchers from these institutions provided nothing in writing that could be summarized for other members. With clinical trials ongoing, they were unwilling to comment until the scientific results were clear. According to respondents, no physician from Mayo testified during the debate, and one physician from the University of Minnesota testified that the procedure should only have been offered through clinical trials until effectiveness could be proven. Insurers criticized the medical community for not being more critical of their colleagues' use of HDC/ABMT. The medical community, it seemed to them, had allowed the insurers to be made the scapegoats instead of taking a more forthright position against an unproven and possibly unsafe technology.

Opponents, led by the insurance industry, focused on HDC/ABMT's experimental status. Arguing that coverage was premature, the industry said that clinical trials were necessary to determine whether the procedure was more effective than conventional treatment. The industry also contended that women could very well be worse off with HDC/ABMT because of the high toxicity and some evidence that survival times were longer with conventional therapy. Insurers were also concerned that paying for HDC/ABMT would raise insurance premium costs for everyone and would undermine legitimate cost containment decisions.

The legislators who spoke for the insurers argued that if the procedure were of proven effectiveness, the industry would cover it; it would make no business sense to fight coverage for an effective breast cancer treatment. Most raised this issue in relation to Minnesota managed care: "Minnesota MCOs deliver the care if it works—they don't stop based on cost" (Minnesota 2004). None of the mandate's proponents took the MCOs' profession of good faith at face value.

Finally, the industry argued that it would be unethical to provide HDC/ABMT coverage outside well-designed clinical trials.[8] It argued that most studies showed increased harm from the procedure. One respondent said succinctly: "It would be cruel and unusual punishment to put a stage IV patient through it" (Minnesota 2004). Before paying for it, the industry wanted to be certain that it worked.

The insurance industry was not entirely united, limiting its political ability to oppose the mandate. A major player in the Minnesota managed care market, although opposed to the procedure and the mandate, decided not to oppose the mandate actively. Support for the mandate seemed politically irresistible, and public opposition could only harm the company. Perhaps more important, our respondents consistently said that the industry's presentation was ineffective. One leading insurance industry spokesman said, "If we pay for ABMT, pretty soon you'll want it for ovarian cancer" (Minnesota 2004), a statement not well received by legislators. In addition, the business community, which opposed health care mandates on principle, did not actively oppose this legislation.

Within the legislature, opposition to the mandate existed but did not run entirely along partisan lines. In general, Republican Party legislators oppose mandates and did so in the House committee on this proposal, but we also spoke to Democrats who were similarly opposed. By the time the proposal reached the floor of the respective chambers, however, opposition was no longer practical. Our interviews indicate that the debate was very one-sided. Most opponents simply said that the debate was "not winnable." This pessimism stemmed from the insurers' public image, already battered, and the proponents successful framing of the debate as a woman's issue. Moreover, the issue was raised, debated, and enacted very quickly. According to one legislative opponent, the issue arose so quickly that he never had a chance to organize the opposition, even to lobby his fellow legislators. As a result, there was never any sustained opposition.

From all accounts, the debate was highly emotional. Our respondents portrayed a mixed picture of the role of women's and patient advocacy groups. Some indicated that advocacy groups played a leading role in transforming the debate into a women's issue, but others suggested that these groups were more significant behind the scenes. Advocates arranged for individual patients to present their stories. During legislative hearings, a breast cancer victim was always present, often accompanied by her family. When the floor vote was taken, family members and cancer patients were prominently seated in the gallery. A vote against the mandate became politically risky, especially as the final outcome was clear. Clearly, the women's groups were lined up ahead of time, along with the American Cancer Society, to support the mandate. One respondent recalled that transplantation centers, such as Response Technologies, favored the mandate.

Advocates won the public relations battle handily by portraying the industry as concerned only about money, not about patients. According to one legislator, "No one loses an election bashing insurance companies." Against this, the insurance industry was unable to present its side of the story. Insurance industry respondents complained about inflammatory newspaper headlines and the media's pro-patient bias. In part because it had already lost in court, the industry lacked credibility in opposing the mandate. To the public, the media portrayal featured a woman who had challenged the HDC/ABMT denial in court, had survived, and was effective on camera. The complex nature of the insurance industry's case made an alternative media strategy difficult to develop and present.

Our interviews strongly suggest that science was subordinated, if not altogether ignored, for several reasons. At best, the debate focused on the need for clinical trials rather than the efficacy of the procedure itself.[9] Most respondents indicated that legislators expressed limited interest in the details of the scientific debate. Although the science was mentioned in the House committee hearings, legislators displayed considerable indifference to the data, in contrast to the captivating emotional testimony from affected women. As one legislator put it: "The effort to demonstrate that the data were not in and the fact that the preliminary data were not great didn't cut it in relation to the women's testimony. The average legislator ignores statistics in favor of a kid in a wheelchair" (Minnesota 2004). Conflicting testimony from physicians also raised doubts about relying on the science. Third, legislators are always overwhelmed with information, so it is difficult to get them to evaluate science and statistics. Most are driven by anecdote, especially identifiable individuals. In a debate such as that concerning HDC/ABMT, it is difficult for science to obtain a hearing. Finally, one respondent noted the tendency of legislators to undervalue scientific uncertainty and to give more credence to potential benefits, ignoring the possibility that potential benefits could be offset by higher mortality.

Technology assessment was ineffective in challenging the mandate. Under prior legislation, Minnesota had established the Health Technology Advisory Committee (HTAC) to advise the legislature on the costs and benefits of controversial health care technology. HTAC was advisory only. Its conclusion that additional clinical trials of HDC/ABMT were needed played no apparent role in the debate. Our interviews suggest why HTAC was ineffective: The legislature was too overwhelmed with information to listen; the full HTAC report was unavailable until after the mandate was enacted and then made no recommendations; and there was no link between its findings and legislative decisions. Moreover, either mandate proponents or opponents could use it. Absent a mechanism forcing the legislature to take an HTAC report into account, the emotional nature of this legislative debate virtually ensured that the report would be ignored.[10] Finally, the referral process from HTAC to the legislature would have required an extra session before voting on the legislation, an unacceptable delay. The Minnesota experience is not reassuring about technology assessment as a way to inform the legislative process. That HTAC has now been disbanded marks the legislature's tepid support.

The February 1995 ECRI technology assessment became a side issue in the debate. Opponents of the mandate referred to it, but Hatch and Grow publicly disparaged it. Although ECRI exchanged letters with various public officials regarding how their assessment was being portrayed, neither the organization nor its report played a direct role in the legislative debate.[11]

The Repeal Effort

In 2002, following reports that the HDC/ABMT procedure provided no significant benefit compared to conventional treatment, opponents of the mandate sought its repeal. The legislative sponsor was a woman. Repeal failed, but the debate revealed both some interesting differences from the 1995 debate and how little actually changed. Republicans now controlled the Senate, ensuring that the opposition would have a hearing. More important, increasing health care costs and premium increases meant that the 1995 focus on access without regard to cost would not be repeated. Surprisingly, the Minnesota Medical Association, not normally supportive of managed care, led the repeal effort. It had presumably decided that, on the basis of the evidence, HDC/ABMT was ineffective compared to standard therapy.

Nevertheless, the political calculus did not favor repeal. Health care costs played a more prominent role than earlier but still did not command sufficient attention to favor repeal. The fact that 1999 reports from NCI-sponsored randomized clinical trials showed no benefit also did not favor repeal. One mandate opponent had sent materials critical of the procedure's effectiveness to his colleagues every year after the mandate; no one responded.

Again, the debate was framed as a woman's issue. Repeal was seen as "ganging-up on women." Even though very few women were then receiving HDC/ABMT, respondents on both sides of the issue asked what would be the political benefit in supporting repeal? After all, the same factors that favored the mandate in the first place (i.e., antagonism to managed care and sympathy for breast cancer victims) were still present. Voting for repeal would have little political benefit and considerable potential for antagonizing women's groups. Equally important, one woman elected representative on the committee that conducted the hearing was herself a breast cancer survivor. She made it very clear that supporters of the mandate were prepared to mount an aggressive media and advocacy strategy to retain it.

By all accounts, the repeal hearing was emotional and turned on anecdotes. Despite scientific evidence to the contrary, the committee chair relied on the fact that two of her friends had won HDC/ABMT cases in court and survived. "When women get HDC/ABMT, they survive" (Minnesota 2004). She pointed to unspecified European studies showing some benefit. Supporters of repeal found it difficult to counter her personal statements as a cancer survivor (e.g., "Have you ever had cancer? How can you know?"). Women who had received the procedure testified against repeal, including one with a crying baby. Emotional testimony dominated the proceedings.

In the hearing, insurers, especially managed care providers, were again vilified. The primary argument against repeal was that the patient and the treating physician should make the choice. The mandate's supporters again framed this as a woman's issue, a view reinforced by the fact it was mostly men who testified for repeal.[12]

In the end, repeal was still seen by most legislators as a losing proposition. "Why get involved?" Although a legislator indicated that Republicans were generally prepared to support repeal, he added that an election year was not the right time to push the issue. In the end, the insurers backed off, deciding that they had little to gain by pushing repeal.

Although few, if any, physicians now recommend the procedure, the legislative mandate still stands. As one legislator who opposed the original mandate said about the subsequent repeal effort: "It is hard to move even now because of the industry's public image. If we can't repeal the mandate now, imagine the emotion at the time."

Minnesota Lessons

The 1995 Minnesota legislative session occurred long after many factors had influenced the use of HDC/ABMT for treating breast cancer. The oncology community had sanctioned it as standard of care; Peters had presented data numerous times before his medical colleagues, to state insurance commissions, and elsewhere arguing the superiority of the procedure over conventional treatment; litigation had been under way for over 5 years and the *Fox v. HealthNet,* no. 219692, Superior Court of California, 1993, decision had resulted in an award of $89 million to the plaintiff; more than 10,000 women would have received the procedure nationwide; the federal OPM had required all health plans participating in the FEHBP to cover the procedure; and at least 10 other states had enacted similar mandates.

Under such circumstances, what lessons can be drawn from this case? First, state legislatures may be even less equipped than state and federal courts to weigh issues of access to experimental treatment against the need to evaluate thoroughly a treatment's effectiveness. This is perhaps truer for breast cancer than for many other diseases, given the intensity of emotions surrounding the disease. The argument by opponents of the mandated benefit that the scientific evidence did not yet indicate the superiority of HDC/ABMT was weak. It did not refute the view, expressed by many supporters, that the absence of evidence of effectiveness did not constitute evidence of ineffectiveness. The promise of the treatment, clearly articulated, reinforced hope.

Second, proponents of the mandate controlled the legislature, the framing of the issue as a women's health issue, the timing of the hearings and floor debate, and the media reporting of the issue. They were also heirs to a legacy of mandated health benefits, legislative "fixes" to a beleaguered health care system.

Third, advocacy took many forms and was persuasive. Community oncologists testified in support of the procedure. Patient advocates were present at all critical events, provided compelling human interest stories, and reportedly operated behind the scenes in important ways. The press crusaded for the mandate. One prominent advocate staked his campaign for governor on support for HDC/ABMT

Fourth, the speed with which the mandate debate occurred caught opponents by surprise. Among the opponents, the insurers not only lacked credibility, but also were divided in their willingness to enter the political fray. Those in the medical community who might have resisted the mandate were silent.

Finally, the cost of the HDC/ABMT procedure and its potential impact on insurers' premiums was dismissed quickly in favor of arguments for access to HDC/ABMT in both the 1995 debate and the subsequent repeal effort.

The enactment of the HDC/ABMT coverage mandate in Minnesota was organized, directed, and led by politicians, with advocates playing a supporting role. Emotion dominated science, which is not a new story. As one commentator noted:

> Science may speak in terms of probabilities, but politics does not. The tearful testimony of women with both breast implants and disabling disease, relayed by congressional committees or by television newscaster[s], . . . was understandably captivating to the public and its representatives. Whether it is "Megan's Law" or the Ryan White Care Act, personal experiences are more compelling to politicians and voters than are statistical analyses. (Sage 1996, p. 208)[13]

Mandates: Comparative Lessons

Events in Washington, D.C., in 1994 and the Minnesota statehouse in 1995 provide evidence that initial conditions matter. The fateful branching described in chapters 1 and 2, which was basically complete by 1990, drove subsequent developments for the better part of the decade. They certainly drove events such as these mandates in the mid-1990s. Breast cancer patient advocacy, in its multifaceted manifestations, contributed strongly to the momentum behind mandated benefits. The lack of coverage for HDC/ABMT was a symptom of the same bias that had undervalued breast cancer research.

A critical factor was how the issue was framed. Looking back from our analytical vantage point, we have framed the story as one of access to an experimental procedure versus the need for its evaluation by randomized clinical trials. But at the time, the issue was framed primarily as insurers denying potentially lifesaving treatment for financial reasons. Overlaid on this view was the powerful, even dominant, viewpoint that this was a women's issue, which was reinforced by the emotionally charged nature of breast cancer. In both cases—the Congressional effort to overturn OPM policy and the Minnesota mandate—a feminist interpretation dominated. The key actors were either women or their close allies, including elected officials, their spouses, their local constituents, clinician-researchers and treating physicians, victims of breast cancer and their families, and the press.

The legislative venue is poorly suited to parse conflicts between the intense concerns of individuals and the more distant, abstract issues of clinical science. Legislators are purposeful and approach legislative strategy with an eye to the effective use of time, often the scarcest resource, and to outcomes. So, considerations about scheduling hearings, sponsorship of legislation, choice of witnesses, control of the agenda, and advance preparation of basic arguments all enter the legislator's calculus and receive careful attention. Timing, a key ingredient of legislative strategy, is determined in part by advance preparation: The buildup to the OPM policy change began as early as 1992; that to the Minnesota mandate began with the litigation involving the wife of the House Speaker. By contrast to an often-lengthy run up, legislative action often occurs swiftly, as it did in both instances. Strong bonds of friendship and personal experience often link legislators and those across from them at the hearing table in cases such as breast cancer. Legislators are less suited than judges to parse questions of science, especially those on which experts disagree.

The case for evaluation of HDC/ABMT by rigorous clinical science was clearly secondary in importance, very complex, and inherently weak. Skeptics did argue that it was not known whether the procedure was better than conventional therapy. Clinical trials were needed. The skeptics' argument evoked two responses. First, authoritative voices countered that superiority had been demonstrated in prior research, and although coin-flip trials would be necessary to confirm this definitively, enough was known to move forward. Second, the procedure was the last best hope of those willing to risk it as they had little to lose.

The argument for evaluation was not only an extremely weak one in the legislative arena, but also skeptical clinical researchers spoke for only a segment of medicine. The situation of insurers was even weaker. They were advancing a weak argument, and they lacked the societal legitimacy to speak on behalf of patients or effective medical care. Always vulnerable to the charge of acting in their financial self-interest, few legislators and fewer patients listened to their arguments. Absent entirely in the congressional hearing of OPM, they were peripheral to the debate in Minnesota.

The two case studies highlight how politics can override scientific considerations. In both cases, determinations were made based on emotional arguments without reference to scientific uncertainties. The terrifying nature of breast cancer in young women allowed physicians and patients to frame the debate according to the emotional difficulty of denying a dying woman possibly lifesaving treatment and obscured the lawmakers' ability to see the significance of obtaining clear evidence of clinical effectiveness.

Part III

The Struggle for Evidence-Based Medicine

7

Technology Assessments

As they say in Chicago, we don't shave here. We just lather. You get the shave on the other side of the street.
—Saul Bellow

Technology assessment (TA) emerged in the late 1960s, concerned mainly with anticipating and mitigating the secondary effects of major technological innovations, such as supersonic transport and nuclear power stations. In medicine, TA focused on the clinical and cost-effectiveness of new medical innovations, a result largely of the rapid diffusion of expensive new technologies before the evaluation of their benefit, cost, or cost-effectiveness (Institute of Medicine 1985; Rettig 1991). The "big ticket" items of dialysis and kidney transplantation in the early 1970s, computed tomography in the late 1970s and early 1980s, and magnetic resonance imaging later in the 1980s highlighted the need for such evaluation.

Various initiatives sought to remedy this need. Congress in 1972 established the Office of Technology Assessment, and in 1975 a health program was created within the Office of Technology Assessment (Banta et al. 1981). Also in 1975, consensus development conferences were established within the National Institutes of Health. In 1976, Congress amended the Federal Food Drug and Cosmetic Act and gave the Food and Drug Administration authority to regulate medical devices. In 1978, Congress established the National Center for Health Care Technology (NCHCT) in the U.S. Department of Health, Education, and Welfare. NCHCT's statutory mission was research and evaluation of medical technology, but it was delegated authority to advise Medicare on coverage decisions. As Medicare provided no coverage for outpatient pharmaceuticals, NCHCT focused mainly on coverage of medical devices and procedures. The agency was not equipped politically for this highly charged task.

When the Reagan administration came to office in 1981, the medical device industry prevailed in its opposition to NCHCT: no funds were requested or appropriated for fiscal 1982; the agency expired, and its functions were transferred to the National Center for Health Services Research.[1] The demise of NCHCT revealed the political vulnerability of federal government TA in medicine and prompted advocacy for a public–private entity (Bunker et al. 1982a, 1982b). This led Congress to authorize a Council on Health Care Technology within the Institute of Medicine of the National Academy of Sciences, which functioned from 1986 until the early 1990s.

The weakness of centralized TA was apparent to many. Political support for a quasi-regulatory governmental effort that challenged medical innovation on effectiveness and cost grounds was very weak. By contrast, political opposition to the assessment of a given technology was intense. These halting public efforts stimulated a shift of TA to the private sector, to health insurers that had to decide about coverage of new technologies, often without any clear evidence of medical effectiveness; to medical societies concerned about effective medical care; and to independent organizations (Rettig 1997). The primary concern was to evaluate new medical technologies, including procedures, for evidence of clinical effectiveness. Prominent among the private organizations engaged in TA have been the American Medical Association (AMA), the American College of Physicians, the Blue Cross Blue Shield Association (BCBSA) in conjunction with Kaiser Permanente, Aetna, Prudential, the HMO Group, Group Health Cooperative of Puget Sound, Health Partners of Minnesota, and ECRI of Philadelphia (Rettig 1997).

Technology Assessments of High-Dose Chemotherapy with Autologous Bone Marrow Transplantation

Autologous bone marrow transplantation (ABMT) was evaluated in 1988 by the National Center for Health Services Research. Its report, which focused mainly on the leukemias and lymphomas, said this about solid tumors: "The available evidence suggests that using ABMT for solid tumors, with the exception of neuroblastoma, has not shown meaningful increased survival time" (Handelsman 1988, p. 11). Breast cancer was mentioned only in passing: A second-line study of 36 patients with stage IV breast cancer had found "no meaningful long-term survival." Absent any direct comparison of ABMT with conventional therapies in phase 3 trials, its role in treating most solid tumors continued to be "undefined."

Blue Cross Blue Shield Association

The BCBSA began its TA efforts in 1977 with a Medical Necessity program to identify obsolete medical procedures still widely used but lacking clear supporting evidence of effectiveness and to help member plans determine whether to continue covering such procedures.[2] It added a Technology Evaluation and Coverage (TEC) program in the early 1980s to assist member plans in making coverage decisions about new medical technologies. Until then, the BCBSA had relied on a committee system to generate coverage advice to plans, but this system lacked standardization and documentation about how decisions were made and often based advice merely on surveys of what plans were reimbursing. As the methodology of these two programs converged, they were merged into the single TEC program (Gleeson 1996). During this period, the BCBSA also actively supported the Clinical Efficacy Assessment Project of the American College of Physicians, financed two college publications, *Common Diagnostic Tests: Use and Interpretation* (Sox 1987, 1990) and *Common Screening Tests* (Eddy 1991), and supported the Institute of Medicine's Council on Health Care Technology.

The initial BCBSA TA challenge was to develop a standardized process for generating consistent advice to individual plans to aid coverage decisions and reduce coverage variability among the member plans. Sue Gleeson, head of TEC, asked Dr. David Eddy to develop criteria to help its medical advisory panel formulate advice based on evidence of medical effectiveness (Gleeson 2002). The TEC program did not wish to be in front of the plans, but once these criteria were developed, its TA role changed from support to leadership. It began to act early in the coverage decision process so plans would view it as a resource. It also wished to dampen comparison shopping among plans by those seeking coverage. If a new medical procedure was effective, however, the BCBSA wanted to pay for it and do so quickly. The criteria are listed in table 7.1.

The TA program of the BCBSA was in place and functioning by the mid-1980s. Then, high-dose chemotherapy (HDC) with ABMT for breast cancer hit the fan, and the BCBSA Medical Advisory Panel would review the procedure no fewer than four times between 1988 and 1996. A December 1988 review concluded that ABMT was clearly investigational. HDC/ABMT was reviewed again in November 1990 after an

Table 7.1 Blue Cross and Blue Shield Association Technology Evaluation Center Criteria

The Blue Cross and Blue Shield Association uses the five criteria below to assess whether a technology improves health outcomes such as length of life, quality of life, and functional ability.
1. The technology must have final approval from the appropriate governmental regulatory bodies.
   - This criterion applies to drugs, biological products, devices and any other product or procedure that must have final approval to market from the U.S. Food and Drug Administration or any other federal governmental body with authority to regulate the use of the technology.
   - Any approval that is granted as an interim step in the U.S. Food and Drug Administration's or any other federal governmental body's regulatory process is not sufficient.
   - The indications for which the technology is approved need not be the same as those that Blue Cross and Blue Shield Association's Technology Evaluation Center is evaluating.
2. The scientific evidence must permit conclusions concerning the effect of the technology on health outcomes.
   - The evidence should consist of well-designed and well-conducted investigations published in peer-reviewed journals. The quality of the body of studies and the consistency of the results are considered in evaluating the evidence.
   - The evidence should demonstrate that the technology can measure or alter the physiological changes related to a disease, injury, illness, or condition. In addition, there should be evidence or a convincing argument based on established medical facts that such measurement or alteration affects health outcomes.
   - Opinions and evaluations by national medical associations, consensus panels, or other technology evaluation bodies are evaluated according to the scientific quality of the supporting evidence and rationale.
3. The technology must improve the net health outcome.
   - The technology's beneficial effects on health outcomes should outweigh any harmful effects on health outcomes.
4. The technology must be as beneficial as any established alternatives.
   - The technology should improve the net health outcome as much as, or more than, established alternatives.
5. The improvement must be attainable outside the investigational settings.
   - When used under the usual conditions of medical practice, the technology should be reasonably expected to satisfy TEC Criteria #3 and #4.

Source: Blue Cross Blue Shield Association, Chicago, Illinois. Reprinted by permission from BCBSA Technology Evaluation Center, Technology Evaluation Criteria. Available at http://www.bcbs.com/tec/teccriteria.html

August meeting with its advocates. The BCBSA again concluded that the procedure did not meet its TEC criteria. This conclusion, which was advisory, was transmitted to BCBS plans initially by memorandum and later through publication and dissemination of the updated TEC assessment. Although the BCBSA ceased making coverage recommendations to plans in 1993 when it expanded its Medical Advisory Panel and collaborated with Kaiser Permanente, TEC assessments have remained influential in coverage decisions. David Eddy's 1992 *Journal of Clinical Oncology* article (see chapter 2) reinforced the conclusion that no compelling evidence existed that the health outcomes of HDC/ABMT were better than standard therapy for metastatic breast cancer. Randomized trials were needed.

The third assessment of November 1994 expanded the scope from metastatic breast cancer to include adjuvant therapy for stage II breast cancer with more than 10 nodes involved and stage III breast cancer (Aubry 2002). The treatment again failed to meet the evaluation criteria. Ongoing litigation did not force revision in either the rigorous process or in the conclusion reached by that process. But, as advice from the BCBSA to individual Blues' plans is advisory only, plans were free to act independently. Many chose to leave their policies unchanged but to respond to patient demands by actually covering the procedure.

The BCBSA would not formally consider HDC/ABMT again until early 1996. From the late 1980s, then, through the mid-1990s, the BCBSA policy toward HDC/ABMT for breast cancer rested on three closely related arguments: Existing data did not provide compelling evidence of effectiveness of the procedure and did not satisfy the BCBSA criteria; randomized clinical trials were needed to determine whether the procedure was better than standard therapy; and a demonstration project had been established to provide support for randomized trials sponsored by the National Cancer Institute (NCI).

The challenges of HDC/ABMT to the national BCBSA were also confronting the Blues' plans at the state and regional levels. Wade Aubry, then medical director and senior vice president for medical affairs of Blue Shield of California (BSC) recalls that that the first requests for ABMT coverage were received in late 1988 (Aubry 2002). Initially, they were not recognized as ABMT: some were seen as HDC, some as harvesting of bone marrow, some as a transplant. In mid-1989, requests for ABMT coverage began increasing dramatically. Blue Shield of California received letters from physicians, mostly in southern California, associated with the Kenneth Norris Cancer Center of the University of Southern California, City of Hope, University of California at Los Angeles (UCLA), Stanford, Scripps, and University of California at San Francisco. Most requests were for harvesting; some were for treatment, mostly for patients with metastatic breast cancer and some for poor performers (i.e., women who had failed other treatments).

These initial coverage requests were turned down as investigational, and the decisions were not challenged. Blue Shield of California was challenged in late 1989 through internal grievance procedures but not yet in litigation. Similar challenges were occurring nationally, with some plans being sued, as indicated in chapter 3. In February 1990, the Blue Shield Medical Policy Advisory Committee met in Los Angeles to review the early studies of HDC/ABMT (Aubry 2002).[3] There was evidence of tumor response but a lack of convincing evidence of an effect on the important health outcome of survival. The results showed treatment-related mortality of 20%–25% in nonrandomized trials. Transplanters from UCLA, Kenneth Norris, and City of Hope argued that a dose–response relationship existed, that higher doses of chemotherapy would lead to higher complete response (CR) rates, and that the procedure should be covered. The transplanters were not persuasive, and the committee turned down their request.

Blue Shield would review HDC/ABMT again in November 1991, October 1992, March 1994, and October 1994. Although litigation was occurring across the country (e.g., Blue Cross Blue Shield of Virginia had been sued in the *Pirozzi* case (*Pirozzi v. Blue Cross–Blue Shield of Virginia,* 741 F. Supp. 586 [E.D. Va. 1990].), BSC confronted mostly injunctions against coverage denials, which allowed treatment to go forward. It faced the first jury trial in California, the weeklong *Klopert* case (*Francine Klopert v. Los Angeles Unified School District and California Physicians' Service dba Blue Shield of California,* No. BC 033741, Superior Court, State of California for the County of Los Angeles [1992]), in the summer of 1992 in the Los Angeles Superior Court. Although BSC prevailed, the judge awarded $25,000 to the plaintiff because a utilization review company had erred in preauthorizing the harvest. Notwithstanding increasing pressure to cover HDC/ABMT for breast cancer, Blue Shield's policy remained unchanged.

Early in discussions with advocates for HDC/ABMT, the BCBSA concluded that randomized clinical trials would be necessary to determine whether the procedure was better than conventional therapy. Its TA program gave it both the confidence and competence to pursue this objective. Consequently, the BCBSA spent considerable time in 1990–1991 to design a demonstration project by which its member plans could support phase 3 trials. The key was to avoid challenging the traditional Blue Cross insurance business model. Gleeson (2002) described the development of the demonstration project in this way:

> On a business basis, the Blues could have paid for the HDC/ABMT procedure. It would have been good PR [public relations]. It would have avoided litigation. Patients would have had access to the procedure. The downside was that we would have undermined the technology evaluation process. We would never get the data this way. We would never answer the question. Alternatively, we could have refused to pay. This would have been bad PR, would have encouraged litigation, and would have stimulated mandates. And we would not have gotten data this way either.
>
> So we thought about the HDC/ABMT procedure differently. What do we need? We need data. We need to be part of getting the data, part of the solution. We also had to consider litigation, mandates, public relations, and assistance for the plans. The big thing was to come up with a solution without setting a bad precedent. We still had to make it happen. We came up with the demonstration project, in which we did everything just the opposite of coverage. We went from an abstract discussion to something real. We developed an entire mechanism for the support of clinical trials. We faced a crisis situation, a very immediate challenge, and we were aggressive in taking it on. We created a foundation for funding clinical trials. (Gleeson 2002)

The major differences between the standard coverage process of an individual Blue Cross plan and the BCBSA demonstration project were the following: Payment for patient care costs of participation in randomized trials was made centrally through

Table 7.2 Comparison of standard Blue Cross & BCBSA demonstration coverage

Standard BC plan coverage process	BCBSA demonstration project
Included as part of reimbursement	Excluded from reimbursement
Paid by individual Blue plans	Paid by BCBSA
Paid for the procedure afterward	Prepaid for the procedure
Used existing contracts	Created new contracts
Paid from premiums	Paid from other sources

the BCBSA, not by individual plans; payment was made before the procedure, not afterward; new contracts were developed; and payment was made from sources other than premiums. These differences are indicated in table 7.2. The BCBSA demonstration was designed to achieve two objectives: to provide a mechanism to support the NCI randomized clinical trials to determine whether HDC/ABMT was better than, worse than, or the same as conventional treatment; and to insulate the existing coverage processes of member Blue Cross plans.

American Medical Association

The AMA established the Diagnostic and Therapeutic Technology Assessment (DATTA) program in the early 1980s (Institute of Medicine 1985). This program, in analyzing the clinical effectiveness of new medical technologies, considered the scientific literature but relied mainly on surveys of physicians expert in the clinical issue being evaluated. A designated panel would be asked to rate any given procedure as established, investigational, unacceptable, indeterminate, or no opinion (p. 297).

In early 1990, the DATTA program assessed ABMT (AMA DATTA 1990). The question posed was this: "Are the harvesting, cryopreservation, and reinfusion of autologous bone marrow (A) safe and (B) effective methods for managing posttreatment ([after] chemotherapy or irradiation) bone marrow hypoplasia/aplasia in patients undergoing treatment for cancer?" (p. 881). The assessment focused exclusively on these techniques and on three hematologic cancers: acute lymphocytic leukemia, acute myelogenous leukemia, and lymphoma. Forty-five physicians responded that ABMT was an "appropriate" posttreatment, and an "overwhelming majority" rated ABMT as "established or promising" (AMA DATTA 1990).

The DATTA report did not discuss solid tumors. That did not deter Dr. Elizabeth Brown, the program director, from entering the fray regarding investigational treatments. In late February 1990, she responded to an inquiry from California about "the interpretation of the term investigational" (p. 1) as used by third-party payers, physicians, and patients (Brown 1990). The term was often "the key determinant" of coverage eligibility and, therefore, "of critical importance" to physicians wishing to offer "the most up-to-date treatment" to their patients and to individual patients receiving such treatment (p. 1). Brown's letter delineated clearly the issues at stake between insurers and the medical profession regarding HDC/ABMT:

> This intense focus on the term investigational is problematical, particularly if the term is interpreted rigidly. For example, many third party payors require evidence from well-controlled clinical trials published in peer-reviewed medical literature to

support the non-investigational status of a medical service. This type of interpretation does not recognize the fact that the literature often lags at least one year behind actual clinical practice and that for many medical services these types of controlled studies may never be available. Furthermore, medicine is always in a state of evolution. Constant refinement and investigation move the practice of medicine forward. A rigid interpretation of the term investigational is particularly problematic for gravely ill patients who have very limited treatment options. If a treatment is considered investigational and thus not eligible for coverage by a third party payor, the patient may be denied access to the only available potentially curative treatment option. From the patient's point of view a medical service is not investigational if there is no reasonable alternative. We would encourage third party payors to be flexible in their interpretation of the term investigational, to acknowledge that the medical literature does not always reflect current clinical practice and to recognize the physician's and patient's perspective, particularly in the case of terminal illness, when making a coverage determination. (Brown 1990, p. 1)

The AMA DATTA report that ABMT was safe and effective was limited to hematologic malignancies. When coupled with Brown's widely circulated letter, it gave implied endorsement to HDC/ABMT for breast cancer treatment. It was certainly used this way by plaintiffs' attorneys. It was no small matter that the AMA appeared to be on record supporting the use of this promising new procedure for treating desperately ill women with breast cancer.

Aetna and the Medical Care Ombudsman Program

William McGivney joined Aetna Health Plans in June 1991 as vice president for clinical evaluation and research responsible for conducting TAs to inform Aetna coverage decisions (McGivney 2002). McGivney, trained as a pharmacologist, had directed the AMA DATTA program before Elizabeth Brown. He remembers "some involvement" with ABMT: "We had a breast cancer forum with Martin Abeloff, Karen Antman, William Peters, and I think someone from Nebraska. Ninety insurers showed up, all DATTA subscribers. We [then] did an evaluation of HDC/ABMT and called it 'promising' and added it to the DATTA assessments. DATTA wrote the assessment very carefully. This was not for any indication. ABMT was not the treatment; HDC was the treatment. I took this to Aetna" (McGiviney 2002).

McGivney recalls vividly his Hartford arrival:

I got to Aetna on June 24, 1991, and lived [ABMT] day and night during the entire time I was there. The focus was coverage decisions. ABMT was so important to Aetna. On Wednesday of my first week I met with a Senior Vice President who said that on the following Sunday *60 Minutes* would feature Aetna denying a BMT for testicular cancer. My first week, I dealt with two heart transplants, two liver transplants, and one bone marrow transplant. It didn't let up until I left. (McGivney 2002)

How should Aetna handle "promising" treatments? That was the question with which McGivney wrestled. He had established the promising category while at AMA and had persuaded Aetna to consider "promising investigational technologies" as eligible for coverage of life-threatening diseases. He had three concerns: the cost of the procedure, the absence of outcomes data, and the plight of the individual patient. On cost, he would write the following:

> The high expense of HDCT-ABMT is a major reason for the attention that has been given decisions regarding its clinical application. Charges for the process of bone marrow harvest, high-dose chemotherapy, and bone marrow reinfusion range from $75,000 to $150,000, with most being in the vicinity of the latter. The cost of an individual procedure is magnified by the approximately 1 million new cases of cancer each year, including 135,000 new cases of breast cancer. The potential for high-volume use of HDCT-ABMT is being realized by an expanding list of indications and by the application of HDCT-ABMT earlier in therapeutic regimens. (McGivney 1992a, p. 45)

McGivney was also concerned about the absence of outcomes data indicating whether the procedure was safe and effective: "The debate over the expanded use of HDCT-ABM is only accentuated by lingering and justifiable concerns over whether HDCT-ABMT improves final health outcomes (i.e., survival) in comparison to standard chemotherapeutic regimens" (McGivney 1992a, p. 45). In this regard, he supported very strongly randomized clinical trials as the most effective way to generate definitive outcomes data, but population-based data from clinical trials did not address the dilemma of the individual patient. "Coverage was binary—Go or No Go," McGivney would say. "But patients facing the clinical situation confronted a risk–benefit calculus" (McGivney 2002). How should they balance the risks of an expensive, highly toxic, experimental treatment against the potential benefit of a cure for cancer when standard treatment offered little hope? How should one align these competing views? The "desperate situation of the patient" would create a dilemma for insurers as well. Coverage decisions for highly expensive, investigational treatments such as HDC-ABMT were "among the most difficult decisions to which payers must respond" and were often hampered by the lack of data on safety and effectiveness. Coverage denials generally resulted in adverse decisions by the courts and adverse portrayals of payers by the mass media. Thus, he would write: "Payer denials have often lacked clinical, legal, and societal defensibility" (McGivney 1994a, p. 112).

McGivney spoke to a number of people about this issue. From these discussions came two things: the Aetna terminal illness policy and the Medical Care Ombudsman Program (MCOP). The terminal illness policy dealt with patients having less than a year to live, for whom Aetna was prepared to consider coverage for innovative therapy. "Aetna no longer automatically denies the use of these investigational technologies in terminally ill patients," McGivney said in a 1993 Institute of Medicine workshop (McGivney 1994a, p. 112). If an investigational treatment for terminally ill patient was promising, then it was eligible for coverage. Promising was deliberately defined in a circular way as a treatment that was "effective for that disease or shows promise of being effective for that disease as demonstrated by scientific data" (McGivney 1994a, p. 112). This provided broad latitude to the outside reviewer to determine if a treatment was "effective or likely to be effective." A procedure identified by NCI as worth evaluating in a phase 3 randomized clinical trial also met the definition. Aetna policy, then, rested on a determination by NCI of promising procedure and on the judgment of an outside reviewer about effectiveness. The insurer controlled neither.

The concrete embodiment of this policy was the advice-seeking program that Aetna established in collaboration with Grace Monaco, which would evolve into the MCOP. If an Aetna plan received a coverage request for HDC/ABMT, which the plan's medical director regarded as inappropriate on the grounds that the treatment was experimental, then the individual case would be sent to Hartford before a coverage decision had been made. Aetna would then send the individual's file, including the complete medical record, to the MCOP for review. Three expert physicians would provide their independent judgment of whether the treatment was likely to be effective for the particular patient. Unanimity among the consultants was required to deny a request, but if just one physician favored treatment, that became the Aetna decision (McGivney 2002).

The MCOP developed as a result of a visit by McGivney to Grace Monaco in July 1991. Monaco, a lawyer and a cancer patient advocate, had lost a daughter to leukemia in 1970. She had organized Candlelighters as a volunteer ombudsman organization for parents of children with cancer.[4] In that capacity, she had assembled "a cadre of people in law, medicine, social services, and all the disciplines related to children with cancer. We provided feedback to families regarding protocols, informed consent, etc." (Monaco 2003). McGivney asked her to consider external review of cancer patients. The MCOP became the commercial venture created to administer such reviews (McGivney 1994b).[5] Monaco assembled a panel of physicians, mostly oncologists as cancer treatments were the most contentious, to whom cases would be sent. The initial 20 adult and 30 pediatric oncologists would eventually increase to 300. In addition to Aetna, the clients of the MCOP included Prudential, MetLife, Provident (now Cigna), and Lutheran.

Aetna and other insurers would pay for the reviews, but Monaco picked the reviewers, who would provide "tight and truthful" reviews (Monaco 2003). "We interacted [with HDC/ABMT] continuously," Monaco recalled (2003). "The facts were needed. Insurers became aware of HDC, not just chemotherapy, in the mid-1980s. It was a shock when they discovered it was being billed as standard chemotherapy." Dr. Raymond Weiss, who became a reviewer in 1993, would recall: "The [MCOP] effort was moving strictly due to breast cancer, to ABMT. I got lots of breast cancer cases, about two per week. Most of the time I said that the evidence of effectiveness came from phase 2, uncontrolled studies on highly selected patients, that randomized clinical trials were ongoing, and that we don't know if HDC/ABMT is better or not" (Weiss 2002).

McGivney remembers that Aetna turned down approximately 15% of about 200 cases in the first year alone, evenly divided between ABMT and non-ABMT procedures. Most turndowns were for requests from community hospitals. The procedure was beginning to take off in 1992 and to move to the outpatient community setting, driven by Response Technologies. "They [Response] sent us a significant percent of patient requests for coverage. We turned down the first two cases from a Tampa doctor. Early in the development, our docs [medical directors and MCOP reviewers] were horrified at what they were seeing. We got excoriating reviews [from the MCOP]" (McGivney 2002). In time, the Aetna process would provide the model for state-legislated independent medical review programs for appeal of coverage denials based on medical necessity or experimental/investigational exclusion clauses.

(In California, both the California health maintenance organization [HMO] association and the California Medical Association supported the Aetna model, which became the basis for the Friedman-Knowles Act.) Such programs have now been enacted in more than 40 states and the District of Columbia (Chuang et al. 2004).

In May 1992, Michael Friedman and Mary McCabe of NCI advanced a "modest proposal" for dealing with the patient care costs of oncology research: "All third-party payers of health care (private and public) should cover the clinical care costs (within the financial agreements of policy provisions) but not the research costs associated with patient participation in NCI-sponsored therapeutic clinical trials" (Friedman and McCabe 1992, p. 761–762). This proposal extended the argument about who should pay for oncology clinical research advanced by Wittes in 1987. McGivney, responding in an invited editorial, found the proposal potentially "acceptable" as "a logical and orderly mechanism" for introducing new, expensive medical technologies (McGivney 1992b). Dr. John Cova, representing the Health Insurance Association of America, reiterated the traditional opposition of insurers to coverage of experimental or investigational procedures (Cova 1992).

In both his writings and in Aetna policy, McGivney was searching for an institutional mechanism for obtaining outcomes data on new medical procedures, while simultaneously arguing that exclusive reliance on data from randomized clinical trials "will not suffice" because of the exigencies of patients with life-threatening illnesses. In 1993, he proposed a "national advisory body to oversee evaluative outcomes research on important new technologies" (McGivney 1993, p. 50). The use of these new technologies would be limited to "a network of designated academic health centers." Reimbursement would be provided but restricted to the protocol under study. Outcomes data would be collected and analyzed under the auspices of the independent national body, whose judgment of safe and effective would be required for a technology "to diffuse into practice."

The Institute for Clinical Systems Integration

In the early 1990s, several Minnesota health management organizations (Health Partners, Park Nicollet Health Services, Blue Cross Blue Shield of Minnesota, the Mayo Clinic, and others) sponsored the creation of the Institute for Clinical Systems Integration (ICSI) to generate clinical practice guidelines and conduct TAs. A single page description of the organization's TA reports indicated that the latter were "designed to assist clinicians by providing a scientific assessment, through review and analysis of medical literature, of the safety and efficacy of medical technologies" (ICSI n.d., p. 1). They were not intended as substitutes for a physician's judgment "or to suggest that a given technology is or should be a standard of medical care in any particular case" (ICSI n.d., p. 1).

The ICSI prepared an initial assessment of HDC/ABMT in July 1993, which was published in 1994. It updated this assessment first in July 1996 and again in April 2002. The 1993 assessment described the treatment, the staging of breast cancer, the rationale for high-dose programs, and the treatment process. The efficacy section discussed the importance of growth factors, stem cells, and marrow contamination, and the procedure's application to stage II (high-risk) and to stage IV (metastatic) breast cancer. The discussion of metastatic breast cancer relied heavily on Eddy's 1992 analysis and observed that: "There are no published, randomized controlled trials that compare any outcomes in patients with Stage IV metastatic breast cancer treated with HDC with ABMT versus conventional-dose chemotherapy," although such studies were under way (ICSI 1994, p. 6). The report examined clinical trials with respect to single-agent pilot studies, studies of refractory metastatic breast cancer, untreated metastatic breast cancer, and responding metastatic breast cancer, as well as indications, contraindications, risks and limitations of treatment, and alternative treatments. It concluded that HDC/ABMT was "an investigational procedure." "In the absence of conclusive clinical data," the 14-page report said, "it is not known whether high-dose chemotherapy with autologous stem cell support is more effective than standard therapy for the treatment of breast cancer" (ICSI 1994, p. 1).

The 1994 report also listed cost data for 4 years: 1988–1989, 1989–1990, 1990–1991, and 1991–1992 (ICSI 1994, p. 10). Length of stay fell during this time from 42 to 27.5 days. Total charges (outpatient, inpatient, and physician charges) for each year were $110,770, $110,950, $87,250, and $95,270, respectively. Total costs ranged from $81,945 in 1988–1089 to a low of $62,010 in 1990–1991. Costs per inpatient day for the 4 years were $1233, $1463, $1259, and $1779, respectively.

The ICSI reviewed the experience of several HMO plans around the country. Of 18 plans in the HMO Group, 13 reported that 12 patients had been considered for HDC/ABMT treatment of breast cancer, of whom 7 were approved, 2 were denied, and 3 were pending.[6] In Minnesota, North Western National Life and Aetna covered the procedure on a case-by-case basis, Medica covered the procedure, but Blue Cross and Blue Shield of Minnesota did not. Among the ICSI sponsors, neither MedCenters Health Plans (MHP) nor Group Health, Inc., covered the procedure. The MHP patients denied coverage for stage II breast cancer were participating in one of two randomized clinical studies of HDC/AMBT versus standard-dose chemotherapy; six MHP patients had requested coverage for stage IV breast cancer; all had been denied; five had received ABMT through "alternative mechanisms." An appendix listed the phase 3 NCI clinical trials, as well as institutional research at the Twin Cities Regional Cooperative Bone Marrow Transplant Group, the University of Minnesota, and United Hospital. The 1996 update evaluated more recent clinical literature, including the publication of the South African trial of metastatic breast cancer, and concluded that "the results of these latest studies do not warrant a change in the overall conclusion" of the 1994 report (ICSI 1996, p. 3). The ICSI reiterated that conclusion in 2002.

The ICSI 1994 report preceded both the September 1994 OPM mandate and the June 1995 mandate by the Minnesota legislature. Even so, neither ICSI nor any of its sponsoring organizations, save Blue Cross Blue Shield of Minnesota, played a role in opposing the Minnesota mandate. Its report was not considered in that debate.

The National Comprehensive Cancer Network and Clinical Practice Guidelines

Clinical practice guidelines received national attention in the 1989 legislation authorizing the Agency for Health Care Policy and Research. The agency's sponsorship of guidelines under its own aegis threatened its existence in the mid-1990s and led to the creation of a dozen contract Evidence-based Practice Centers. Many medical specialties later assumed responsibility for guidelines development as a way to distill the continuing flow of scientific literature into useful summaries of what was known and not known. Although not the same as TA, the methodologies of both efforts relied on systematic review of the medical literature.

In oncology, the National Comprehensive Cancer Network (NCCN) led the way in guidelines development, with cancer-specific guidance that is reviewed and updated annually. The American Society of Clinical Oncology (ASCO) is also active in guidelines development (T. J. Smith and Somerfield 1997). In its 1996 breast cancer guidelines, the NCCN concluded "that high-dose therapy with rescue was appropriate only within the confines of an appropriately designed, peer-reviewed prospective clinical trial." It did so for all stages, I–IV (NCCN 1996, pp. 55, 61, 63). The NCCN 1997 guidelines again referred to high-dose chemotherapy three times. In the discussion of stage I, IIA, and IIB breast cancer, the guideline panel considered "dose-intensive chemotherapy . . . for patients at very high risk (i.e., those with 10 or more involved axillary lymph nodes)" but concluded "the data do not yet warrant the inclusion of high-dose therapy with rescue in the guidelines" (NCCN 1997, p. 213). Similarly, for stage III breast cancer, the panel stated that it had reexamined "high-dose chemotherapy with rescue . . . for inclusion in the guidelines" but "the available data do not yet warrant the inclusion of high-dose therapy with rescue in the guidelines" (NCCN 1997, p. 215). Finally, in discussing stage IV breast cancer, it said:

> The panel felt that enrollment of women with metastatic breast cancer into clinical trials of high-dose chemotherapy with bone marrow or peripheral blood stem-cell rescue was especially appropriate. As elsewhere in the guidelines, this recommendation has generated controversy and discussion between the panel and institutional members who are experts in high-dose chemotherapy. . . . The panel fully supports the ongoing randomized trials comparing full-dose with high-dose chemotherapy plus rescue and is prepared to modify this recommendation based on the results of these prospective trials. (NCCN 1997, p. 217)

ECRI

Technology assessment was not solely the province of health insurers, health plans, and government agencies. Independent organizations also evaluate medical innovations. ECRI of Plymouth Meeting, Pennsylvania, a not-for-profit organization, established itself in the 1970s as an engineering and economic evaluator of medical devices and technologies for small and medium-size hospitals that lacked the capacity to perform their own evaluations.[7] In the 1980s, it built a TA capability on the basis of its substantial analytical competence and developed a subscription market for its evaluations among insurers and provider organizations. By continuous monitoring of the scientific literature and interactions with potential clients, it acquires information about which technologies, procedures, and innovations to evaluate.

A distinguishing ECRI belief is that evaluation of medical technologies should be separated from coverage decisions of insurers. Therefore, it has adopted a policy of not making coverage recommendations and restricts itself to evaluating the evidence of effectiveness of medical innovations. It eschews the use of the terminology of experimental and investigational and uses instead the language of harms (or risks), benefits, efficacy, and effectiveness (Lerner 2002).

ECRI concluded in the early 1990s that an evaluation of HDC/ABMT for treating metastatic breast cancer was needed. It issued an initial report in 1993, which was reviewed in *The Lancet* (Triozzi 1994). The report received a "decent response," according to Jeff Lerner, then ECRI vice president for strategic planning and now president. But, reviews led ECRI to conclude that an updated study was needed as clinical use of HDC/ABMT for breast cancer was increasing rapidly and new studies and abstracts were appearing. "It was a moving target," Lerner recalls: "An elusive new subgroup [of patients], a new regimen, was always emerging" (Lerner 2002).

A second ECRI report, written in 1994, received unfavorable reviews from external experts. This led ECRI to adopt an entirely new approach focused on treatment outcomes, which asked whether HDC/ABMT was "better than, worse than, or the same as" standard therapy. Using only studies that reported response rates of 40% or better and 50% or better, ECRI compared HDC/ABMT to conventional-dose chemotherapy for duration of response and disease-free survival rates. This study faced severe data limitations, as did all assessments done in the period. There were no randomized clinical trials; therefore, no meta-analyses of trials could be done. The literature still consisted of reports of phase 1 and 2 studies as it had when Eddy had done his earlier review.

Data was sought from all available sources, including not only peer-reviewed journal articles but also abstracts of studies presented at professional meetings. ECRI used regression analysis in which multiple independent predictor variables were identified (age, estrogen receptor status, etc.) and statistical models of the effect of these variables on patient outcomes were developed. Data from various sources were introduced into these models and correlated with the treatment outcome variables. Lerner described the process in this way:

> We did a series of multiple regressions, 400–500 regressions, comparing HDC to standard chemotherapy. We dumped in every predictor variable we could imagine. We also broke one of our rules: we included abstracts in the literature review. That had never been done before in evidence-based medicine. The problem was that no one would believe us if we excluded the abstracts. We made a policy decision that whatever evidence existed, we would consider it, not just RCT-based evidence. This was radical at the time. We were interested in the "best available" evidence. (Lerner 2002)

ECRI reached five conclusions, summarized in the executive summary. First, there was "no evidence of any prolonged disease-free or overall survival benefit from the use of any reported HDC/ASCR [autologous stem cell rescue] therapies compared with conventional chemotherapy under any circumstances" (ECRI, 1995a, p. 2). Second, patients in typical studies were "more likely to have a shorter disease-free and overall survival time" than if treated conventionally (p. 2). Third, there was "*evidence of harm* [emphasis added] with reported HDC/ASCR therapies for all outcome measures, except the response rate" (p. 2). In this respect, the report differed from other assessments with which it shared the "no benefit" conclusion. Fourth, there was "substantial evidence for decreased median response duration, median survival time, and 1-year overall survival" reported for HDC/ASCR compared to conventional chemotherapies (p. 2). Finally, the literature was "inadequate" in identifying a subset of patients likely to benefit in long-term survival (p. 2).

The report, published in February 1995, was previewed in draft at ECRI's annual conference in November 1994, just 2 months after the controversial OPM mandate had been issued (ECRI 1994). Ron Winslow, in the *Wall Street Journal,* summarized the issues raised by the two events (Winslow 1994, p. A1). After the OPM decision, he noted, 20 plans of United HealthCare had received fax letters requiring them to cover the procedure, giving them 24 hours to reply, and prohibiting them from raising their premiums to cover the cost of this expensive therapy. Winslow quoted Lee Newcomer, medical director at United HealthCare and an oncologist, as saying that more troubling than procedural details was that "the [OPM] decision wasn't based on medical science at all. It was 100% political." HDC/ABMT, he wrote, "has set off a high-profile but hardly unusual confrontation between science and politics over who can get experimental treatments." On the one hand, proponents of access to the procedure had hailed the OPM order as a victory "for patients and academic medical centers seeking reimbursement for experimental treatments." Roy Jones of Colorado was quoted saying: "If insurance companies don't pay for this kind of treatment, we're going to have 1990s health care in the year 2020." On the other hand, critics complained that the OPM order showed what happens "when politics writes medical prescriptions. It encourages dangerous, unproven procedures and undermines efforts to determine whether they really work." The ECRI study reinforced the critics:

> For the average woman with the most advanced form of breast cancer, the high-dose procedure is not only worthless but also likely to shorten her life. Other reports have questioned the effectiveness of ABMT, but the finding that it is likely to harm many women raises tough questions about both its widening use and the federal health-program decision. (Winslow 1994, p. A1)

In Winslow's account, Lerner acknowledged the need for randomized clinical trials but argued that the OPM decision "threatens the progress of those very trials by preventing health-care plans from requiring affected federal employees to participate in the experiments. 'If they offer the technology outside of experimental situations, few people will want to be in the experiments,' Dr. Lerner says. 'That undermines the process of getting to the truth'" (Winslow 1994, p. A1).

The scientific director of the Autologous Bone and Marrow Transplant Registry (ABMTR), Dr. Mary Horowitz, also attended the conference and according to Lerner was impressed with the report. ECRI had arranged previously to obtain a limited set of ABMTR data; this was supplied by September 1994, for which ECRI paid $5,000 (Nugent 1994). ECRI wished to determine whether ABMTR data differed from what it had examined. If ABMTR data showed HDC/ABMT to be substantially better or worse than literature data, then the ECRI analysis might not reflect the current status of research. If the literature data were representative, however, then ECRI expected the majority of the studies it had reviewed to fall within the 95% confidence intervals of ABMTR data. ECRI's analysis found no indication that 1- and 2-year disease-free survival rates in the literature differed from patient outcomes reported to ABMTR, reinforcing its original conclusion that HDC/ABMT was "no better" than conventional therapy (Coates 1995).

ECRI wished to include its analysis of ABMTR data in its report. Vivian Coates, ECRI vice president, sent Horowitz the section of the report dealing with ABMTR data, which had been reviewed internally, indicating that the data would be referred to nowhere else in the report and requesting permission to publish (Coates 1995). In a February 1995 response from Horowitz, ECRI was informed that that the ABMTR board had denied permission to use the data or publish its analysis; the $5,000 was returned (Lerner 2002).

The ECRI report was released in February 1995. The conclusion that the treatment of metastatic breast cancer by HDC was "no better than conventional chemotherapy" was well received by health plans and insurers who remained skeptical of the effectiveness of HDC/ABMT, but it was not well received within the oncology community. ECRI had virtually no profile or reputation within oncology, it was not an academic institution, and it controlled its own review process, both producing and reviewing its own products. Moreover, it sold its reports to subscribers for a high annual fee intended to cover the costs of producing its reports. Subscribers were entitled to four reports each year; nonsubscribers could buy individual reports at prices comparable to what market research firms charge for-profit customers, but that were extraordinarily high for oncologists accustomed to paying for journal subscriptions from research grants or practice revenues. The price to nonsubscribers for the ECRI report was $5,000.

ECRI was a late entrant into the HDC/ABMT controversy. But, as its report became public, it became the focus of some discussion. The report was interjected into the OPM discussions, but only after the Norton hearing and after the OPM had acted. In the Minnesota legislative debate, both Mike Hatch as an advocate and Doug Grow in the *Minneapolis Star Tribune* would criticize the report (Grow 1995). In neither case, however, did the ECRI report affect the diffusion of HDC/ABMT for breast cancer. For that matter, none of the other TAs had any effect. Perhaps ECRI's most important long-term contribution would be a guide that put information about the procedure and its scientific basis into the hands of intelligent women.

Patient Information

Dr. Sheryl Ruzek, an epidemiologist from Temple University, spoke on health insurance in July 1994 at a women's health conference in Chicago, as she was then writing a chapter on the subject for a book on women's health issues. She argued that women health advocates should be paying attention to evidence, partly because she had become alarmed that people were advocating that insurance should pay for everything without regard for evidence. She was also concerned that the World Health Organization's prerequisites to good health were getting short shrift in favor of advanced medical technology. "My talk did not go over well," she recalled (Ruzek 2004). "The sentiment of the hour was that women had been short changed. There was a lot of objection to my talk. [But] Cindy Pearson steadfastly supported me."

Ruzek knew of ECRI's assessment of HDC/ABMT, and that the results did not look good. As a result of the controversy at the conference, Ruzek said later, she called Jeff Lerner from the conference and, on her return to Philadelphia, went to see Lerner and Joel Nobel (then ECRI president). " 'This report will make the front page of the *New York Times* and it will be interpreted as men trying to take things away from women,' she said" (Ruzek 2004). She urged ECRI to share its data and analysis with patients. So, at ECRI's invitation and expense, a select group of women with scientific training and inclinations, including representatives from the National Women's Health Network and the National Breast Cancer Coalition, attended a day and one-half meeting at the organization's suburban Philadelphia facility. Although ECRI was anxious about its outcome, the meeting went "extraordinarily well." "The message was that the report should get out and ECRI should communicate to women," Ruzek said. "The idea for a patient brochure came out of this meeting" (Ruzek 2004).

ECRI decided to pay for such a brochure, which actually became a 45-page patient-oriented guide. It was drafted by an ECRI staff member, Diane Robertson, with input from ECRI analysts and from the women who had came to the meeting. ECRI, accustomed to expert feedback on substance, was now getting feedback on how to communicate with an intended audience. As part of a conscious communication strategy, "the guide was written for the well-educated woman as a way to get information to doctors," Ruzek would recall (Ruzek 2004). "The ECRI patient guide was later criticized as being pitched to too high a literacy level. [But] this was consciously written for a 12th or 13th grade level, for the well-educated patient, for women who are actively engaged in seeking information regarding their medical treatment, and as a way to reach doctors." Lerner would say that the "Patient Reference Guide to HDC/ABMT" was written for two groups of "attentive patients": the highly educated patient and the highly interested patient (Lerner 2002). ECRI distributed the guide free to patients, later putting it on the Internet and thus available at no cost to users. It became one of the few public documents available to women that raised serious questions about the benefit of the HDC/ABMT procedure for treating metastatic breast cancer (ECRI 1995b). In 1996, the patient guide would receive the Rose Kushner Award for breast cancer communication from the American Medical Writers Association.

Conceptually, the audience for the guide was information-seeking women who monitor medical developments closely. "They have been the mainstay of the women's health advocacy movement," Ruzek said. "The whole literacy issue [by contrast] involves putting information into a form at the level appropriate to the audience, usually a 6th or 7th grade level. But writing for a high level of literacy involves the strategic intent of reaching physicians" (Ruzek 2004). Subsequently, ECRI prepared a general patient guide, "Should I Enter a Clinical Trial?" This was financed by the American Association of Health Plans, which had received an unrestricted educational grant from Pfizer (ECRI 2002).

Blue Cross Blue Shield Association Revisits High-Dose Chemotherapy with Autologous Bone Marrow Transplantation

Fox v. HealthNet (No. 219692, Superior Court of California [1993]) altered the legal landscape in 1993. Peters's presentation to ASCO that year, followed by his *Journal of Clinical Oncology* article, powerfully reinforced the clinical momentum behind

HDC/ABMT (Peters et al. 1993). OPM's action in 1994 radically changed the health insurance situation. Events in 1995 would alter the TA landscape. In a Point–Counterpoint argument published in *Important Advances in Oncology* in 1995, Garret Smith and Craig Henderson argued with Bill Peters over the value of HDC/ABMT for breast cancer. Smith and Henderson noted the dichotomy between insurers and HMOs and physicians. The former had conducted extensive reviews of the literature and had concluded that "there is insufficient evidence to consider high-dose chemotherapy and bone marrow transplantation as effective as conventional treatment for either metastatic or early breast cancer" (p. 201). By contrast, a recent survey had revealed that fully 80% of physicians believed that "women with metastatic disease should be treated with a bone marrow transplant despite inconclusive evidence that this approach is superior to standard chemotherapy" (p. 291). Although the article reviewed carefully the literature related to both metastatic and high-risk breast cancer, the authors wasted no time in stating the issues:

> ABMT has generated an intense medical-legal debate centered on the expense of a procedure of unproven benefit and the controversy regarding third-party insurance coverage for investigational treatments. The resulting media attention has further augmented public expectations of this procedure. Medical researchers have continued to generate significant enthusiasm for HDC/ABMT in the absence of data to support their claims. Moreover, the popularity of HDC/ABMT has hindered patient enrollment in properly controlled trials comparing ABMT to standard chemotherapy. According to the North American Autologous Bone Marrow Transplant Registry, despite a dramatic increase in the number of transplants performed each year for women with breast cancer, the vast majority are not components of controlled clinical trials. Only the results of such randomized trials will determine if ABMT is truly a reasonable treatment for women with metastatic disease, or if HDC/ABMT is an appropriate strategy for women in the high-risk adjuvant setting. (G. A. Smith and Henderson 1995, pp. 201–202)

Smith and Henderson had concluded by dividing "current medical opinion" into optimists and pessimists, listing David Eddy as a pessimist, but categorizing Bill Peters and Karen Antman in both categories—supporting randomized clinical trials but fully expecting those trials to confirm the effectiveness of HDC/ABMT.

Writing in the affirmative, Peters observed that breast cancer was now the most common disease for which HDC/ABMT was performed (Peters 1995). Over 900 patients had been registered with the ABMTR in 1993. Increasingly, the procedure was being used in the high-risk setting. Toxicity had rapidly decreased, and "in experienced hands, with the use of colony-stimulating-factor-primed peripheral blood progenitor cells, the acute mortality of the treatment is less than 3–5%, and in some centers, the procedure is largely performed as an outpatient procedure with average lengths of inpatient hospitalization as low as 5 days" (Peters 1995, p. 215). Insurers were facing large overall expenditures for the procedure, notwithstanding the rapid decrease in charges for a given treatment. However, "[a]rbitrary and capricious denial of insurance coverage for some patients has resulted in litigation, sometimes with enormous punitive damages." Randomized, comparative trials were under way, but results would not be reported for 3 to 4 years. "In the absence of prospective randomized data to rely on," Peters declared, "numerous reviews have been published presenting very different views, some based on hypothesis, and little data" (p. 215).

Standing the argument on its head, Peters claimed that the absence of data of effectiveness provided no basis for concluding that the treatment was ineffective. In the meantime, patients should be referred to centers conducting such trials.

Peters laid out the by-now-familiar rationale for HDC/ABMT, reviewed the development of the procedure, addressed "the importance" of randomized clinical trials, characterized the various data sources of HDC, and reviewed the data. He reported on a survey of 37 centers conducted to answer some of the many questions about the effectiveness of HDC/ABMT. For 1106 patients with metastatic breast cancer receiving induction therapy and then HDC as a primary treatment, overall survival was 37%; for "controls" based on historical comparisons, it was 20% or lower (Peters 1995). Peters concluded by enumerating the issues facing BMT for breast cancer: randomized clinical trials; bone marrow purging; patients with bone involvement; long-term effects of HDC; repetitive high-dose therapy; and improvements in supportive care in the outpatient setting.

In May 1995, at the annual meeting of the ASCO, Peters and colleagues presented two abstracts related to HDC/ABMT involving women with high-risk of breast cancer (i.e., having 10 or more positive lymph nodes). One addressed the "bone marrow micrometastases" (i.e., the small numbers of breast cancer cells that would predispose patient relapse) (Vredenburgh et al. 1995). The significance of contaminating tumor cells was unknown; "characteristics of the tumor" appeared more predictive of relapse and survival. The more significant report was a Duke University study (CALGB 8782) of 85 patients with 10 or more nodes positive (Peters et al. 1995). Through June 1994, 5-year follow-up data showed the median age was 38 years; median number of positive lymph nodes was 14; and treatment-related mortality was 12%. The abstract concluded that high-dose consolidation treatment "was feasible" and indicated that a prospective, randomized trial was under way evaluating the procedure, which "must provide the primary basis for evaluating the value of ABMT" (Peters et al. 1995). Peters made clear his belief that the trial would demonstrate the superiority of HDC/ABMT over conventional-dose chemotherapy.

The major event of 1995, however, was not the ASCO meeting but the publication of a South African randomized clinical trial of HDC/ABMT in the prestigious *Journal of Clinical Oncology* in October (Bezwoda et al. 1995). Werner R. Bezwoda, the most prominent South African oncologist, reported the results of a trial comparing high-dose versus conventional-dose chemotherapy as a first-line treatment of metastatic breast cancer. Ninety patients had been randomized to either two cycles of a high-dose regimen of cyclophosphamide, mitoxantrone, and etoposide (HD-CNV) or to six to eight cycles of conventional-dose cyclosphosphamide, mitoxantrone, and vincristine (CNV). The response rates were "significantly different": Overall response was 95% for HD-CNV compared to 53% for CNV alone; CR was 51% for high dose compared to 4% for conventional dose (2 of 45 patients). Both duration of response and duration of survival were significantly longer for patients receiving the high dose, and toxicity was "moderate" for most. The report concluded, "HD-CNV appears to be a promising schedule that results in a significant proportion of CRs and increased survival with metastatic breast cancer" (p. 2483).

Dr. M. John Kennedy of the Johns Hopkins Oncology Center responded in a 1995 editorial, "High-dose Chemotherapy of Breast Cancer: Is the Question Answered?"

To him, it was, although not without some qualifications. Controversy over the procedure, he wrote, "has been fueled by the absence of data from randomized clinical trials" (p. 2477). He noted that the study was "not a pure study of the dose question," either of dose intensity or total dose, as the two regimens "did not contain identical drugs given at different doses." "Nevertheless," he continued, "this study is an important test of a practical question: is it better to give brief intensive therapy with stem-cell infusions or more chronic therapy with doses of similar drugs that do not require such support?" Kennedy acknowledged the "dangers of drawing firm conclusions" from small, randomized trials, and asked if there was "a biologically plausible explanation for the observed results." He concluded that the differences in the doses of cyclophosphamide and mitoxantrone were "comparable" to prior studies of conventional-dose treatment that suggested a dose–response effect on outcome.

One possible interpretation of prior studies was that of a "shoulder": inadequate doses (too low) would result in a poor outcome, but once an adequate dose was achieved, dose intensification would not improve outcomes. He noted that the poor results of the "conventional" dose arm in Bezwoda's trial might be due to doses that "we [U.S. investigators] would now consider inadequate." Notwithstanding this possibility, "we can say the results for both the high-dose and standard-dose arms are consistent with published experience and are believable" (Kennedy 1995, p. 2478). The high-dose results were "excellent" and "well tolerated," and Bezwoda and colleagues were to be commended for a study with results that were "provocative and encouraging." "It is probably fair to say there is a qualitative superiority to the high-dose regimen," Kennedy concluded (p. 2479).

Although the BCBSA had reviewed the evidence about HDC/ABMT effectiveness for breast cancer on three prior occasions, it felt compelled to reexamine the procedure. The implications of the 1995 ASCO report by Peters, the results of the South African trial, and recent data from the ABMTR showing decreased mortality could not be ignored. The question before the BCBSA Medical Advisory Panel in late February 1996 was this: Did the new data meet the criteria (see table 7.1) that would support a recommendation that coverage of HDC/ABMT was justified? Peters, who had left Duke to head the Karmanos Institute at Wayne State University, presented "new evidence" showing that the procedure was at least as good as conventional treatment for disease-free survival. Roger Dansey, formerly a colleague of Bezwoda's (and coauthor of Bezwoda's 1995 paper) but by then in Detroit with Peters, presented the results of the South African trial. Mary Horowitz presented ABMTR data showing that treatment-related mortality had declined from 20%–25% to 5%, due mainly to the use of human growth factor (BCBSA 2002).

Henderson recalled the discussion beginning at 10 A.M. and continuing until after lunch. "If we had voted before Bill Peters made his presentation, I think it would have been unanimous [in favor of change]. But Peters antagonized practically everyone" (Henderson 2002). The discussion seesawed back and forth for several hours. Peters's data and those of the registry suggested benefit but were not conclusive. But now, a randomized clinical trial had reported significant benefit in the premier oncology journal. The conventional arm of the South African trial was weaker than standard therapy common in the United States, so the advantage of the experimental arm might not be so compelling against the stronger standard treatment common in this county.

Finally, Wade Aubry, chair of the medical advisory panel, called for the vote on whether compelling evidence now existed that the HDC/ABMT procedure was better than standard therapy for treating metastatic breast cancer. Although the BCBSA TEC does not record individual votes (or the total number voting for, against, or abstaining) in the minutes, it was widely known that the methodologists on the panel voted against changing the policy; that Henderson, voting last, voted to change; and that Aubry, as chair, did not vote. By one vote, a majority decided to change the policy.

Then came the task of justifying and explaining why BCBSA changed its views on HDC/ABMT for breast cancer treatment. It did so in February 29 press release, to which was attached a 7-page question-and-answer document from which the following excerpt is taken (BCBSA 1996, attachment, pp. 1–7):

Why has TEC decided to re-evaluate high-dose chemotherapy with BMT at this time?

Two recently completed randomized controlled trials have provided new evidence on the risks and benefits of this therapy for women with metastatic breast cancer. These trials provide data on survival up to 5 years after treatment.

Do these studies show that high-dose chemotherapy with BMT is better than conventional chemotherapy for women who have metastatic breast cancer?

No. This evidence does not demonstrate that **high-dose chemotherapy with BMT** [emphasis in original] is the superior treatment?

The first study, which is from South Africa, showed longer survival for women given one specific regimen of **high-dose chemotherapy with BMT** than for women given conventional dosage of a similar (but not identical) regimen. But survival after treatment with **high-dose chemotherapy with BMT** in this study was no longer than survival usually observed with conventional-dose chemotherapy in this country; and survival for the patients treated with the conventional dose regimen was worse than for most U.S. patients treated with conventional dose chemotherapy. So there is concern that the results of this study do not apply to patients treated with the best conventional-dose therapy used in the United States. Clinical investigators have also published other criticisms of this study.

The second study, from the Duke University Medical Center, studied whether **high-dose chemotherapy with BMT** is best used for first treatment of metastatic breast cancer or reserved for women who have a recurrence after conventional treatment with chemotherapy. This study is interesting, and somewhat surprising, because the results available so far suggest that it is better to save **high-dose chemotherapy with BMT** for a later course of treatment. Patients who had **high-dose chemotherapy with BMT** as their first treatment for metastatic breast cancer had a longer interval until their cancer recurred than did patients who had conventional dose therapy as first treatment. But the patients who had **high-dose chemotherapy with BMT** after their cancer recurred actually lived longer than the patients who had it as first treatment. This study, while encouraging, does not demonstrate that **high-dose chemotherapy with BMT** is a better treatment option than conventional chemotherapy.

Another important point is that mortality from **high-dose chemotherapy with BMT** treatment is now much lower than it used to be and is approaching that of conventional-dose therapy. [This] is demonstrated in the Duke University and South African studies as well as by data from the Autologous Blood and Marrow Registry of North America.

What is the new position of TEC on high-dose chemotherapy with BMT for breast cancer?

Based on the available evidence, the BCBSA Medical Advisory Panel made the judgment that **high-dose chemotherapy with BMT** in the treatment of breast cancer meets the TEC criteria [emphasis added] when administered . . .

- As first treatment after diagnosis of metastatic breast cancer; or
- As first treatment for metastatic breast cancer that has recurred after a period of complete remission.

Does this mean that high-dose chemotherapy with BMT is appropriate for all women with breast cancer?

No. The new position of TEC applies only to specific cases of metastatic disease. And the women in these trials were relatively young and healthy. . . . The clinical trials that address the effectiveness of **high-dose chemotherapy with BMT** compared to conventional treatment in women with earlier stage breast cancer are underway. . . . To date, results of **high-dose chemotherapy with BMT** for women who have refractory breast cancer (cancer that does not respond to conventional treatment) are discouraging.

How soon can Blue Cross and Blue Shield Plans respond to this change in policy?

The Blue Cross and Blue Shield Plans are independent companies and reach coverage decisions independently of other Plans and BCBSA. . . .

What do you say to women who have not had access to this treatment in the past?

Women who had conventional dose chemotherapy should be reassured. The evidence does not demonstrate that **high-dose chemotherapy with BMT** is superior to conventional-dose chemotherapy. . . .

Can any hospital effectively provide this treatment?

High-dose chemotherapy with BMT is a complex and risky therapy. Therefore, it is important that only properly selected patients are offered **high-dose chemotherapy with BMT** and that these patients are treated at centers with extensive experience and a track record of good outcomes.

Should we continue to support clinical trials of high-dose chemotherapy with BMT for breast cancer? Why are such trials important?

Many questions remain unanswered regarding the optimal use of **high-dose chemotherapy with BMT** as a treatment for breast cancer. . . .

Why should patients still participate in clinical trials?

There are two reasons for participating in clinical trials. The first benefits the patient participating in the trial and the second benefits all patients.

- Many oncologist believe that clinical trials offer the best available care. Clinical trials also offer patients the best opportunity to exercise informed consent. There is still much uncertainty as to how to treat breast cancer. In a trial, women are provided the most complete and balance information on the risks and benefits of the options available to them.
- Patients who participate in trials not only benefit themselves, but also benefit others by improving knowledge of the best ways of treating breast cancer. . . .

What does the patient need to know to make an informed decision about high-dose chemotherapy with BMT?

Each patient needs complete information so that she can choose the treatment option that is best for her. . . . When considering **high-dose chemotherapy with BMT**, it is important to keep the following points in mind.

- **High-dose chemotherapy with BMT** has not been proven to be superior to conventional chemotherapy. . . .
- **High-dose chemotherapy with BMT** is simply not appropriate for some women. . . .
- Women choosing **high-dose chemotherapy with BMT** should be treated at experienced centers that have a track record of good therapeutic outcomes and low treatment-related mortality. . . .

What are the implications of the change in the TEC position on high-dose chemotherapy with BMT on the NCI randomized trials?
The NCI states that the NCI-sponsored randomized trials . . . will remain open. . . . The NCI feels that the results of the randomized trials reviewed as part of the TEC re-evaluation did not definitively establish that either approach is superior to the other for metastatic breast cancer. Clinical trials are needed to determine who can benefit from **high-dose chemotherapy with BMT**. The BCBSA continues to support randomized **trials of high-dose chemotherapy with BMT** through the Demonstration Project on Breast Cancer Treatment. (Reprinted with permission from Blue Cross Blue Shield Association Technology Evaluation Center. All rights reserved.)

The carefully nuanced BCBSA position that HDC "meets the TEC criteria" and simultaneously "has not been proven to be superior" to conventional therapy was not interpreted in a nuanced way. Peters was quoted in *The Cancer Letter* both supporting and criticizing it: "The recommendation says that [Blue Cross and Blue Shield plans] can cover it for patients with metastatic breast cancer, but for patients who are enrolled in clinical trials for primary breast cancer, they are still not covering it. And that's where the biggest benefit is most likely to be seen" (Cancer Letter, 1996, p. 5). The NCCN guidelines developers were quite aware of the BCBSA policy change but nevertheless concluded that the evidence still did not support a judgment of effectiveness (NCCN 1996). The 1996 ICSI update review concluded that "the results of these latest studies do not warrant a change in the overall conclusion" of its 1993 study (ICSI 1996). Fran Visco recalled that she and her colleagues in the National Breast Cancer Coalition found Henderson's vote "very disappointing." "We were stunned," she said (Visco 2004).

California

An indication of how the intertwined forces of politics, TA, independent medical review, and the women's health movement came together is provided by an episode that occurred in California in the early 1990s. Several years of interactions had taken place between the staff of the California Public Employees' Retirement System (CalPERS) and participating health plans regarding HDC/ABMT as a treatment for breast cancer. In 1996, the California State controller, Kathleen Connell, a statewide elected official with aspirations to be governor, proposed that CalPERS-participating health plans be prohibited from excluding HDC/ABMT for breast cancer, that they not be allowed to deny coverage on the grounds that the procedure was experimental, and that coverage not be limited to randomized clinical trials. Blue Shield of California, which had administered the self-funded preferred provider organization (PPO) option for CalPERS since 1989, had by this time formally evaluated the procedure four times and found the procedure to be investigational. The PPO plan administered by Blue Shield had also decided to participate in the NCI randomized trials comparing HDC/ABMT with conventional-dose chemotherapy and had initiated its own "pilot project" for nonrandomized phase 2 studies at four major California transplant centers for patients who were ineligible or unwilling to participate in the NCI trials.

The controller's proposal was sent to the California Women's Health Council in early March 1996, where it was proposed that the Council endorse it as an insurable item by CalPERS. Jane Sprague Zones, a member of the council and a medical sociologist who chaired the board of the National Women's Health Network and cochaired its breast cancer committee, argued successfully against such an endorsement (Zones 2004). Following that meeting, Zones wrote the controller on March 13, 1996, on network letterhead stationery, a letter (to which she received no response) explaining her action:

> My opposition to insuring ABMT/HDC outside of clinical trials is because this very harsh treatment has not been demonstrated to be more beneficial than conventional chemotherapy, and there is some evidence that it may actually be less effective. It is possible that increasing access to ABMT/HDC for women with breast cancer may prove to be harmful to the people we want so much to help. Research information on ABMT/HDC's safety and effectiveness is not well established. Only in the past few months, the first randomized clinical trial report was published. This study, though it found ABMT/HDC to be superior to conventional chemotherapy, reported results from the conventional treatment arm that were significantly worse than comparable treatments in other studies. (Zones 1996, p. 1)

Substantial pressure in addition to that brought by the controller was being exerted on CALPERS to cover the HDC/ABMT procedure. The CALPERS Health Benefits Committee originally discussed the issue at its meeting on February 21, 1996 (CalPERS 1996a), but held the issue over to the March meeting (CalPERS 1996b). The February meeting had reviewed Blue Shield of California's TA procedures and its coverage policies for bone marrow transplants, as it administered claims for the self-funded PPO health plans PERSCare and PERSChoice. That information document had reviewed the process by which the Medical Policy Committee of Blue Shield reviewed investigational procedures, the five criteria used in evaluation, the status of BMT, and Blue Shield's participation in a pilot project to evaluate the procedure at Stanford, UCLA, University of California at San Francisco, and City of Hope. It indicated that HDC/ABMT had been approved by Blue Shield of California for neuroblastoma, glioblastoma, multiple myeloma, testicular germ cell carcinoma, leukemia, lymphoma, and Hodgkin's disease, but that its use was considered investigational for "stage IV metastatic breast cancer and stage II-III breast carcinoma with 10 or more involved axillary lymph nodes" (CalPERS 1996a, p. 3).

Out of the March meeting, which was also informational, came a CalPERS Health Plan Administration Division recommendation presented at the April 16 meeting that all participating health plans establish independent medical review on an expedited basis, that they notify CalPERS at the end of their internal dispute process, that CalPERS conduct an expedited review of appeals, that all plans provide care at Centers of Excellence "within reasonable travel distance for the patient," that all plans be notified of the CalPERS expedited review process, and that all plans that previously did not cover the procedure "notify plan physicians and members of the availability of treatment coverage if needed" (CalPERS 1996c, p. 1).

The CalPERS division contrasted its recommendation with that of the state controller. The latter, as indicated, had recommended that health plans be prohibited from excluding HDC/ABMT for breast cancer, that the plans not be allowed to deny coverage on the grounds that the procedure was experimental, and that coverage not be limited to randomized clinical trials. In response, the division recommended that ABMT not be excluded on the basis that it was experimental, but that the procedure for breast cancer be evaluated "on a case by case basis to determine medical appropriateness"; that plans not limit coverage to clinical trials; and the language of self-insured plans be revised to "remove HDC/ABMT exclusions" (CalPERS 1996c Attachment 4, p. 1).

Although the CalPERS recommendation yielded to the controller's at several points, the heart of it lay in the recommendation for independent medical review. It did so because it lacked competence to make medical decisions. In essence, it copied the Aetna policy of several years earlier. If a health plan denied a given patient, then the case would be sent to three reviewers for independent review. If one or more reviewers approved treatment, then CalPERS would approve. If all three denied, then the patient would be informed of the denial. She would also be informed of the availability of expedited review by the CalPERS-authorized Blue Shield process and could then either accept the denial or appeal.

Summary

By the early 1990s, then, the health insurance industry had responded to HDC/ABMT by initiating TAs based on careful reviews of the scientific literature. These assessments failed to support claims of effectiveness. The BCBSA had established a demonstration project for supporting NCI-designated clinical trials. Aetna had laid the basis for independent medical review through support of MCOP. In addition, ECRI, an independent, nonprofit TA organization, had conducted its own assessment that concluded no benefit and potential harm. Perhaps as important, ECRI had published a patient information guide to inform women of ECRI's findings about the procedure, the first publicly available document questioning HDC/ABMT directed to information-seeking women.

All assessments had concluded that existing data failed to support claims of HDC/ABMT effectiveness compared to conventional therapy. All had argued the imperative of randomized clinical trials as the way to obtain such data. Then, in 1996, the BCBSA demonstrated the dependence of TAs on randomized trials. The BCBSA Medical Advisory Panel reviewed the favorable results of a South African randomized trial and concluded that HDC/ABMT for metastatic breast cancer was no worse than conventional chemotherapy. The defensive line of prior TAs had been breached.

The decisive turn of events, however, would occur only in May 1999 at the annual meeting of ASCO. Four trials, including the Philadelphia trial of the use of HDC/ABMT for treating metastatic breast cancer and Peters's trial (CALGB 9082) for high-risk patients, would report no significant difference between the experimental treatment and the control arms. In this controversy would be the reports from the phase 3 randomized clinical trials. Even then, a second Bezwoda trial from South Africa would report dramatic benefit. We turn in chapter 8 to those trials and in chapter 9 to the audits of the South African trials.

8

Clinical Trials

Glen. I can call spirits from the vasty deep.
Hot. Why, so can I, or so can any man. But will they come when you do
call for them?
—William Shakespeare

There are diseases and clinical situations in which randomized, controlled trials
are not necessary or are unrealistic. However, the treatment of breast cancer is
not one of them.
—I. C. Henderson

During most of the 1990s, insufficient evidence existed to support claims that high-
dose chemotherapy with autologous bone marrow transplantation (HDC/ABMT)
was superior to conventional treatment for patients with either metastatic or high-
risk breast cancer. The evidence that did exist came from single-site, phase 2 studies
involving small numbers of highly selected patients compared to historical or no
controls. Decisive evidence about the effectiveness of the procedure required data
from phase 3 randomized clinical trials. In contrast to the rapid diffusion of
HDC/ABMT in the 1990s described in previous chapters, the evaluation of the procedure in randomized trials required a long, slow process of accruing sufficient numbers of patients, conducting the trials, following up patients over an adequate period,
analyzing the data, and reporting results. When, in 1999, the trials reported "no benefit," the news would come like a thunderclap.

The accrual of patients to HDC/ABMT trials was severely complicated by the
widespread availability of the procedure outside such trials. Many factors drove diffusion. The oncology establishment legitimated the procedure very early in the
1990s. Breast cancer patients often saw the treatment as their last best hope. They
tended to defer to their physicians, who often believed that the experimental treatment was superior or who regarded the preferences of individual women as out-
weighing any ambivalence they might have about its effectiveness. In the rare
instances of being offered opportunity to participate in a clinical trial, women often
declined, fearing randomization to standard treatment that was generally considered
inferior. Health insurers, reluctant to pay for investigational or experimental procedures, frequently aided rapid diffusion by provoking strong negative reactions to
coverage denials, at least until litigation made that option unattractive. Plaintiffs'
lawyers obtained some highly visible, even stunning, reversals of coverage denials

before judges and juries. Courts typically dismissed scientific evidence in deciding cases by parsing contract language, scrutinizing insurers' procedures, and highlighting the plight of patients. Entrepreneurial oncology developed the "market" for the procedure. Federal and state government mandates required that HDC/ABMT be covered as a benefit without evidence of treatment effectiveness.

This clinical utilization pathway was the strong arm of a natural experiment that would hamper the clinical evaluation pathway. However, a small cadre of skeptical physician-researchers insisted that the hypothesis emerging from phase 2 clinical studies (that HDC/ABMT was superior to standard chemotherapy for metastatic and high-risk breast cancer) be tested in multisite phase 3 trials. Randomized clinical trials were essential, they believed, because of the high variability in the disease, the wide range of patient responses to treatment, and the uncertain relationship between tumor response and survival benefit. These skeptics could not be ignored forever. Oncology had witnessed too many doctrinal conflicts about effective treatment that were resolved eventually only by rigorous clinical research (Henderson and Canellos 1980a, 1980b; Lerner 2001). Some transplanters, however, believed that clinical trials would confirm what they already knew, or thought they knew, namely, that HDC/ABMT was superior to conventional treatment. The National Cancer Institute (NCI) would place its "high priority" imprimatur on the clinical trials but defined the issues narrowly as scientific. Some insurers and health plans financed trials and pioneered new mechanisms for doing so, differing sharply from those that simply denied coverage or acceded to patient demands. By 2001, in the United States an estimated 23,000 to 35,000–40,000 women had received HDC/ABMT treatment for breast cancer. In the same period in the United States, only 1000 had received the experimental procedure within an NCI-approved clinical trial that had reported results.

Getting Started

In January 1989, Bruce Cheson, Robert Wittes, and colleagues reviewed 160 studies of HDC/ABMT published between 1978 and May 1988, including studies of both hematologic malignancies and solid tumors. ABMT had developed "at a remarkably slow pace," they wrote, and concluded that outcomes could be improved "through systematically developed, carefully designed clinical trials" (Cheson et al. 1989, p. 59). "For more rapid progress," they said, attention should focus on tumors "for which adequate numbers of patients permit completion of a trial in a reasonable time period" (p. 59). Most trials had been done at single centers with limited numbers of patients, but collaboration among centers would be essential in the "eventual Phase III trials" (p. 59). The review noted the "encouraging results" of phase 2 studies for various solid tumors, for which ABMT "results in response rates that are probably superior to the best available results with conventional therapies in comparable patient groups, although not yet associated with improved survival in most diseases" (p. 61). A single paragraph on breast cancer noted that interest in ABMT was "relatively recent," and that "more extensive evaluation of combination chemotherapy regimens seems warranted" (pp. 56–57). The review showed little awareness that breast cancer treatment by HDC/ABMT would soon explode into wider clinical use in ways that would complicate the conduct of clinical trials.

Within a year, however, the NCI would commit itself to sponsor phase 3 randomized trials of HDC/ABMT for breast cancer, an outgrowth of discussions with investigators, health insurers, and the NCI. A critical meeting, convened by the Blue Cross Blue Shield Association (BCBSA), took place in August 1990 at the Chicago O'Hare Hilton, as discussed in chapter 2, where David Eddy argued strongly for a randomized trial (Aubry 2002; BCBSA 2002; C. Henderson 2002). According to participants, Michael Friedman, who had followed Wittes as head of the Cancer Treatment Evaluation Program, indicated that the NCI was willing to sponsor such trials and to collaborate with the BCBSA (Aubry 2002). This agreement was a critical turning point, the beginning of collaboration among the researchers and between researchers and insurers.

It took a year to get the breast cancer trials off the ground. In late 1990, Friedman discussed with the National Cancer Advisory Board the decision "to test whether the expensive and arduous treatment [HDC/ABMT for breast cancer] is cost effective and to better define which patients it would most benefit" (*Clinical Cancer Letter* 1991a, p. 5). "Does it work, for which patients, and at what cost?" were the questions that the studies were intended to answer. The proposed study of patients with stage II breast cancer (poor prognosis, node positive) would randomize patients to the best conventional treatment or to conventional plus ABMT. Patients with metastatic breast cancer would receive conventional therapy and then be randomized to further conventional therapy or ABMT. Endpoints would include survival, disease-free survival, short-term costs, quality of life, and long-term economics. Necessarily, this decision had involved discussions between the NCI and the oncology cooperative groups, especially Cancer and Leukemia Group B (CALGB), the Eastern Cooperative Oncology Group (ECOG), and the Southwest Oncology Group (SWOG). A major concern was reimbursement for the procedure, but breast cancer patients had been successful, Friedman noted, in forcing insurers to pay for the experimental treatment.

The 1990 NCI decision would be sealed in June 1991. The Forum on Emerging Treatments for Breast Cancer was convened at the National Institutes of Health (NIH) to discuss four clinical trials already approved or under active consideration (*Forum Proceedings* 1991). Friedman began by noting the convergence of scientific and clinical issues (dose intensity, the effect of growth factor, and mechanisms of drug resistance) and social and economic issues (access to treatment and insurance coverage) that were of concern to patients, insurers, and the general public. He repeated his concern that "[j]udges and juries have been asked to decide the merits of a medical treatment" in nine cases since early 1990 and had decided against insurers in all nine (*Clinical Cancer Letter* 1991b, p. 1). He noted that the BCBSA had recently agreed to consider paying for the patient care costs of the procedure.

Andrew Dorr, the NCI program director for breast cancer clinical trials, laid out the rationale for considering four trials as "high priority."[1] The poor survival of patients with stage II, III, and IV breast cancer provided "a compelling reason." Learning whether increasing the dose of chemotherapeutic agents would overcome drug resistance was a second reason. The fact that HDC/ABMT applied mostly to younger women was also important (*Forum Proceedings* 1991). He would comment later, "There's a real sense of urgency about these trials" (*Clinical Cancer Letter* 1991b, p. 1). Friedman reinforced this: "How often do we see so many issues converging in a single topic: efficacy of a new methodology, access to health care, economics. Patients, clinicians, investigators, and insurers care about this topic deeply" (*Clinical Cancer Letter* 1991b, p. 1).

The forum focused on four clinical trials: a CALGB trial already under way of HDC in high-risk (stage II or IIIA) women; an Intergroup/ECOG trial about to begin, also for stage II or IIIA women; a trial under discussion within CALGB for women with stage III breast cancer; and a proposed SWOG trial under discussion for patients with metastatic breast cancer. The meeting also discussed issues of bone marrow contamination, drug resistance, patient concerns about endpoints, measurement of health status and quality of life, and evaluation of the costs of treatment and costs to patients in clinical trials. Each of these trials is discussed briefly here.

William Peters of Duke presented the first trial, which was designed to test HDC in high-risk patients, defined as women with stage II or stage IIIA breast cancer and 10 or more positive axillary nodes (*Forum Proceedings* 1991). This trial had been recommended by the CALGB breast cancer committee and approved by the NCI before the conference. Earlier discussions between Peters and Craig Henderson, then chair of the CALGB breast committee, had resulted in a trial design focused on dose, not on transplantation per se or on the specific chemotherapy regimen. Enrollees were to receive primary treatment by surgery but would not have had prior chemotherapy or radiotherapy. The study involved standard induction chemotherapy with four doses of CAF (cyclophosphamide, doxorubicin, 5-fluorouracil; see table 1.2, chapter 1), after which women would be randomized to either the high-dose Solid Tumor Autologous Marrow Program (STAMP) I regimen with ABMT or a lower dose of STAMP I that was still higher than conventional therapy without ABMT. Target enrollment was 500 patients, with an anticipated annual accrual rate of 120 patients, which was to be achieved by the end of 1994. The trial had begun enrolling patients in late 1990 and by the time of the conference had registered 27 patients, of whom 9 had been randomized.

This CALGB trial was notable in several respects. First, both arms were experimental: After induction treatment, a patient would be randomized to either HDC or intermediate-dose chemotherapy. Thus, a patient might benefit from either arm: "We had true equipoise," Henderson would say later (Henderson 2002).[2] Second, Peters insisted that all eligible patients at Duke, which would enroll the bulk of the patients, were required to participate in the trial to have a chance at receiving the procedure. If they were unwilling to be randomized, then they would have to go elsewhere. Not all institutions insisted on this. Finally, every transplanter in the trial was required to undergo a run-in period, conducting three transplants safely under supervision. (We note that treatment was available "on protocol" in phase 3 randomized clinical trials, in nonrandomized phase 2 trials in some institutions, and "off protocol" in many places.)

The second trial, an intergroup trial, would be approved by the NCI within 3 weeks of the conference. ECOG had the lead, but CALGB and SWOG institutions would also participate and provide patients. Nicholas J. Robert, MD, of Fairfax Hospital,

Virginia, presented the study, which would be chaired by Martin Tallman, MD, of Northwestern University Medical School. The trial was designed to evaluate conventional adjuvant chemotherapy (CAF) administered every 4 weeks for six courses versus CAF followed by bone marrow harvest and HDC (cyclophosphamide and thiotepa) followed by transplantation. The initial accrual objective was 429 patients within 3 years (*Forum Proceedings* 1991).

The third trial discussed was for women with inflammatory or stage III breast cancer, of which Karen Antman, then of Dana-Farber Cancer Institute, was to be principal investigator. Patients responding to induction treatment involving doxorubicin and granulocyte colony-stimulating factor would be randomized after restaging, Antman said, "to either of two high-dose arms of cyclophosphamide, thiotepa, and carboplatin, with peripheral blood stem cells harvested as well as the marrow," or to the same total dose "over four to six cycles" (Forum Proceedings 1991, p. 55). This trial was to be a dose-rate study and Antman indicated discussions about it were under way within CALGB.

The fourth trial presented at the forum was a proposed intergroup study of stage IV metastatic breast cancer (*Forum Proceedings* 1991). Robert Livingston of the University of Washington, and a SWOG investigator, would be principal investigator. Patients with no prior chemotherapy were to receive conventional chemotherapy of CAF followed by CMF (cytoxan, methotrexate, 5-fluorouracil) over a 6-month period. Those with complete or partial responses would then be randomized to one of three arms: continuation of induction therapy; two doses of CEP (cytoxan, etoposide, platinum) plus granulocyte-macrophage colony-stimulating factor growth factor; or CTC (cytoxan, thiotepa, carboplatin, i.e., STAMP V) plus ABMT plus granulocyte-macrophage colony-stimulating factor. Livingston indicated that 585 patients would need to be entered in the trial from SWOG and ECOG members to randomize 130 patients to each of its three arms.

Rebecca Gelman of Dana-Farber Cancer Institute sounded a prescient warning. This "clutch" of trials would be decisive, she said, because "there's not going to be a second chance" (*Forum Proceeding* 1991, p. 20). The randomization, expense, and "hardening of medical opinion" would mean that "the cohort [of patients] we are talking about now is going to be it." Reviewing differences among the active and proposed protocols, she found three different induction therapies, three different ABMT regimens, five different standard therapies, and three patient groups," all of which would complicate efforts to draw conclusions. The various endpoints also posed problems prospectively about what could be concluded from results: Time to relapse and relapse-free survival both suffered from definitional ambiguity and subjectivity of evaluation and from the fact that time to relapse did not count toxic and other non–breast cancer deaths against the treatment while relapse-free survival did. She argued strongly against the former and for the latter. Her remarks highlighted the complexities of the scientific issues in these trials.

Not discussed at the forum was the Philadelphia trial, which would only later receive the NCI high-priority designation. In 1990, U.S. HealthCare, then one of the country's major health insurers (and since merged with Aetna), initiated a trial (PBT-01) of metastatic breast cancer a full year before the NCI trials began because it faced coverage inquires about BMT (*Cancer Letter* 1991). Hyman Kahn, MD, chief medical officer, saw the issue through the lens of whole organ transplantation. "Kidney transplantation [coverage] was clear-cut," he said. "If you had kidney failure and were on dialysis, there was no question about the benefit of a transplant. It was the same with liver transplantation; there were not many in number and the indications were clear-cut" (Kahn 2003). However, ABMT for breast cancer was different:

> From a health insurance company's view, bone marrow transplantation to support high-dose chemotherapy was very costly and just beginning to get underway. It became very clear that there was problem with coverage and how to make a proper coverage decision. Very apparent that we would soon leave evidence-based decision-making and would be heavily influenced by emotional factors. (Kahn 2003)

Kahn convened a meeting of the Philadelphia breast cancer doctors, bone marrow transplanters, and radiotherapists in late 1989 (Stadtmauer 2002). "Who should we cover? What's the consensus?" were the questions that he and Robert Gordon, vice president for medical affairs, asked. "We don't know," was the response. "A clinical trial is needed." Kahn recalls the meeting in the following way:

> They all came—from Penn, Temple, and Hahnemann. We met in the basement auditorium of U.S. HealthCare in Blue Bell [Pennsylvania]. The question was what criteria should be used for HDC/ABMT for breast cancer. We had a discussion that lasted several hours. At the end of the discussion, I had not received much help. Everyone agreed that the procedure should be used, if at all, only for metastatic breast cancer. But they all agreed that we'd never know [if the procedure worked] unless we did a randomized clinical trial. John Glick was especially vocal. I said to him, John, it's obvious what needs to be done. Why don't you write a proposal for a randomized clinical trial? Then we'll move forward. (Kahn 2003)

How would a trial be financed? The group consisted mainly of academic physicians, not community-based oncologists. "There was lot of sensitivity among them about dealing with an insurance company. The question was how they could use U.S. HealthCare money in a way that didn't appear tainted," Kahn (2003) recalled. The insurer agreed to make an unrestricted educational grant of $1.5 million to finance administrative costs of the trial, including data management, at $500,000 a year for 3 years. It also covered the patient care costs for those in both the transplant and non-transplant arms of the trial. Had the decision required a lot of internal discussions within the company? "About 4 minutes," Kahn replied. "The clinical decisions were totally controlled by physicians at U.S. HealthCare at that time. Len Abramson, the CEO [chief executive officer], was very interested in breast cancer. His wife had had breast cancer. He would do anything to build the knowledge base. He put $100 million into the cancer unit at Penn, for example" (Kahn 2003).

Kahn noted that this was the first time a health maintenance organization had "officially provided coverage on an exception basis in order to support experimental therapy in a randomized clinical trial" (*Cancer Letter* 1991, p. 7). "I recognized," he said:

> that because of the prevalence of breast cancer and the fact that bone marrow transplantation is increasingly popular around the country, there would be a lot of demand for this, and whether it should be covered is not agreed upon. Most insurers don't cover it up front, and a lot have been under coercion, if you will, to cover it. It is a

toxic treatment; it has a certain mortality of its own. But one should have good statistics. If we don't do something like this, it is going to be anecdotal for another 10 years. (*Cancer Letter* 1991, p. 7)

Ironically, although Kahn could not have foreseen it at the time, it would be 10 years before randomized clinical trial data would be available. Although Kahn invited a number of other health insurers to join in financing this trial, none responded.

Of the five trials described above, two (CALGB 9081 and INT 1021) would be initiated as NCI high-priority trials and would eventually report results; two (the Antman and Livingston trials) would fail to accrue sufficient patients; and one (the Philadelphia trial) would be initiated by an insurer, transferred later to a cooperative group, and designated high priority by the NCI.

Randomized Clinical Trials

Randomized clinical trials are routinely described as the gold standard of modern medical science, generating the only reliable data about treatment effectiveness. They have the intrinsic merit of neutralizing implicit and explicit observer biases, patient selection biases, and biases arising from comparing experimental to historical results. However, not all procedures are evaluated by randomized trials, and the medical profession weakly embraces the gold standard on many occasions.

Randomized clinical trials confront many challenges (policy, organizational, methodological, analytical, and ethical), all of which have numerous mundane technical details. Policy issues include establishing agreement that a trial is needed, then identifying a principal investigator, and securing financial support. Organizational issues include assembling an advisory group to the trial; organizing a coordinating center and a data center; recruiting nurse coordinators and other trial personnel; enlisting the clinical centers with the potential to enroll patients; identifying potential patients and recruiting them to participate; and creating a data safety monitoring group to review interim results and stop the trial if the data demonstrate clear superiority or inferiority of the experimental arm.

Methodological issues include designing the trial to test the key hypothesis; formulating the critical questions; selecting the endpoints or health outcomes of the study; determining the criteria for including and excluding patients; calculating the statistical power required to determine the number of patients who need to be enrolled and randomized; adopting a randomization procedure; and incorporating all of these factors into a protocol that will guide all centers as they enroll patients.

Analytical issues involve collecting, cleaning, and validating data and analyzing it in terms of "intent to treat" and preparing abstracts, presentations, and journal manuscripts for reporting results in formats specified by professional societies, cooperative groups, and scientific journals.

Ethical issues turn on whether true equipoise exists (i.e., whether it is known that the experimental treatment is better or worse than conventional treatment) and on patient informed consent.

Here, we comment on organization; endpoints; equipoise and randomization; on-protocol and off-protocol treatment; trial; and patient enrollment.

Organization

An extensive network of NCI-financed oncology cooperative groups exists to conduct phase 3 multisite cancer clinical trials. The cooperative groups were created in 1959. The NCI cancer chemotherapy program had generated a number of compounds that had been tested in animals for their effects against various cancers. Congress, impatient with the slow translation of these compounds to useful chemotherapy interventions, insisted that a program be created to test the most promising compounds in humans. The cooperative groups resulted from this initiative.

A cooperative group consists of an affiliation among a number of institutions, typically tertiary medical centers and specialized cancer centers, a number of clinical investigators associated with these institutions, and a supporting infrastructure. The institutions and investigators constitute resources-in-waiting; the infrastructure has an ongoing existence that actively supports ongoing trials. In table 8.1, we list the adult cancer cooperative groups as of 2003.

Decisions about any given clinical trial emerge from discussions between NCI and the cooperative groups. These discussions involve prospective investigators, the relevant cooperative group committees and officers, and NCI officials, and lead to the preparation, circulation and review of a proposal and a formal submission to NCI for approval or disapproval. A decision to conduct a trial is accompanied by the commitment of funds to support the specific trial. Cooperative groups are financed by an annual NCI contract of approximately $150 million that is independent of specific trials but from which specific trials are funded. The entire process may take several years from the initial proposal to enrollment of patients.

The most important cooperative groups conducting clinical trials of HDC/ABMT for breast cancer have been CALGB, ECOG, and SWOG, although the Mayo Clinic and Canadian groups have also been involved. All NCI high-priority phase 3 trials of HDC/ABMT were intergroup trials, involving institutions and investigators from several groups. Such trials increase the number of participating centers, each of which enrolls patients according to a common protocol. The complexity of an intergroup, randomized phase 3 clinical trial is substantial. Each participating group has a chair, various committees (e.g., breast, transplantation, radiation) reflecting the

Table 8.1 United States and Canadian cancer cooperative study groups

American College of Radiology Imaging Network (ACRIN)
American College of Surgeons Oncology Group (ACOSOG)
Cancer and Leukemia Group B (CALGB)
Eastern Cooperative Oncology Group (ECOG)
European Organization for Research and Treatment of Cancer (EORTC)
Gynecologic Oncology Group (GOG)
National Cancer Institute of Canada Clinical Trials Group (NCIC)
National Surgical Adjuvant Breast and Bowel Project (NSABP)
North Central Cancer Treatment Group (NCCTG)
Radiation Therapy Oncology Group (RTOG)
Southwest Oncology Group (SWOG)

Source: National Cancer Institute, http://www.cancer.gov/cancertopics/factsheet/NCI/clinical-trials-cooperative-group.

specialties involved, and a study coordinator (or coordinators). Although all groups, centers, and investigators enter patients according to the same protocol, a trial will carry the number of the primary group, an intergroup number, and a different number for participating groups. The CALGB 9082 trial, for example, was an intergroup trial (INT-0163); the principal investigator was William Peters of Duke University; the coordinating center was located at Duke; and the chairs of the CALGB committees were involved. Other participating groups were the National Cancer Institute of Canada Clinical Trials Group and SWOG.

In early 1995, there were 35 transplant centers enrolling patients in the CALGB 9082 trial: 24 from CALGB institutions, 10 from SWOG, and 1 from the National Cancer Institute of Canada Clinical Trials Group (Hurd and Peters 1995). In the trial for which ECOG was the lead (INT-0121/E-2190), all 29 ECOG centers were participating; 20 SWOG BMT centers were participating; 34 CALGB institutions were added in 1995, but only a few were actually participating (ECOG 1995).[3] In the Philadelphia trial, the initial institutions were the University of Pennsylvania, Hahnemann University, Temple University, and the Fox Chase Cancer Center; the Mayo Clinic and Tufts University joined later in 1990; in 1995, this would be transferred to ECOG auspices.

Endpoints

The endpoints or measured outcomes constitute the second area of importance. All HDC/ABMT trials have reported three major endpoints: treatment-related mortality; overall survival; and progression-free, event-free, or disease-free survival. Treatment-related mortality was very high in the early years of the procedure, a factor leading critics to call for clinical trials. For example, the initial phase 2 trial by Peters reported treatment-related mortality of 22% in the women receiving HDC/ ABMT (Peters et al. 1988). The introduction of growth factor, facilitating the reconstitution of rescued bone marrow or stem cells, helped decrease treatment-related mortality from about 20% in the 1980s to 3%–5% by the mid-1990s. The report by the North American Transplant Registry to the Medical Advisory Committee of BCBSA in early 1996 that treatment-related mortality had fallen contributed to that organization's decision to modify its position on the procedure (Aubry 2002).

Overall survival from treatment until death is a classic endpoint of clinical trials in all of medicine. The failure of HDC/ABMT to prolong life in a significant way has been its Achilles' heel. David Eddy emphasized this in 1992, and it continues to be argued today. Against its limited effect on overall survival, advocates for the procedure have pointed to disease-free survival. (For high-risk breast cancer, disease-free survival means no current evidence of disease; for metastatic disease, this means no new events or no evidence of progression of disease and is therefore called event-free, disease-free, or progression-free survival.)

Other health outcomes are sometimes measured. For example, the Philadelphia trial reported results for both quality of life and costs. Many studies also report the time to relapse or time to death (median survival data). Some report survival curves with hazard ratios. The lack of standard terminology and of a system to enforce standard definitions in phase 3 clinical trials makes comparing the results across trials difficult and potentially limits performing a meta-analysis to combine the results of all trials; it also means that investigators often select outcomes to measure what they believe a priori will support favorable results of their studies.

Equipoise and Randomization

Patient recruitment to a randomized trial begins with the judgment that equipoise exists between the old and new treatments. What does *equipoise* mean? It is not part of the average patient's vocabulary. It means that sufficient uncertainty exists about whether the experimental treatment is better or worse than existing treatment, uncertainty that only a clinical trial can eliminate. Equipoise is also an ethical precondition for randomization. If a new treatment is known to be better or worse than existing therapy, then it is unethical to conduct a randomized trial.

Who determines whether equipoise exists? The determination is made by physician-investigators collectively and by individual physicians. The collective decision is reached by discussions involving clinical researchers, cooperative groups, and the NCI in the case of oncology procedures. This judgment is not authoritative and binding but represents prevailing thinking within the research community. The judgment by an individual physician may agree or disagree with the collective judgment by researchers. The determination that equipoise exists depends on the interpretation of data, which depends in turn on the values brought to bear on the issue. Physicians' judgments about equipoise are subjective, and physicians often differ among themselves about whether it exists and about the ethics of randomization. As we have seen, subjectivity clearly existed among oncologists regarding whether a randomized trial was needed or ethical.

Further complicating the situation, the individual physician who suggests to a patient that she enter a randomized clinical trial is saying, in effect, "I don't know what you should do. Instead, I suggest you let a computer (with a randomization sequence) make the decision. And it would be unethical for me to favor either arm of the trial." So a physician not only must determine that equipoise exists, but also must be prepared to admit ignorance about the appropriate course of action for the patient and must justify randomization as the ethical course under the circumstances. This is a long way from the image of the physician as an all-knowing guide to patient decision making, an image held by many patients and not always disowned by physicians.

Moreover, even though a great deal of literature justifies randomized clinical trials, the literature provides precious little guidance on when such a trial is necessary and when and under which conditions one can be bypassed. Andrew Kelahan (2002) recalled a bifurcated discussion of this issue in the late 1980s with advocates and critics of HDC/ABMT on opposite sides: "We are beyond equipoise; the procedure saves lives," argued the advocates. "No," responded the critics, "there are not enough data; we must do a randomized clinical trial" (Kelahan 2002).

Even when a trial has been determined to be necessary, the physician-investigator has two roles that often conflict: One is the obligation to care for the patient; the other is to ensure the integrity of the scientific research (Fox and Swazey 1978). Enrolling patients in a randomized trial requires that a physician-investigator obtain a woman's informed consent. This requires discussing with a patient why, given the limitations of existing treatment, she should agree to being randomized. It means persuading her that the limits of existing treatment must be balanced against the unknowns of the experimental treatment. This takes time, often many hours. This time is often uncompensated, as physician reimbursement is based mainly on doing something to the patient, not on conversation with the patient, regardless of how central such talk is to enrolling patients in a trial. John Glick (2002) characterized the problem this way: "The fact that insurers don't pay [for patient care costs of clinical trials] accounts for only a small part of the problem. Explaining a BMT trial often required 3 hours and three visits to persuade a metastatic breast cancer patient to go on a trial. Many refused" (2002). Glick's colleague, Edward Stadtmauer (2002), said: "Randomization depends on patient preferences and physician preferences. The experience of terminal breast cancer patients is 2–3 years survival. A subset of patients want the new treatment; a subset of doctors want the new. A subset of patients don't want to be killed; a subset of doctors don't want to kill patients" (2002).

Gabriel Hortobagyi, MD, at the M. D. Anderson Cancer Center of the University of Texas in Houston, said this in 2002 about the physician time required to randomize patients:

> We have a number of mechanisms in place to protect physician time. In 1977, for example, I hired my first research nurse, who has been with me 28 years. She is highly paid and has a role in all trials. She explains the procedure to the patient in advance of me seeing the patient. It saves an hour or two of my time. Also it gives the patient the same message from two sources, one of whom speaks in terms more understandable to the patient. The time cost of accrual is enormous. Also the nature of patient education requires that the message be repeated several times. Patients often tune out what they don't want to hear. It's very important to get the full message across.

Hortobagyi (2002) commented on an institutional dilemma of randomization:

> We are a tertiary center, a referral center [in oncology]. So we became a "center of excellence" for insurance companies. If a physician and an insurer send a patient to us, it is very difficult for us to randomize. Patients who come here are highly selected. They are not disposed to be randomized. They are strongly motivated to treatment. For example, if a patient comes with lung cancer and the choice is between treatment and supportive care, it is impossible to persuade many to sit around and wait to die. It's the same at Memorial Sloan Kettering and the other major centers. It took us 8 years to randomize 78–80 patients [in a 1989 trial]. It easily takes a couple of hours [to explain the appropriateness of randomization to a patient]. These are very difficult discussions. [For HDC/ABMT] you had to explain why your colleagues who were doing the procedure outside a randomized trial were misguided (without saying they were dumb). Then you had to explain why it was important to randomize. You had to walk a very fine line. This was at a time when the procedure was spreading like wildfire.

On-Protocol, Off-Protocol Treatment

Patient enrollment became a central issue for the HDC/ABMT trials, largely because the procedure was widely available outside randomized clinical trials. This availability eroded the willingness of women to enter randomized clinical trials, reflected the weak physician commitment to trials, and undermined the ability of investigators to collect data systematically about the procedure's effectiveness. The procedure was available both on protocol and off protocol. A protocol can be thought of as a recipe that specifies various factors (patient eligibility, treatment regimen, study endpoints, informed consent procedures, etc.). Both phase 2 and phase 3 studies can be on protocol. We have emphasized the differences of single-site versus multisite studies and numbers of patients. The basic difference is randomization: Phase 2 trials seldom involve randomization; phase 3 trials nearly always require randomization. *Off protocol* means that treatment is provided entirely outside of any study.

Response Technologies, for example, characterized the treatments provided by its IMPACT centers as clinical trials. In fact, they were phase 2 clinical trials, but the protocols did not involve randomization; thus the trials lacked controls, and Response did not participate in any of the cooperative group trials. All women who came to them received the HDC/ABMT procedure. The protocol in this case was a recipe for treatment. The firm did have a centrally managed data collection system and generated substantial reports in the literature, but gave priority to the wishes of the individual patient without regard to the requirements of systematic evaluation of the procedure and technically provided treatment on protocol.

Response Technologies was hardly alone. Many other cancer centers provided the treatment outside the phase 3 clinical trials. For example, in 1995 Andrew Pecora, director of the BMT program at Hackensack Medical Center in New Jersey, indicated that he gave women a choice of entering a national trial or getting the procedure outside a trial. Only a few of the 60 women receiving the procedure at Hackensack in the past few years had opted for the trial (Kolata 1995).

The experience among major cancer centers engaged in trials was mixed. Committed trialists believe that it is necessary that a woman agree to randomization if she is to receive treatment at a center engaged in a clinical trial. This requirement is needed to protect the scientific integrity of a trial and reflects a judgment that the desires of individual patients must be subordinated to a population-oriented scientific evaluation of a procedure. Peters insisted, for example, that no breast cancer patient eligible for CALGB 9082 could receive HDC/ABMT at Duke unless that resulted from randomization. Other academic centers, however, simultaneously entered some women in randomized clinical trials and acceded to the request of those women who refused randomization by granting access to the experimental treatment in a phase 2 trial.

Patient Enrollment

Recruiting patients is one of the central challenges of phase 3 clinical trials. Table 8.2 presents enrollment data on the NCI high-priority clinical trials. We comment briefly on the experience of each trial.

The Philadelphia trial enrolled its first eight patients in 1990 and maintained decent accrual rates through 1993. By 1994, however, enrollment had begun to slow as the pool of potential Philadelphia area patients was exhausted (Stadtmauer 2002). The failed ECOG efforts to mount a metastatic breast cancer trial led to discussions in 1994 among the Philadelphia group, ECOG, and the NCI, which led to the transfer of the trial's coordinating center and data center to ECOG. In 1995, the trial became an

Table 8.2 Annual and cumulative study accruals for U.S. clinical trials of HDC/ABMT from activation to closure by year and study

Study	1990	1991	1992	1993	1994	1995	1996	1997	1998	1999	2000	2001	Total
PBT-01/E/PBT01													
Annual	8	54	78	79	62	100	104	68					553
Cumulative		62	140	219	281	381	485	553					553
CALGB9082/INT-0163													
Annual		95	170	162	174	169	127	108	31				1,036
Cumulative			265	427	601	770	897	1,005	1,036				1,036
E2190/INT-0121													
Annual		9	64	82	97	86	95	74	34				541
Cumulative			73	155	252	338	433	507	541				541
S9623													
Annual							33	210	194	103	50	12	602
Cumulative								243	437	540	590	602	602

Source: CTEP (Cancer Therapy Evaluation Program), NCI.

ECOG intergroup trial and was designated as an NCI high-priority trial (E/PBT-01). Patient enrollment from 1995 through closure in 1997 occurred at a respectable pace.

The CALGB 9082 trial began in January 1991 and closed accrual at the end of May 1998. The initial projected accrual was 170 patients to each of two arms, at an estimated accrual rate of 75 eligible patients each year (Hurd and Peters 1995). Patients were entered into the trial rapidly, however, and the accrual goal was met 1 year ahead of the original plan. The initial enrollment target was calculated to have a 90% power to detect an expected 50% increase in disease-free survival, one of the study's primary endpoints. As a result of the rapid accrual, the protocol was modified, and the target was raised to an estimated 380 patients per arm, with an anticipated accrual rate of 120 patients annually. The trial accrued a total of 1036 patients for the years 1991 through May 1998 (Peters et al. 1999).

By contrast, the INT-0121/E-2190 trial accrued patients far more slowly. Its initial target was enrolling 536 patients by January 1996, but it had only enrolled 377 patients by May of that year. So, the date for completing enrollment was slipped to November 1997, by which time 500 patients had been enrolled. The trial was finally closed to new patients on August 3, 1998, at which time it had enrolled 541 patients (NCI 1998). It met its target but 2 years late.

S9623 began late, in 1996, a response to the enrollment crisis of 1994–1995 discussed in the next section. It had a target enrollment of 1000 patients with stage II and III breast cancer and 4–9 nodes positive. It enrolled 33 patients in its first year, 210 in 1997, and 194 in 1998, but the impact of the May 1999 American Society of Clinical Oncology (ASCO) meeting can be seen in the figures for 1999 through 2001 (103, 50, and 12, respectively). The fall-off in accrual that began in 1999 led to opening the trial to all patients with four or more nodes involved, but this was to no avail. The study terminated accrual in 2001, having enrolled only 602 patients, far short of its initial target.

Enrollment data tell only part of the story. The power of clinical trials derives from the number of eligible participants who are randomized and for whom results are analyzed, which is often far less than the number enrolled. Enrolled patients may drop out before randomization as a result of trial design or for other reasons. Even after randomization, women may be deemed ineligible or may refuse to participate and be lost to follow-up. Women found to be ineligible after randomization may or may not be included in the data analysis: If the protocol violation is trivial, then they may still be included. Although for various reasons many women in these trials did not receive the treatment to which they were allocated, results were analyzed on an "intent-to-treat" basis, which research generally accepts as the most valid approach. This means that all women for whom outcomes are known are analyzed in the groups to which they are allocated, regardless of which treatment they actually receive. Data relating the number of patients randomized in the studies of interest are presented in table 8.3.

The differences between the number of patients enrolled and those randomized in PBT-01 and CALGB 9082 is largely a consequence of the trial designs: Enrolled participants were reevaluated after induction chemotherapy and were randomized only if their response to the initial conventional-dose treatment met predetermined inclusion criteria. In E2190, there was no such reevaluation, as women were randomized before any chemotherapy treatment began.

Table 8.3 Study enrollment and randomization by study

Study	Total enrolled	Randomized	HDC arm	Control arm	Analyzed
PBT-01/E/PBT01	553 354 not randomized: 208 insufficient response to induction chemotherapy 57 ineligible 48 withdrew consent 41 other reasons	199	110 Of these: 9 ineligible (excluded from analysis) 5 minor protocol violations (included in analysis) Of the 101 analyzed: 6 refused HDC (1 had alternative HDC, 5 had no HDC)	89 Of these: 6 ineligible (excluded from analysis) 4 minor protocol violations (included) Of the 83 analyzed: 14 refused treatment (10 had HDC, 3 had no therapy, 1 no data) 3 had HDC after relapse	184 HDC 101 CDC 83
CALGB 9082/ INT-0163	1,036 151 preliminary patients 100 of these not randomized: 26 primary or metastatic cancer 25 insurance denied 25 had no insurance 15 withdrew 14 removed for medical reasons 10 never received treatment 8 reasons unknown 5 ineligible 3 removed for unknown reasons 2 died of CAF toxicity 2 died from induction therapy	785	394	391 Control arm was an intermediate dose without transplantation (numbers do not correlate in all publications; no figure given in 2001 abstract)	785 HD 394 ID 391

E2190/INT-0121	540	540	270	270	511
			Of these:	Of these:	
			16 ineligible (excluded from analysis)	1 had no data (excluded from analysis)	
			45 minor protocol violations (included)	12 ineligible (excluded)	
			Of the 254 analyzed:	49 minor protocol violations (included)	
			51 did not have study HDC:		
			22 refused	Of the 257 analyzed:	
			4 insurance reasons	18 eventually had HDC elsewhere	
			19 removed for medical reasons		
			2 ineligible		
			4 removed for unknown reasons		
			18 had HDC elsewhere		
S9623	539	539	271	265	539

Source: Cynthia Farquhar

Abbreviations: PBT-01, Stadtmauer et al. 2000; CALGB 9082, Peters et al. 2005; E2190, Tallman et al. 2003; Bearman et al. 2005. CDC = conventional-dose chemotherapy; HDC = high-dose chemotherapy.

Midcourse Adjustments

Midcourse adjustments were required in 1995. Although the court battles had actually seesawed back and forth (see chapter 3), the *Fox v. HealthNet* (No. 219692, Superior Court of California [1993]) punitive damages award dominated perceptions that litigants were prevailing and insurers were giving ground. Patients, physicians, and patient advocates (with few exceptions) were pressing for treatment outside clinical trials. The Office of Personnel Management decision of September 1994 had laid a coverage requirement on 300 health plans in the country, at least for their enrollees who were federal government employees, and state legislatures were following suit.

Two of the original NCI high-priority trials of HDC/ABMT for breast cancer remained in business: the trial led by Peters at Duke and the ECOG trial. Both of these dealt with high-risk breast cancer patients. The trial presented by Antman in 1991 had not gotten off the ground. The SWOG trial of metastatic breast cancer had been "closed without results" due to low enrollment (NCI 2001). This failure created the possibility for a time that there would be no high-priority trial for metastatic breast cancer, a prospect that provided a major reason for NCI authorizing the transfer of PBT-01 to ECOG.

The NCI high-priority trials, with the exception of CALGB, were losing steam. A *New York Times* story by Gina Kolata in February 1995 laid out the problem in detail. Noting that scientists were skeptical about the efficacy of the HDC/ABMT procedure, the article discussed the NCI trials undertaken to determine whether the procedure was preferable to standard treatment. "But so many women," Kolata wrote, "turn to this grueling, risky and expensive treatment that they [NCI] are having a hard time enrolling patients" (p. C8). The problem involved randomization to conventional or experimental treatment: "Many women, faced with the unencouraging survival rates associated with conventional treatment, are unwilling to take the chance that they will be assigned to this group." The article noted that Karen Antman, who had arrived at Columbia-Presbyterian Medical Center in 1993, had been "eagerly looking forward to playing a major role in one of the [NCI] advanced breast cancer studies. But she has been bitterly disappointed. So far she has not enrolled a single woman in the national study."

The HDC/ABMT experience, Kolata wrote, was "emblematic" of one of the most difficult issues in clinical medicine: "Must patients be forced to join clinical trials by being denied new treatments unless they participate?" (1995, p. C8). Researchers had been confident when the NCI started the trials in 1990 that they would be completed by this date. But one trial had already "fallen by the wayside" due to low enrollment; two others had enrolled only half of the women needed. "One, [for] women whose cancer has spread beyond the lymph nodes, was begun in 1990 and needs 549 patients. It has 271. The study Dr. Antman is involved in began in 1991 and needs 429 patients but has only 234." Only the fourth study, the CALGB study by Peters at Duke, had "filled its rolls fairly well." However, it was testing a slightly different regimen, and the study directors had recently decided that 800 patients were needed to "get a decisive answer"; it currently had enrolled 459 patients.

The *Times* story juxtaposed the views of Craig Henderson against those of Andrew Pecora of Hackensack, New Jersey (Kolata 1995). For too many high-tech treatments,

Henderson said, the issue became "intuition versus scientific evidence." Pecora, by contrast, had difficulty providing the therapy only in a clinical trial: "As important as the clinical trial is—and my institution will continue with it as long as it's open—I don't feel that I have the right not to offer a transplant to a woman who wants one" (p. C8). Abrams of the NCI defended the ethics of NCI sponsorship of the trials. "We feel," he was quoted, "that if you believe that this is a question that is unanswered then you should not also be offering this procedure outside of a clinical trial."

One month later, on March 30, 1995, Abrams convened a meeting, High-Dose Chemotherapy with Stem Cell Support for the Treatment of Breast Cancer, the focus of which was "how to increase accrual to BMT trials" (NCI 1995a). Nearly 60 attendees included patients, lay advocates, investigators, reimbursers, and research sponsors. The three active NCI high-priority clinical trials were reviewed.

Tallman reported on INT-0121, begun in August 1991 with an accrual goal of 429. Actual accruals at that date were 202 patients from ECOG institutions and 63 from SWOG participants, for a total of 265; closure of the trial was projected for February 1997. The projected accrual rate had been 143 patients annually; the actual rate had been 86 patients per year.

Stadtmauer reviewed the Philadelphia experience. Enrollment had been "remarkably stable" at 60–80 patients per year; 305 patients had been enrolled, but only 90 had been randomized. The discrepancy was attributed to the fact that patients had to respond to induction treatment before randomization, and thus a long lag time to randomization inhered in trial design.

Peters reported on CALGB 9082. One conclusion that emerged was that the CALGB design might have been more acceptable to patients and doctors as both arms were experimental: After induction treatment, patients were randomized to either high-dose chemotherapy with transplantation or an intermediate-dose regimen without transplantation. Both arms used the same drugs.[4]

The minutes record that "the agenda was amended" for a brief presentation by Dr. Lerner of ECRI, who was actually an uninvited guest (NCI 1995a). In 10-minute remarks at luncheon, he reported that ECRI's assessment had found no evidence of benefit and some evidence of harm. ECRI recommended informing the public of the absence of benefit, making the procedure for metastatic disease available only through clinical trials, evaluating the validity of HDC/ABMT for stage II and III patients in trials, and improving the quality of the oncology literature from which the study data were derived. His remarks were met with criticism verging on hostility, especially as ECRI reports were not peer reviewed in the traditional way and were distributed on a subscription basis, and this report cost $5000. Moreover, the mood of the meeting was one of crisis. Receptivity to more bad news from an outside source was not welcome.

In the afternoon, Roy Jones and Gabriel Hortobagyi squared off in a point–counterpoint session (NCI 1995a). Jones claimed that HDC yielded survival rates of 70%–80% in stage II patients compared to 25%–40% historically with standard treatment. Hortobagyi cautioned that patient selection and disease staging might affect outcomes; that there was no difference between high-dose and standard regimens; that randomized trials were required to answer "the question"; and that the procedure should not be offered outside trials until then. William Vaughn argued that comparisons of high and low doses for metastatic breast cancer were not needed, but better phase 1 and 2 studies were needed; for stage II breast cancer patients, randomized clinical trials should be considered standard of care.

Craig Henderson compared the HDC debate to that over the Halsted radical mastectomy. He noted that lower doses reduced response rates, but no evidence showed that increased doses provided benefit. Single institution studies often had better results than multi-institution trials, suggesting patient selection bias. He concluded by saying that if HDC/ABMT was better, then the trials should soon be showing that benefit to the data safety monitoring boards. If not, then it might be a long time to wait for answers.

Tallman asked if the NCI could reduce the number of competing phase 2 studies. Abrams responded that the NCI "should not control all research, but that they can, and do, exercise considerable powers of moral persuasion. To that end, there seems to be consensus that randomized clinical trials are an ethical way to answer these questions in both the adjuvant and advanced settings" (NCI 1995a, p. 11).

Fran Visco expressed concern that some physicians were conveying the message to their patients that BMT was necessary to survive. She asked at one point how many in the room were providing treatment off protocol. No one raised a hand. As she left the meeting, someone pulled her aside and said, "They're lying." Later, she realized that she should have asked how many were treating patients in phase 3 randomized trials and how many in phase 2 nonrandomized trials (F. Visco, personal communication, September 2, 2004). The distinction between randomized trials and nonrandomized trials that had been clear in the congressional hearing of August 1994 was not clear in this gathering of scientific researchers.

Ten patient advocates had been invited to the meeting, and one session was devoted to "patient perspectives." One patient, Ms. Nancy Havens, had been diagnosed in June 1992 with stage II breast cancer with 10 positive nodes, then randomized in the CALGB trial and treated with HDC/ABMT. She "experienced life-threatening lung changes, . . . and was only now beginning to feel that she has her strength back" (NCI 1995a, p. 11). Patient advocates voiced the concern that a good deal of misunderstanding existed among patients about the failure of induction treatment as the difference between the metastatic and adjuvant settings were substantial; in the former, no response usually meant no benefit from HDC. They urged that the consent forms address these issues thoroughly. The concluding paragraph of the minutes of the day session deserves mention:

> Dr. Friedman stressed the importance of finishing the adjuvant trials, and devising strategies to enroll more women. In response to a question whether the trials should be mandated, Amy Langer answered yes for high-risk patients with 4–9 and 10+ nodes; but she felt it was hard to deny women with multiple sites of metastatic disease access to treatment. Hortobagyi disagreed and said that desperate situations didn't necessarily benefit from desperate remedies. HDC and BMT were most likely to benefit better prognosis women. Ultimately the burden of deciding the best treatment falls to the physician and the patient. (NCI 1995a, p. 14)

In addition to the daylong event, an evening session was held to develop strategies to increase accrual (NCI 1995a, Evening Session, pp. 1– 4). The 25 participants included a high proportion of patient advocates. The organizing questions dealt with the following: the level of support for the trials among patient advocacy groups, professional organizations, and health insurers; barriers to the support of trials; strategies to increase participation; development of a comprehensive plan for the media, newsletters, and public meetings; and coordination through the NCI. "Concern was expressed," the minutes read, "that patients and their doctors were receiving mixed messages regarding the efficacy of BMT for breast cancer. If the group of experts gathered at today's meeting could not reach consensus, how would patients and private physicians perceived this?" (NCI 1995a, Evening session, p. 2). James Armitage provided a laundry list of barriers: unavailability of payment for study; a patient's belief that one treatment was best; a physician's belief that one treatment was best; a physician's financial interest; a physician's time and expense for study participation; a patient's wish not to be a guinea pig; a physician's lack of knowledge of choices and of data; an institution's financial interest; the need for academic clinical investigators to get credit; and patients who did not meet eligibility criteria (NCI 1995a, Evening Session, pp. 2–3).

Most of the possible actions identified by the discussants fell under better communications. Recommendations included the following, with an express or implied "the NCI should": develop a network of professional and advocacy organizations to disseminate information about the three trials; develop better physician and patient materials about the trials, including a videotape for each and a consensus report about what is known and unknown about BMT for breast cancer; facilitate discussions among physicians about the procedure, including regional meetings; consider a national marketing campaign about the importance of completing the three trials; unify behind the message that "the best treatment is enrollment in a clinical trial"; find someone like the surgeon general to convey the message, targeted to the grass roots level; and encourage women who have breast cancer to communicate to those considering their treatment options (NCI 1995a, Evening Session, pp. 3–4). Other suggestions included reviewing the trials to see which modifications might make them easier for patients and physicians to accept; conduct research "to better understand" physician nonparticipation; offer incentives to oncologists for enrolling patients; and streamline the paperwork needed to obtain approval from insurers.

This 1995 meeting led the NCI to engage in enhanced education and promotion efforts to promote the trials. "We wanted the trials to be completed or we would never get an answer to the question [of superiority]," Abrams said (2003). The NCI's Office of Cancer Communication conducted a project to determine the reasons for low enrollment in the three HDC/ABMT trials. One part involved a focus group study of oncologists' attitudes and perceptions of the trial; a second part was qualitative study of patient decision making regarding participation in HDC/ABMT clinical trials (NCI 1995b, NCI 1996). The patient decision-making study involved 29 women, 15 who had been randomized to the transplant arm, 11 to standard treatment, and 4 who had declined participation. The main conclusion was that: "From the patient's perspective, physicians are key to trial accrual" (NCI 1996, p. v).

The report added that ABMT trials appealed to women seeking aggressive treatment of their cancer who saw the trial as their "best chance" for survival. Although women were largely unfamiliar with clinical trials at diagnosis, they had little difficulty understanding the ABMT trials; they "generally accepted and understood" randomization; informed consent was not a barrier to participation; and the primary value of participation in a trial was its contribution to survival, but contribution to science was an important secondary value. The patient report recommended that physicians present ABMT in the context of a clinical trial, not introduce it as an available treatment option, as was often done, which implied a potential bias against trials.

The March meeting also led to another SWOG trial (S9623), which had originated at Duke in 1993 as an effort by Peters to study high-risk patients with four to nine-nodes positive (NCI 2001). At a July 1995 meeting, Peters proposed this trial to CALGB but met resistance. The NCI wished this to be an intergroup trial, but as the CALGB 9082 trial was ongoing and the Philadelphia metastatic trial had been transferred to ECOG by this time, it was given to SWOG to administer. Scott Bearman, a transplanter at the University of Colorado and an active SWOG investigator, became principal investigator. The basic outcome of the March meeting was to put everyone on notice that the widespread availability of HDC/ABMT was severely complicating the ability of the NCI high-priority randomized trials to recruit and randomize patients.

International Trials

Although clinical practice varies from one country to another, medical research is international. It is appropriate, then, to ask about the international clinical trials of HDC/ABMT, most of which were European. What, if any, influence did international trials have on U.S. trials and U.S. clinical use?

European investigators began phase 3 clinical trials later than did those in the United States, but did so with some sense of priority (Antman 2001). In June 1993, Bertrand Coiffier and Thierry Philip in Lyon, France, convened a 3-day consensus conference on "intensive chemotherapy plus hematopoietic stem-cell transplantation in malignancies" (Coffier et al. 1994, p. 226). Their purpose was "to evaluate this therapy and to identify the diseases for which intensive HDC/ABMT [we substitute our term here] could be considered as standard treatment, those diseases for which it should remain in prospective trials, and those diseases that do not benefit from this therapy" (p. 226). France, Belgium, the United Kingdom, Germany, the Netherlands, Italy, and the United States were represented.

The consensus panel focused mainly on the role of HDC/ABMT for hematologic malignancies, but it also considered solid tumors: "Although HDC has a good theoretic basis," the panel wrote, "it has not been established as superior to conventional therapy for any stage of any adult solid tumor" (Coffier et al. 1994, p. 229). On breast cancer, the Europeans said: "Although there is currently insufficient evidence to justify the use of HDC/ABMTs HSC [hematopoietic stem cells] transplantation outside the setting of a clinical trial for any stage of breast cancer, there is ample scientific background for vigorous clinical investigation in this important area" (p. 229). Their "reasonable" priorities for clinical study were (1) phase 3 adjuvant studies in high-risk operable breast cancer (10 or more nodes or 4–9 nodes plus receptor negative); (2) phase 2 studies in locally advanced disease "with proper stratification and tissue or biologic correlations of responsiveness or non-responsiveness"; (3) the development of more effective cytotoxic regimens for metastatic disease that should be introduced into phase 3 studies as newer approaches were shown to be "feasible, safe, and active"; (4) studies of cost-effectiveness, quality of life, and intermediate and late toxicities; and (5) "careful consideration" of incorporating surgery, radiotherapy, and hormone therapy into these studies (Coffier et al. 1994, pp. 229–230). In short, the European view was rather conservative compared to both the U.S. perspective and accumulating experience.

What were the major European trials? In the Netherlands, the Dutch Health Insurance Council, a public agency for the insurance companies and the Ministries of Health and Science, funded a phase 2, single-site pilot and a larger phase 3 study (Schrama et al. 2002). The phase 2 trial began in 1991, randomized 81 women, and in 1998, became the first randomized trial to publish survival data on high-dose therapy in the adjuvant setting. No differences in survival rates were reported between the two treatment groups. Seven-year results published in 2002 showed no significant difference in survival between the two groups, but this could have been expected given the few patients involved (Schrama et al. 2002). The primary purpose of the study was "to develop a practical approach" to the larger multisite study (Rodenhuis et al. 1998).

All Dutch university hospitals, two cancer institutes, and one large regional hospital participated in the larger study, which began in 1993. Every eligible patient in the Netherlands could participate. The original plan for this phase 3 study called for a sample size of fewer than 300 women, but the investigators later realized that a much larger sample would be needed to detect a true relapse-free survival benefit of 15%–20%. Eventually, this trial randomized 885 women, making it the largest trial to date. The Dutch Health Insurance Council had agreed to finance this study on the condition that an interim analysis would be reported in 2000 and would justify continuation. The analysis was presented at the ASCO 2000 meeting (Rodenhuis et al. 2000). Five-year results, published in 2003, showed a benefit to the high-dose group of borderline statistical significance for relapse-free survival but no significant difference between groups in overall survival (Rodenhuis et al. 2003). The investigators suggested that 5–10 years of additional follow-up might be required before a definitive conclusion could be drawn about overall survival. The principal investigator of these trials, Sjoerd Rodenhuis, estimated that fewer than 10 women in the Netherlands received high-dose treatment outside a clinical trial in the 10-year period 1993–2003 (S. Rodenhuis, personal communication to J. Majoribanks, July 17, 2003).

In Scandinavia (Sweden, Norway, and Denmark), a large multicenter trial for women with high-risk primary disease was begun in 1994. Comparison was made of HDC with transplantation to an experimental regime without transplantation that used higher-than-standard doses of chemotherapy individually titrated to give a similar degree of hematological toxicity between participants and supported with growth factor (granulocyte colony-stimulating factor). When the study was designed in 1993, the investigators felt it unethical to assign women to a standard-dose control arm in view of the reports from uncontrolled studies of a 30%–40% survival benefit from high-dose treatment. The target sample size was increased from 320 to 500 during recruitment to increase the power of the study from 80% to 90%, and recruitment was planned to continue until the first interim analysis at the end of 1998. However, accrual was stopped in March 1998, after reports of secondary leukemia in the nontransplantation arm, and the chemotherapy regimen in that arm was shortened from 9 to 6 cycles. At the time, 525 women had been randomized. Bergh presented preliminary results at the ASCO meeting in 1999, and an article was published in *The Lancet* in October 2000 (Bergh et al. 2000; Scandinavian Breast Cancer Study Group 1999). In the nontransplantation group, relapse-free survival was significantly better, and there were fewer deaths, but there were also several cases of secondary acute myeloid leukemia and myelodysplastic syndrome in this group. The interpretation of this study's results has been limited by the study design as it did not test HDC against conventional chemotherapy. It would reinforce, as we shall see in the next section, the perception of "no benefit" from HDC/ABMT.

In France, a national cooperative group (the Programme d'Etude de la Greffe Autologous dans les Cancer du Sein [or PEGASE]) was set up in 1994 after the Lyon conference had recommended that phase 3 adjuvant studies be large enough to detect survival differences of 10% to 20%. The group received financial and logistic support from the Ligue National Contre le Cancer, the Health Ministry, and some pharmaceutical companies.

Five clinical trials were conducted between 1994 and 2000; these included two phase 3 trials for stage IV disease (PEGASE 03 and 04), one for stage III disease (PEGASE 01), and two phase 2 trials of differing chemotherapy regimens for inflammatory breast cancer (PEGASE 02 and 05). PEGASE 02 was successfully completed and demonstrated that high-dose treatment was feasible. PEGASE 05 was suspended after the first interim analysis due to the toxicity of the chemotherapy regimen. Among phase 3 trials, the two largest trials (PEGASE 01 and 03) found it necessary to extend their 3-year recruitment periods by 1 and 3 years, respectively, to meet accrual targets of more than 300 women each. PEGASE 04 failed to meet its accrual target.

Preliminary results of these French trials were presented at the ASCO meetings in 1999 and 2002, and the full results of all of them were published in 2003 (Roche et al. 2003). Overall, they showed improved disease-free survival for women on the high-dose arms, but no evidence of improved overall survival except in the tiny PEGASE 04 trial, in which accrual had failed, and only 61 women were randomized. The five published trials accrued a total of 808 patients, of whom 555 were randomized: This comprised 80% of all women in France who received HDC for breast cancer during the relevant period (Roche et al. 2003). Two other trials continue: PEGASE 06 for nonmetastatic disease and PEGASE 07 for inflammatory breast cancer.

In Germany, several trials of HDC have been conducted and completed but have yet to publish final results; some are still in progress. All were summarized in 2001 (Kroger et al. 2001). Two of the completed studies involved women with stage III disease. One randomized 302 women between October 1993 and October 2000 and reported preliminary results at the ASCO meeting in 2002 (Zander et al. 2002). The first published results of this trial appeared in June 2004: After a median follow-up of 3.8 years, no statistically significant difference in survival was found between the two groups. Another study randomized 403 women between 1995 and 2002 and presented preliminary results at the ASCO 2003 annual meeting, reporting a statistically significant benefit in event-free survival for women in the high-dose group but no such benefit in overall survival (Nitz et al. 2003). In both cases, recruitment dropped off after the ASCO 1999 meeting.

Another trial involving 98 women with metastatic disease was conducted between 1998 and 2001 in Germany and Austria. In reported preliminary results reported at the 2002 ASCO meeting, the high-dose group had a benefit of borderline statistical significance in time to disease progression, although it showed no statistically significant overall survival advantage. From 1993 to 1999, German insurance companies funded high-dose treatment regardless of whether the recipients were enrolled in studies.

In Italy, a multicenter trial for women with high-risk disease randomized 398 women between 1993 and 1998. Results presented at the ASCO 2001 conference showed no difference in either relapse-free or overall survival between the arms (Gianni and Bonadonna 2001).

In addition to these European trials, three other international trials for women with high-risk primary disease have been based in Europe or Australasia. A collaboration of eight cancer centers in England, Italy, Spain, and Australia randomized 281 women between 1993 and 2001. Results were presented on a poster at the ASCO meeting in 2003 and showed no overall or disease-free survival benefit from high-dose therapy (Bliss et al. 2003). Another collaboration among 17 centers in Australasia, Switzerland, Hong Kong, Slovenia, and Italy randomized 344 women between 1995 and 2000. Preliminary results were presented at in 2003 at the ASCO conference; again, there was no statistically significant advantage to the high-dose groups (Basser et al. 2003).

A large international trial by the Anglo Celtic Oncology Group, led by John Crown from St. Vincent's University Hospital in Dublin, included 34 centers in the United Kingdom, Ireland, Belgium, and New Zealand. Recruitment began in February 1995 with a target of 300 women. Rapid accrual made a more ambitious study possible, and the accrual target was increased to 450 in November 1996 and to 600 in March 1998. Eventually, 605 women were randomized, and the study was closed in June 1999. Results were reported at the ASCO conference in 2002 and 2003: There was no statistically significant difference between the groups in terms of deaths or relapses (Crown et al. 2002).

There was also an international trial for women with metastatic disease, again led by John Crown and involving 18 centers in Ireland, Switzerland, the United Kingdom, Spain, Greece, Italy, Poland, South Africa, Bulgaria, and the United States (Crown et al. 2003). Randomization began in August 1997, but accrual fell short of the target, and the study was closed in June 2001 with only 110 of the 263 planned participants. Low accrual was attributed partly to the presentation of negative results at the ASCO meeting in 1999, along with the publication of the audit of the Bezwoda trial in January 2000. This trial reported results at the ASCO conference in 2001, at a median follow-up of 19 months; the disease-free survival rate was significantly better for women on the high-dose arm, but overall survival rates were not significantly different.

A small multi-center trial was also held in Japan, which randomized 95 women between 1993 and 1999. Preliminary results were presented at the ASCO meeting in 2001 but showed no survival difference between the groups (Tokuda et al. 2001).

Although the Europeans initiated randomized clinical trials of HDC/ABMT for breast cancer later than U.S. investigators, it appears that they accrued patients more rapidly and reported results in a more timely manner. Why? In response to this question, Canadian investigators commented that "accrual was slow . . . [i]n the United States (because) this promising treatment was offered to patients outside of clinical trials long before enough evidence became available to support such decisions. European and Canadian institutions demanded more evidence to justify the rather toxic and potentially dangerous treatment" (Glück et al. 2001, p. 2).

A major reason for accrual differences lay in the much greater difficulty for patients to obtain access to high-dose treatment outside a randomized trial in Europe. By 1997, the European Group for Blood and Marrow Transplantation database had data on nearly 90% of all autologous transplants carried out in Europe. In a 1998 survey of member institutions, they identified 162 centers in 20 countries that regularly carried out transplant procedures for the treatment of breast cancer. Eighty percent used high-dose treatment and transplantation for breast cancer mainly or only on patients enrolled in clinical trials (Neymark and Rosti 2000). In Germany, however, the situation was apparently different. One leading clinical trialist, Professor A. R. Zander, estimated that for every one patient entered into a trial protocol, two patients received treatment off trial (A. R. Zander, personal communication to C. M. Farquhar, July 25, 2003).

Between August and November 1998, *The Lancet* published the views of European and U.S. trialists regarding off-trial treatment, responding to the report of the Dutch pilot study results. Rodenhuis had written: "We strongly believe that this therapy should be given only in the setting of a randomised clinical trial" (Rodenhuis et al. 1998). In the same issue, Pusztai and Hortobagyi agreed "that HDC as adjuvant therapy for high-risk breast cancer should not be used in routine clinical practice" (Pusztai and Hortobagyi 1998a, p. 502). In subsequent letters, Pedrazzoli et al. of Pavia, Italy, agreed "with Rodenhuis and colleagues in that high-dose adjuvant therapy should be given exclusively in the framework of a randomised clinical trial" (Pedrazzoli et al. 1998, p. 1220). However, Price at the U.K. New York Chemotherapy Foundation dissented: "The idea that such treatments should only be given as part of a randomised controlled trial is naïve. . . . I believe it is unethical to enter such patients into a randomised clinical trial because if assigned the standard treatment only, they would die" (Price 1998, p. 1551). Pusztai and Hortobagyi responded that "only 11% of these patients (i.e., those on ABMT registry who had HDC in North America between 1989 and 1995) received treatment in randomized studies. If 50% of these patients had received treatment as part of a randomized clinical study, we would be closer to knowing which group of patients benefits to what extent from which type of HDC" (Pusztai and Hortobagyi 1998b, p. 1552).

It is hard to gauge whether European women are more willing to participate in clinical trials than their American counterparts, although a study of all cancer patients clinically eligible for NCI-sponsored clinical trials in the southeastern United States in 1997–1998 reported that patient refusal accounted for the nonenrollment of nearly 40%, which was twice the refusal rate of a similar study in the United Kingdom (Corrie et al. 2003; Klabunde et al. 1999). One could speculate that American women are less deferential to their doctors, but the evidence suggests that the people most likely to agree to participation in a clinical trial are those who are active and information-seeking partners in the doctor–patient relationship (Ellis et al. 2001; Siminoff et al. 2000). A national probability sample of attitudes of American adults toward participation in cancer clinical trials suggested that patients ultimately base their decision on the recommendation of the physician (Comis et al. 2003).

The reluctance of many clinicians to encourage eligible patients to enter clinical trials appears to be a problem on both sides of the Atlantic: A 1997 survey of 3578 oncologists in Britain found that 75% entered fewer than half of eligible patients for clinical trials, and comparison with U.S. data showed the situation to be broadly similar (Fallowfield et al. 1997). Presentation of the clinical trial option to patients requires very substantial time and effort on the part of clinicians, often without appropriate reimbursement (Corrie et al. 2003; Comis et al. 2003).

Funding mechanisms are critical to the discussion of differences between U.S. and European studies. The above-mentioned study in the southeastern United States in 1997–1998 found that patients with fee-for-service coverage were more likely to be enrolled in clinical trials than those with other types of coverage, including managed care (Klabunde et al. 1999). Of the European transplant centers in the 1998 European Group for Blood and Marrow Transplantation survey, 85% were public institutions, mostly either university hospitals or specialized cancer centers, and the majority of the private institutions were nonprofit organizations: Only 3% of the 162 centers were "profit-maximizers" (Neymark and Rosti 2000). The Dutch trials suggest a working relationship between insurers and investigators, acting through the Dutch Health Insurance Council, a public agency.

American Society of Clinical Oncology 1999 Meeting

The May 1999 meeting of ASCO was pivotal in the development and use of HDC/ABMT for breast cancer, as were the months before the meeting. In January 1998, the Clinton White House announced a 3-year demonstration program of Medicare coverage of patient care costs for cancer clinical trials (ASCO 1998a). Throughout 1998, ASCO would lobby Congress to make this support for clinical trials permanent (ASCO 1998b). In July, Allen S. Lichter, the ASCO president, warned that cancer treatment was threatened by a "crisis in clinical research" (ASCO 1998c). Participation in clinical trials was at a "dismally" low rate, and financial pressures in health care were forcing both practicing and academic oncologists to devote more time to reimbursable procedures, leaving less time for research. ASCO proposed increased funding for the NCI, enactment of legislation to require Medicare coverage of cancer clinical trials, establishment of a clinical research study section at the NIH, and an NIH program to train clinical researchers. Its advocacy of various clinical research initiatives would continue up to and through the 1999 annual meeting.

Other developments bore more directly on HDC/ABMT. In February 1998, the *Journal of the National Cancer Institute* published a review of the HDC/ABMT literature by the NCI officials responsible for breast cancer clinical trials. Entitled "Much Ado about Not . . . Enough Data," the review identified more than 600 English language papers or abstracts published between 1966 and 1997 on HDC with autologous bone marrow or stem cell rescue. It found only one randomized phase 3 trial comparing HDC/ABMT with conventional therapy in the treatment of metastatic breast cancer, the 1995 South African study that had influenced the policy change by the BCBSA in early 1996 (Bezwoda et al. 1995). Completion of U.S. and international trials, they wrote, "is urgently needed to establish definitively the role of HDC/ABMT in the treatment of breast cancer" (Zujewski et al. 1998, p. 200).

The urgency that NCI officials had expressed in early 1998 came to fruition dramatically in the months before the May 1999 ASCO meeting. The NCI learned that "preliminary results" of two U.S. and two foreign trials would be presented at the ASCO meeting (NCI 1999a). Richard Klausner, the NCI director, called a meeting in February ostensibly "to determine how soon data analysis could be completed and the preliminary findings released,"[5] but the NCI knew that those preliminary findings would be negative. The actual purpose of the meeting was to determine how to release these negative trial results and explain what they meant for women who had had the procedure or were considering it. Wade Aubry, representing the BCBSA, remembers this occasion as the first time he heard that "no benefit" would be the reported outcome (Aubry 2002).

The news of the meeting spread quickly. The preliminary results were the subject of a March 9 report on *NBC Nightly News,* which prompted a single-page NCI press release the following day. The press release reflected the dilemma in which NCI found itself. On the one hand, it had to be true to the science. "After discussing a full range of issues, particularly the importance of data accuracy and completeness, the [February] group decided that more work was needed before the results would be ready for release" (NCI 1999a). Representatives of the patient advocacy groups, the release noted, joined in this opinion.

On the other hand, NCI faced an urgent the need to inform the public, especially women with breast cancer. The press release indicated that the NCI was "eager that the results be made public as soon as possible" (NCI 1999a). It continued: "The NCI recognizes the need for women and physicians to have information that will reliably guide treatment choices." Then, veering back toward NCI's role as a research agency, the press release stated: "The imperative need for information about the benefits of various treatments can only be satisfied by well-designed and well-conducted clinical trials. A final but absolutely necessary aspect of clinical trials is the need to assure the correctness of data and the soundness of their analysis" (NCI 1999a).

How would NCI' dilemma be resolved? The press release indicated that: "The investigators are now in this final phase: assuring that the data and the analysis are correct and complete. The results of this analysis have not been provided to NCI. NCI expects that preliminary analysis will be completed by April 15 and made available at that time. Data that have been more fully analyzed will be presented at the ASCO meeting" (NCI 1999a).

The *Wall Street Journal,* on March 11, reported that after the February meeting, "rumors that some of the data showed the procedure wasn't effective rippled through the oncology community," building pressure to release the data early (Jeffrey and Waldholz 1999, p. B2). The story quoted Fran Visco as saying "'I think the data should be available as soon as it is ready'" (p. B2). "Ms. Visco," the story continued, "said she long has been upset that the trials have taken years to produce any data at all. That is because many women, convinced by their doctors that the transplants were better than conventional treatment, received them from doctors not participating in the trials. 'I'm outraged that physicians were recommending bone-marrow transplants to women outside of clinical trials,' she said" (p. B2).

The *Cancer Letter* of March 12 devoted extensive coverage to the debate over early release of data (*Cancer Letter* 1999). Sources to whom it had spoken said that the ECOG-Philadelphia trial was unlikely to show benefit for stage IV breast cancer "either in terms of increased time to progression of disease, the primary endpoint of the study, or long-term survival, a secondary endpoint" (p. 2). But it was unclear whether some subgroups would benefit or whether the statistical power was sufficient to resolve the issue of benefit. The CALGB 9082 trials was also "unlikely to produce definitive answers" about the procedures efficacy for high-risk patients, but officials at the NCI, ASCO, and the cooperative group refused to comment on the preliminary results. Jeff Abrams was quoted saying: "I would not have confidence in preliminary data in terms of accuracy or interpretation. The investigators have not completed the analysis of the data, and we at NCI don't have anything we would consider credible" (*Cancer Letter* 1999, p. 2).

What lay behind the release of "preliminary data"? *Cancer Letter* (1999) opened a small window onto a process that is normally shielded from public view. Writing abstractly, it reported:

> After the statisticians present the results for analysis to the scientific leadership of the cooperative groups, the real analysis of the data begins. Generally, scientists go through the data, patient by patient, verifying the endpoints, and drawing conclusions. When that process is completed, the data are sent to NCI and submitted for peer review. In this case, ECOG and CALGB investigators submitted preliminary data to ASCO in order to present the data and informed NCI about potentially important findings. (p. 3)

Data safety monitoring committees for clinical trials are charged with periodic review of the data to determine whether the experimental treatment is sufficiently better or worse than the control arm to warrant stopping the trial. "Since the trials were not stopped early, the results do not involve either a major detriment or a major benefit," the *Cancer Letter* reported in 1999 (p. 2). "Generally, at the time when the data are released by the data safety monitoring committees, the committees know the answers on the major endpoints of the studies" (*Cancer Letter* 1999, p. 2). The ECOG-Philadelphia trial principal investigator, Edward Staudtmauer, on April 15 said that it was "very unlikely that the results would change over time" (*Clinical Cancer Letter* 1999, p. 3). In the case of the CALGB trial, the data safety monitoring committee had determined that the preliminary data were unlikely to change over the remaining follow-up period and forced the release of the data (Berry 2003). Peters had resisted this step.

Reactions differed. Dr. Allen Lichter, professor of radiation oncology at the University of Michigan and then the ASCO president, had participated in the February meeting but favored further analysis of the data before public release. "I feel that when something is practice-altering, it merits consideration for a clinical alert, early release, and wide dissemination. We have tried to look at these trials under that standard, and I can say—without trying to prejudge the final data and what the discussants are going to say—that these results will not be practice-altering. . . . This is not the end of the story; this is the beginning of the story" (*Cancer Letter* 1999, p. 3).

Barbara Brenner, of Breast Cancer Action in San Francisco, which had not been a participant in the February meeting, took a diametrically opposed view: "If NCI has data on the effectiveness or non-effectiveness of a treatment, to not release that information to the public that needs that information [is] outrageous" (*Cancer Letter* 1999, p. 3). Fran Visco suggested that this was not "top secret information." She was quoted as saying: "We've known for years that there were no data to support this intervention, and the delay in getting the answer is the result of the medical community and patients demanding transplants outside randomized clinical trials" (p. 3). Susan Braun, president of the Susan G. Komen Breast Cancer Foundation, came down on both sides of the early release issue: "As patient advocates, we believe it is imperative that this information be made available to patients at the earliest possible time. However, when patients who are faced with the difficult decision of whether to undergo stem cell transplant rely upon incorrect or incomplete information to make that decision, it is worse than having no information at all" (p. 3).

The NCI anxiety about the forthcoming presentation of trial results led it, with ASCO concurrence, to issue two press releases on April 15, 1999. "For the first time since the introduction of high-dose chemotherapy for breast cancer with bone marrow or stem cell transplants," one release read, "patients and their physicians have data from large scientific studies comparing this treatment to standard therapies" (NCI 1999b, p. 1). Four randomized studies (two from the United States, one from Sweden, and one from South Africa) would be presented in plenary session, and a smaller French study would be presented in a poster session. Casting the results in the best possible light, Klausner was quoted as saying: "The hypothesis going into these trials, our hope, was that the more aggressive approach would prove clearly superior to standard therapy. But based on these studies, high-dose therapy has not yet been shown to be superior to lower-dose treatment. These studies do suggest that it is at least equivalent in terms of overall survival, but the added toxicity and costs of high-dose treatment required that it be superior if it is to become a standard of care" (NCI 1999b, p. 1). Klausner noted, however, that the positive results of the South African study should not be disregarded.

Robert Wittes, who had returned to the NCI from a tour in the pharmaceutical industry, reiterated Klausner's cautious response. The five trials had "added greatly to our knowledge," he said, and women now had "more reliable information" than smaller studies had provided. But follow-up was still relatively short, and results might change with time. Moreover, results applied only to women with metastatic or high-risk breast cancer and might not apply to other high-dose regimens. Even though many women had received the procedure outside of clinical trials, NCI was continuing to support ongoing phase 3 studies. Rather lamely Wittes added, "NCI strongly encourages the use of well-designed clinical trials wherever possible" (NCI 1999b, p. 2).

For the working press that would cover the ASCO meeting, the NCI issued a detailed, 14-page, 23-item "Questions and Answers" document (NCI 1999c). This document provided background on HDC and BMTs and their purposes; cited an estimate of 12,000 women who had been treated for breast cancer; indicated that such transplants had become standard treatment for other cancers; highlighted the danger of damage to the marrow and its capacity to produce red cells, white cells, and platelets; explained the clinical trials; and presented the evidence from the three adjuvant trials for women at high risk of relapse and the two trials of metastatic breast cancer. The document also noted that two other small trials (one Dutch, the other South African) had been reported previously. What could be concluded from the five trials? "The results at present are not clear-cut," read the press release (NCI 1999c, answer to question 12). In the adjuvant setting, three studies (Sweden, Netherlands, and United States) had yet to show superiority to lower-dose treatment, but the results of the fourth, the South African study, "should not be disregarded." For metastatic breast cancer, the U.S. study had shown no survival benefit, but the French and another South African study had shown positive results. Importantly, the document noted, the results of the trials were preliminary. The subsets of patients "in which the therapy is especially effective" had not been identified.

Question 15 of the NCI "Questions and Answers" (1999c) asked: "Why did it take so long to accrue patients to the U.S. trials?" The response was as follows:

Patients and physicians in the United States had easy access to this new technique as many academic and community hospitals opened transplant centers in the early 1990s. Many of these centers either did not participate in clinical trials or performed pilot, non-randomized trials. Thus, patients could have transplant outside of the randomized trials. Unlike the constraints placed on new anti-cancer drugs that are under the supervision of the FDA, no such regulations exist for this technique.

Many physicians recommended high-dose chemotherapy based on the widely disseminated results of pilot studies that found this approach superior to historical comparisons with conventional-dose treatment. Thus, during the 1990s, many thousands of patients (estimated to be over 12,000) received transplants in the United States for breast cancer, but fewer than 1000 of these women took part in randomized trials (p. 11).

The concern of the NCI about how to inform the public about the trials was shared by ASCO. Professional societies prefer to bask in the news of research-based "medical breakthroughs" presented at their annual meeting rather than present bad news beforehand. ASCO placed a cautious interpretation on results that were basically unfavorable. Contrary to its usual policies, it posted a summary of the five studies on its Web site before the meeting "because of the significant public interest" in HDC/ABMT for breast cancer. The summary read as follows:

The information posted on this site represents preliminary data that have not yet been fully analyzed and are yet to be reviewed and discussed in the scientific community. However, because of the important nature of the research, ASCO and the investigators have worked to make information about these studies available to the public before the Annual Meeting.

The investigators will continue to review and analyze their data, and the full presentations at the ASCO meeting will be the first time the data will be presented for discussion. The studies will then be further analyzed for peer review and publication in the scientific literature. It should be stressed that follow-up is not complete and, no doubt, these studies will be the subject of future reports. (ASCO Online 1999, p. 1)

The National Breast Cancer Coalition (NBCC) was not as cautious as ASCO or NCI. On the April 15, it issued a statement "on bone marrow and stem-cell transplants" for immediate release. It read, in part:

> While we have not seen the study results, it has become clear that the results will not show that this treatment benefits women with breast cancer. NBCC's position has always been that there are no data to support Autologous Bone Marrow Transplants for breast cancer and that the procedure should only occur within a randomized clinical trial. For years now, some women have made the decision to have bone marrow or stem cell transplants regardless of the fact that little or no data are available, because they were told that this treatment was their only hope. Unfortunately, because so many physicians performed this procedure outside of a clinical trial setting, we do not know how effective it is. *Had these procedures been performed within a randomized clinical trial we would have had the answers some time ago* [emphasis in original]. So let's not lose sight of the real issue on this story. This experience clearly illustrates the important of conducting quality, randomized clinical trials and educating both physicians and patients. In the future, we need to make certain that women have the appropriate scientific evidence before making important decisions about breast cancer. It is time to move beyond the infrastructure created around ABMT. It is time to look at something better. (NBCC 1999, p. 1)

Denise Grady, in a front-page story in the *New York Times,* suggested that the announcement might not resolve the issue of whether "the drastic and costly treatment" would be worthwhile. Instead, it may "fuel the longstanding disagreement between the procedure's advocates and its detractors, and do little to help women decide whether to undertake the treatment" (Grady 1999a, p. A1).

The ASCO annual meetings are gigantic events. Attendance at the 35th Annual Meeting in Atlanta, May 15–18, 1999, was estimated to have 20,000 registrants from 70 countries. The meeting proceedings tome that every registrant receives includes all abstracts presented at the meeting (in plenary sessions, in smaller symposia, and posters) and is nearly 1000 pages long. The plenary session at which four of the studies were presented on May 17 was held, according to the *Times,* "in a vast, echoing hall the size of a football field at the Georgia World Congress Center" (Grady 1999b, p. A19). In plenary sessions, a series of six to eight huge screens, perhaps 12 feet by 12 feet, are hung in three parallel rows from the front to the back of the cavernous hall so the thousands of attendees, wherever they are sitting, can see the speaker on the center screen and the speaker's data slides on the screens to either side.

The plenary session abstracts for HDC/ABMT for breast cancer were numbered 1, 2, 3, and 4 in the 5-pound proceedings volume, indicating the importance that ASCO attached to these reports. Edward Stadtmauer (1999) presented the results of the ECOG-Philadelphia trial (Stadmauer et al. 1999). The trial, which had opened in 1990, had treated 553 women with metastatic breast cancer with four to six cycles of conventional induction therapy (CAF, 507; CMF, 46). There were 303 women (54%) who responded, 56 complete responses and 247 partial responses. Of these, 199 women agreed to be randomized, and 180 were actually randomized and analyzed, with 101 to HDC and 79 to low-dose chemotherapy. Analysis at a median follow-up of 31 months showed no difference in overall survival and no difference in toxicity between the two arms. Analyses of time to failure, quality of life, and economic costs were in progress. So much, then, for the use of HDC/ABMT for treating metastatic breast cancer, the primary application of the procedure a decade earlier. John Glick (2002) would comment later: "We showed 'no difference' between HDC and standard therapy for metastatic breast cancer. This changed the standard of care. BMT was stopped overnight" (Glick 2002).

The use of the procedure had already shifted away from metastatic to high-risk breast cancer, as the data in chapter 5 indicate. William Peters, the foremost advocate for HDC/ABMT in the United States, made the second presentation on results of the CALGB 9082 trial for high-risk women with 10 or more axillary nodes positive (Peters et al. 1999). A total of 874 women with stage II or IIIA breast cancer had been treated between January 1991 and May 1998. Following conventional induction therapy, 783 women had been randomized to either HDC with bone marrow or peripheral blood support or to an intermediate dose of the same regimen without transplantation. Median follow-up was 37 months. Based on intent-to-treat analysis, event-free survival was 68% versus 64% for high-dose compared to intermediate dose (EFS [event-free survival]) chemotherapy; and overall survival was 78% and 80%, respectively. Neither outcome showed a significant difference between the experimental and the control arms. Peters also reported fewer relapses for high-dose patients, but higher treatment-related mortality (29 treatment-related deaths occurred in the high-dose group but none in the intermediate dose group). However, the study design called for an additional 3 years of follow-up, so with only 60% of the expected events, he gamely announced, "The outcome data are currently inconclusive for policy decisions" (p. 21b). A press release from the Barbara Ann Karmanos Cancer Institute at Wayne State University in Detroit, where Peters was president, also put a positive spin on results.

The effect of these two U.S. reports was palpable. Not only had the Philadelphia trial reported no benefit for metastatic breast cancer, but also the CALGB report by the procedure's foremost advocate was stunning. Peters's advocacy of the procedure, including his 1993 *Journal of Clinical Oncology* paper showing dramatic differences in outcomes between the high-dose procedure and historical controls, had persuaded many of his colleagues to embrace HDC/ABMT. His advocacy had influenced judges, brow-beaten insurers, influenced the Office of Personnel Management, and cajoled state legislatures. Notwithstanding the preliminary nature of the trial results, the report was a dramatic comedown from expectations. Contrary to Peters's admonition, the decisions that counted were not policy decisions but what patients would decide on the basis of their doctors' recommendations. Those decisions, as we shall see in the following chapter, led to a dramatic decline in the number of procedures conducted as patients and doctors walked away from the procedure.

Two international trials reported results in the plenary session. A Scandinavian trial of 525 high-risk patients had compared HDC with conventional therapy "tailored" to the individual patient (NCI 1999c, answers to questions 7 and 8). Thus, it was not a direct comparison of HDC versus conventional chemotherapy. With 20 months of median follow-up, this trial showed no difference in overall survival and a greater recurrence of breast cancer in the high-dose group. This trial reinforced the verdict of no benefit (Scandinavian Breast Cancer Study Group 1999).

The only trial reporting positive results was a South African trial. Werner Bezwoda, University of Witwatersrand, reported that 154 high-risk breast cancer patients with seven to nine nodes positive had been entered into a randomized trial of HDC with peripheral blood stem cell rescue versus standard dose CAF chemotherapy (Bezwoda 1999). Median follow-up exceeded 5 years. The women receiving HDC had fewer relapses than patients who received a standard dose (25% compared to 66%) and had lower mortality (17% compared to 35%). In 1995, Bezwoda's article reported the use of a conventional dose lower than the standard conventional dose used in the United States, which had subjected the study to serious question in the literature. In 1999, then, he reported conventional treatment comparable to that used in the United States.

On Saturday, the 17th, the same day as the plenary session, an Op-Ed piece by David Eddy and Craig Henderson appeared in the New York Times. In "A Cancer Treatment Under a Cloud," they wrote that based on the summaries of the four trials released two days earlier, HDC/ABMT "is not a miracle cure" and the results "do not show the leap in survival rates that had been predicted" (Eddy and Henderson, 1999, p. A17). They pointed to "an equally compelling fact: we should know whether treatment works before we routinely pay for it." "We should also recognize," they wrote, "that insurers are generally justified in withholding routine payments for a new treatment until its effects are known," not for bottom line reasons but for quality of care. However, they added, insurers could also "take the initiative" to finance important clinical trials that will "answer critical medical questions quickly."

The fifth trial, presented at a poster session, was a smaller French trial of HDC/ABMT (Lotz et al. 1999). Sixty-one patients had been randomized after induction treatment, 29 to standard treatment and 32 to intensive HDC. Although progression-free survival was 15.7 and 26.9 months for the standard and experimental groups, respectively, and 2-year relapse rates were 52% and 27%, respectively, there was no statistical significance between the two groups in overall survival. This was one more trial involving small numbers of patients.

Bezwoda's positive findings lacked the force of the negative results of the other trials, but his results would hang there in clinical mid-air, so to speak, suspended until they could be replicated elsewhere. The following year, however, would clarify the meaning of this trial as dramatically as the other four trials had done, as we discuss in the following chapter.

A full decade after the NCI had agreed to sponsor high-priority randomized clinical trials, the results of the promising HDC/ABMT procedure for breast cancer were finally being reported. The procedure had been used initially with women with metastatic breast cancer, for whom there were few good therapies, but it had increasingly been applied during the decade to high-risk breast cancer patients. Contrary to the hopes of many women and their physicians, the 1999 reports—although preliminary—pointed to no benefit. There were some positive results, but no overall survival benefit. Nothing would shake the general pessimism of the moment. Indeed, subsequent events would deal even more harshly with the high expectations many had for HDC/ABMT.

9

Dénouement

To be in Error and to be Cast Out is also part of God's Design.
—William Blake

The one beneficial outcome of this saga may be the acknowledgment that experimental treatment must be assumed to be experimental until sound, ample evidence is reviewed and presented
—Jane Sprague Zones

Utilization of high-dose chemotherapy with autologous bone marrow transplantation (HDC/ABMT) for breast cancer plummeted after the negative reports at the 1999 American Society of Clinical Oncology (ASCO) meeting. The two U.S. trials reported by Stadtmauer and Peters influenced American clinical practice most strongly, but Scandinavian and French trial reports reinforced that effect. The Philadelphia trial had concluded that HDC/ABMT was no better than conventional treatment for metastatic breast cancer. William Peters, the foremost advocate for the procedure, had reported that it was no better for high-risk patients in overall survival. The Autologous Blood and Marrow Transplant Registry stopped indicating breast cancer in the total number of transplant procedures it counted. Response Oncology suffered revenue losses and steadily closed a number of its centers. Finally, some insurers acted on coverage policy to withdraw what had been extended earlier. In mid-February 2000, for example, Aetna/US HealthCare informed physicians that it would no longer reimburse HDC/ABMT treatments of breast cancer for its 1.6 million members (Kolata and Eichenwald 2000). Left unanswered, however, was how two South African trials, the first reported in 1995 and the other presented at the 1999 ASCO meeting, had produced positive results.

The seeds for decline in the use of HDC/ABMT had been planted before the ASCO meeting. Litigation after *Fox v. HealthNet* (No. 219692, Superior Court of California [1993]) had not produced an unbroken string of plaintiffs' triumphs but rather a set of seesaw results, quite different from what many had assumed. Many technology assessments had concluded that the data did not support claims that HDC/ABMT was superior to conventional therapy, and ECRI in 1995 had concluded both no benefit and potential harm. Although its effects are unknown, the ECRI patient guide of 1996 led some patient advocates to caution prospective patients. From 1996, the National Comprehensive Cancer Network stated that the data were insufficient to support the development of clinical practice guidelines for HDC/ABMT in breast cancer (National

Comprehensive Cancer Network 1997). Hortobagyi and colleagues had published several papers suggesting that the patient selection criteria for phase 2 studies were a factor that may have biased phase 2 outcome data (Rahman et al. 1997, 1998; Wright-Browne and Hortobagyi 1996). The 1998 Dutch pilot study reported no benefit. By the mid-1990s, it had become increasingly clear to many women that the treatment was very severe, even though treatment-related mortality was declining. Clinicians were seeing more patients with metastatic breast cancer who were relapsing within months after treatment with HDC/ABMT. As a result, clinicians and patients were slowly becoming disenchanted with a procedure that showed few visible benefits and subjected some patients to painful deaths.

South Africa

Werner Bezwoda was the leading oncologist in South Africa. His 1995 article published in the *Journal of Clinical Oncology* had been very influential in the United States as the only randomized trial comparing HDC with conventional treatment of metastatic breast cancer, and it had reported positive results (Bezwoda et al. 1995). But, the 1995 trial had been severely criticized because Bezwoda's conventional regimen included vincristine, a drug not active against breast cancer. This regimen was unique to South Africa, weak by U.S. standards, and not comparable to CAF (cyclophosphamide, doxorubicin, 5-fluorouracil) therapy, which was standard in the United States. In response, Bezwoda's 1999 trial of high-risk breast cancer patients compared CAF conventional treatment directly to HDC/conventional treatment in two tandem cycles to demonstrate the effectiveness of HDC relative to conventional U.S. treatment (Bezwoda 1999). This high-dose regimen involved no induction period and relied on tandem transplant cycles. Perhaps two cycles of high dose were better than one.[1]

The 1999 ASCO meeting abstracts were available several weeks before the meeting, and the contradiction between Bezwoda's results and those reported by others was clear. Some oncologists were openly skeptical. Raymond Weiss, a general oncologist, was seated in the second row of the 1999 ASCO plenary session "taking notes furiously."[2] Weiss is a major figure in cancer clinical trial auditing, having been the chair since 1981 of the Cancer and Leukemia Group B (CALGB) audit committee.[3] In 1993, he had described that group's audit system in the context of trials conducted by the National Cancer Institute (NCI) cooperative groups (Weiss et al. 1993). In 1998, he wrote: "The size of these [cooperative] groups, their geographical dispersion, and the number of studies accruing patients at any one time make it a challenge to ensure that all requirements of institutional oversight, patient consent, protocol compliance, and data submission and quality are met" (Weiss 1998, p. S88). He also chaired the committee that audited CALGB 9082, which involved auditing at least one patient for every investigator who had entered a patient in the trial, conducting a special audit of the Duke patients, and auditing 28% of all patients in the trial.

In February 1999, at a CALGB breast committee meeting, Weiss learned that Peters would report negative results at the ASCO meeting. In mid-March, when

ASCO abstracts became available, he saw that Bezwoda would report positive results. Before the May meeting, he proposed to Jeff Abrams that the NCI audit the South African trial and offered to help organize it. The debate over HDC was so contentious, he argued, that an audit would help clear the air. Abrams showed no enthusiasm for an audit as South Africa was a foreign country, and the NCI had provided no financial support to the trial. "Let's hear the paper," he said. At the end of May, the NCI said no to an audit: The U.S. studies were negative; we believe the U.S. studies; and Bezwoda is a non-U.S. investigator.

In addition to auditing clinical trials, Weiss was skeptical of the benefits of HDC/ABMT. In the 1990s, he was a reviewer for the Medical Care Ombudsman Program (MCOP) of coverage denials for specific patients. In June 1999, he wrote a critical review for MCOP of HDC/ABMT (MCOP Consultants 1999). He reviewed four randomized clinical trials for metastatic breast cancer, concluding that "the results of these trials . . . suggest that transplant does not produce any better overall long-term survival than treatment with chemotherapy given in conventional doses" (MCOP Consultants 1999, p. 18). The single trial suggesting benefit was the 1995 South African trial, but its protocol differed from standard treatment in the United States. The other randomized studies had not shown favorable outcomes. The Eastern Cooperative Oncology Group (ECOG) (Philadelphia) trial "can be considered to be the best assessment of the efficacy of [HDC/ABMT] by U.S. standards" (p. 18). Moreover, it had "on-site auditing" of a large sample of patient records "for verification of patient eligibility for the study and compliance with the treatment" (p. 18). The "preponderance of evidence" was that HDC/ABMT did not produce "a meaningful long-term benefit" over standard chemotherapy. For patients with high-risk breast cancer, "the preponderance of evidence is again against the transplant regimen" (MCOP Consultants 1999, p. 18).

Using Weiss' review as a starting point, the Medical Care Management Corporation, parent of MCOP, established a panel of experts to review the nine prospective, randomized trials of HDC/ABMT that had reported their outcomes (MCMC Consultants 1999). The review concluded that none of the studies showed that HDC/ABMT was superior to standard therapy for women with either metastatic or high-risk breast cancer, that "the previously reported 20%–30% improvement in health outcomes does not exist;" that the treatment was "experimental/investigational" and "cannot be regarded as standard of care at this time;" and that the use of HDC/ABMT for breast cancer "should only be performed within the context of a scientifically adequate clinical trial" (MCMC Consultants 1999, p. 1).

Based partly on his review for the MCOP, and taking the ASCO reports into account, as the MCMC consultants did, Weiss would publish a critique of HDC/ABMT for breast cancer in December 1999 (Weiss 1999). The question he asked was this: "Does such therapy truly provide a benefit to women with breast cancer, and is it therefore a therapy that should be routinely offered to suitable patients?" (p. 450). In succession, he reviewed the 1995 South African metastatic trial, the ECOG Philadelphia metastatic trial, the 1999 PEGASE (Programme d'Etude de la Greffe Autologous dans les Cancer du Sein) 04 metastatic trial, the 1999 Dutch high-risk pilot trial, the 1998 Hortobagyi high-risk trial, the 1999 Bergh Scandinavian trial, the CALGB 9082 trial, the 1999 South African high-risk trial, a 1999 retrospective comparison of four CALGB conventional dose trials with women in the Autologous Blood and Marrow Transplant Registry receiving HDC, the ECOG high-risk trial that had yet to report, and the Intergroup trial that had yet to report. Results of all trials had to be considered preliminary as most had only been published in abstract form, several had not been published at all, and follow-up was "somewhat limited." Even so, Weiss concluded "the overall message for each is unlikely to change" (p. 455). Notwithstanding the 1995 South African results, "the preponderance of scientific evidence is that transplant therapy for metastatic breast cancer has failed to have a significant effect on overall survival" (p. 455). He continued: "The overall results in high-risk early disease also do not demonstrate a strong effect of transplant therapy" (p. 456). Weiss did suggest, however, that the South African regimen of treating high-risk patients without induction therapy was "a scientific point possibly to test further" (p. 456). This is where the discussion stood at the end of 1999.

The Audit of the 1999 Trial

In addition to his skepticism about the 1995 trial, other concerns led Weiss to propose an audit. In January of 1999, he had visited South Africa on vacation with his son. He wished to meet Bezwoda but didn't know him and had no direct entrée to him. He did visit the oncologists at the University of Pretoria, about 20 miles from Johannesburg, several of whom he knew as the university was an ECOG member. What did they think of Bezwoda's work? he asked. "We are not so convinced of it," they responded. "He does not have the follow-up" (Weiss 2002a).

Unexpectedly, in July 1999, Bill Peters called Weiss to say that he had arranged with Bezwoda to audit the high-risk trial in the first week in September.[4] Peters was unaware of Weiss's suggestion that the NCI sponsor an audit but well aware of his audit experience. This was short notice. Roy Beveridge, a Fairfax, Virginia, transplanter in private practice who had been trained at Hopkins, was told to put an audit team together. Beveridge also recruited Alan Herman, a doctor of medicine/doctor of philosophy at Howard University, whom he knew as their children attended Sidwell Friends School in Washington, D.C. Herman, a "colored" South African émigré who had favored the abolition of apartheid while at the University of Southern Africa in Pretoria, had been invited back later by the university to establish a public health unit.[5] He would spend 2–3 months each year in Pretoria but never with the intention of returning permanently. Importantly, he knew the South African minister of health.

Bezwoda then sent word that the audit team could not come in September. The visit was put on hold for rescheduling. In October, Beveridge and Weiss met to discuss the audit, which was to be conducted like a CALGB audit. Weiss said he could make the trip in the third week of January 2000. Weiss then wrote Bezwoda asking for the trial protocol to develop an audit work sheet. He also asked for contact information for the trial data manager. Bezwoda responded that a four-person team would be the maximum size, and only 2 days would be allowed for the audit. The audit team accepted these conditions but wondered how four people could audit a trial of 154 patients in 2 days.

No protocol had arrived by December 1, so Weiss again asked for it by letter and e-mail. It had not come by December 10. Bezwoda then wrote Weiss to say that the audit team could not come. The importance that U.S. investigators attached to the audit was underlined on December 15 at an NCI meeting with the cooperative groups to discuss the next HDC/ABMT breast cancer study. Peters, Weiss, and Beveridge attended. The consensus was to try to replicate Bezwoda's approach using HDC/ABMT with no induction therapy compared to the South African's conventional therapy. After this meeting, Alan Herman called the South African minister of health to express great concern about Bezwoda's effort to block the audit visit. The minister spoke to Bezwoda. Joseph Bailes, then the ASCO president, also called Bezwoda and said that he must permit the audit. Just before the holidays, Bezwoda reluctantly agreed to the visit. Team members were relieved as all had nonrefundable airline tickets.

When Weiss left on January 1 for a 2-week vacation in Israel, there was still no protocol. An audit work sheet could not be developed without a trial protocol. It had still not arrived on Sunday, January 14, when Weiss returned. Beveridge finally received it on Monday, January 15, and Weiss got it the following day before a scheduled Saturday departure on the January 20. In fact, Weiss received two protocols, one for the 1999 trial and the other—unsolicited—for the 1995 trial. These protocols provided the initial basis that something was amiss. They indicated that the 1995 trial had used a conventional regimen, which had been reported, but the protocol cover sheet showed that the second trial had also done so, contrary to what had been reported at the ASCO meeting, although the protocol text said CAF. Moreover, the ASCO-reported dose of Adriamycin differed from that indicated in the protocol. Both protocols had been prepared using the identical type font. Weiss recalls that his immediate suspicion was that Bezwoda had something to hide: the initial trip cancellation, limiting the team to four people and the audit to 2 days, and the second attempted cancellation. He thought there was some reason for embarrassment.

Weiss made up a work sheet for the 1999 trial of the high-risk population. On Thursday, he received the information requested in early October, the name (M. Bezwoda) and phone number of the trial data manager. He called but got no answer. "I wanted to know where we would be working," he said (Weiss 2002a). The team flew on Saturday, arrived in Johannesburg on Sunday morning, and stayed in an inexpensive bed and breakfast in a well-guarded part of town.[6] This was the first time that the team, which included Beveridge, Weiss, Marc Stewart, and Robert Theriault (a neutral breast cancer doctor from M. D. Anderson, not a transplanter), had been assembled. The team also took Lori Williams, a registered nurse, and Robert Rivkin, a computer-savvy physician, for support.

The initial meeting was scheduled for Tuesday afternoon. On Monday, Weiss called the number for the data manager, who turned out to be Sister M. Bezwoda, a nurse, and Werner Bezwoda's wife.[7] She indicated that the team would only be able to get approximately half of the 154 records, all of the HDC arm, but none of the control arm. Many of the controls had been treated in Hillside Hospital, a black hospital, which had been closed after apartheid ended. Charts for the controls were "in a room behind chicken wire" at Hillside. Weiss offered the assistance of the audit team to search for the records, but Sister Bezwoda declined.

The team went to Johannesburg Hospital (1,200 beds, with as many as 12 beds to a room) on Tuesday and met with Bezwoda. He was cold and unsmiling, "very reserved," according to Weiss. Weiss thanked him for the protocols. For the high-risk patients, the protocol indicated that the HDC regimen was conventional, but it was reported as CAF at the ASCO meeting, Weiss noted. That was a "typo," Bezwoda responded. Also, the Adriamycin dose for CAF in the protocol was not the same as that reported at the ASCO conference, and the difference (between 50 and 60 mg) was significant. That also was a "typo." The team was shown the charts. The height of all the charts was approximately 16 cm, about the thickness of a single patient chart for CALGB 9082. Weiss again asked Bezwoda for any of the control charts that were available, but Bezwoda said he had not provided them because Beveridge had not asked for them. Beveridge knew this was untrue as he held in his hand the two letters he had sent Bezwoda making the request. Beveridge chose to remain silent.

On Wednesday, the team was given a list of patients for both the 1995 and 1999 trials. Both lists were written in exactly the same handwriting, which Weiss regarded as strange because a contemporaneous list of entrants would have typically involved several different people entering patients. "Is this a contemporaneous list?" Weiss asked. "Yes," was the response. However, the first four patients on the list got CAF, the next five received HDC treatment, and the final five on the list got HDC. The odds of this sequence occurring if patients were actually being randomized were extraordinarily low.

The audit team, working in two teams of two people, reviewed the patient records. Each thin file had a pathology report and outpatient records. The members finished their review in 4 hours and returned to their bed and breakfast. Williams and Rivkin put all the data into the computer and for each patient wrote questions and comments, such as, Was there a chest X-ray? There is data missing regarding the second dose, etc.? On Thursday, all four auditors reviewed each file. Approximately 90% of the patients were black, whereas the ASCO presentation reported that only 60% were black. Often, there was no signature on notes in the records. Notes were all in the same handwriting. Individual consent forms were not found in patient files, even though a three-page consent form was included in the protocol.

The group now had lots of suspicions. Either Bezwoda had made up the control files or the controls did not receive CAF. An exit interview was held on Friday morning before a Saturday departure. "Could we at least see one control file," Weiss asked? No, Bezwoda answered. Then, the team heard Bezwoda's third excuse: It took 3 months to get the charts together; if they would give him another 3 months, he could get the control records. Weiss then asked the Perry Mason question: "Dr. Bezwoda, Is the reason that you are unable to provide us access to the control files because these patients did not receive CAF?" "No," was his answer. "You have all the records that are available" (Weiss 2002a). The auditors concluded that Bezwoda had written the two protocols shortly before the audit team left the United States for South Africa, that the typos were uncorrected and unnoticed, that it was unlikely that the same type font would have been used for two protocols prepared several years apart, and that both patient lists were made up.

Alan Herman had arrived in South Africa late Thursday evening and had met with the team on Friday morning. They laid out their suspicions. Herman spoke to the chair of the Committee for Research on Human Subjects (the local institutional review board [IRB]) and spoke to the minister of health. On 8:30 A.M., the Monday morning after the auditors had left, a letter from Bezwoda, typed by him, was delivered to all the staff. "I regret to inform you that the study we reported did not use CAF." He was fired from the university the next day for scientific fraud. The university sent a letter to ASCO and posted a Web site release on Thursday of that week.

"My phone started ringing," Weiss recalls. "The pressure was on to put this in print." The University of Witwatersrand had due process procedures that required a hearing within 60–90 days of its action against Bezwoda. Bezwoda's faculty colleagues would judge him at the hearing. These were apparently recent requirements, and only three faculty—none with medical training—had been qualified to conduct hearings under the new process. The hearing, to be conducted by two mathematicians and a professor of English, was scheduled for March 10, 2000.

Weiss inquired whether the *New England Journal of Medicine* would publish the account of the audit, but the request was turned down. The matter had already been "adequately discussed in public" (Weiss 2002a). Simultaneously, *The Lancet* associate editor, David McNamee, wrote (Weiss 2002a) to say that they would be pleased to publish an account of the audit but wanted it for the March 10 issue, concurrent with the Witwatersrand hearing 6 weeks away. By the end of February, the audit team's paper had been e-mailed to *The Lancet.* An electronic peer review took only 48 hours to obtain four reviews, three suggesting minor changes and one expounding on scientific fraud. The coauthors agreed to the suggested changes by March 2 or 3 and received the galleys back by March 4 or 5. The *Lancet* editors knew that the audit report could not be included in the March 10 issue but posted it on the Web by then and printed it in the March 18 issue. Weiss believes that this was the fastest peer-reviewed paper in history, taking only 6 weeks from the start of writing to publication.

The *Lancet* article began by noting the controversy surrounding HDC/ABMT (Weiss et al. 2000). Historical controls suggesting an advantage had not been confirmed by randomized studies, save the two studies by Bezwoda of metastatic and high-risk breast cancer patients. A U.S. audit team had conducted an on-site review of the 1999 high-risk study "to corroborate the study results before starting a large international confirmatory study" (p. 999). The audit report was devastating: Limited numbers of records had been made available, all of the HDC recipients but none of the controls; there was "much disparity" between the reviewed records and the data presented at two international meetings; the reviewers saw no signed informed consents; the institutional review board had no record of approving the study; and after the site visit Bezwoda "admitted scientific misconduct by using a different control chemotherapy regimen from that described in presented data" (p. 999). The somewhat laconic "interpretation" was this: "The Bezwoda study should not be used as the basis for further trials to test the efficacy of the cyclophosphamide, mitoxantrone, etoposide regimen for high-dose chemotherapy in women with high-risk primary breast cancer. This review validates the essential nature of on-site audits, especially in single-institution studies" (p. 999).

In an accompanying commentary, Jonas Bergh (2000) wrote that the Weiss report "necessitates a rethink" of the HDC/ABMT approach to breast cancer. Horton, *The Lancet* editor, drew "four immediate lessons" from the report of Bezwoda's fraud (Horton 2000). First, "a fast and thorough investigation" with timely publication of results was the best way to resolve uncertainty when "suspicion falls on an individual or research group" (p. 943). Second, the "pivotal role" of the IRB was "underlined once again." A recommendation from Duke University, unrelated to South Africa, that the costs for IRB oversight "be recoverable for federally and privately funded research" needed to be applied well beyond the United States (p. 943). Third, scientific societies "must look again at their abstract review procedures" (p. 943) for discrepancies that should raise warning signs. Fourth, the Bezwoda case strengthened the argument for "an international register of randomized trials" (p. 943).

Peter Cleaton-Jones, chair of the University of Witwatersrand Committee for Research on Human Subjects, described the IRB's process in a letter and recounted the events set in motion by the audit. Tellingly he stated: "No record of ethics committee approval for this [Bezwoda's] study was found" (Cleaton-Jones 2000, p. 1001). He indicated that the university had dealt with the audit team with "speed, openness, and cooperation." A formal inquiry into the alleged misconduct had been set in motion within an hour of Bezwoda's acknowledgment of misrepresentation of the control arm of the study. He further noted that the misconduct was "by an individual, not an institution." The university, by contrast, "upholds international standards of research ethics."

On February 4, 2000, at 6 weeks before *The Lancet* publication, the NCI posted the results of the independent audit on its Web site. Jeff Abrams was quoted as saying: "The falsification of the South African study is devastating. However, an even greater tragedy could result if this news causes patients and doctors in the United States and around the world to avoid clinical trials of transplants altogether. The basic research this treatment is based on remains solid, and we urgently need to complete well-conducted, carefully monitored, randomized trials to figure out which breast cancer patients could benefit most from high-dose chemotherapy plus transplants" (NCI 2000).

Also on February 4, ASCO issued this statement: "Although the peer-review of the [Bezwoda] abstract prior to the Annual Meeting revealed no irregularities," an independent U.S. audit team had "found significant deviations from standard conduct in following a research protocol" (ASCO Online 2000). Joseph Bailes, the ASCO president, said "The Society regards these developments with the utmost seriousness" and would cooperate fully with the University of Witwatersrand in its investigation.

At the March 10 hearing regarding his dismissal, Bezwoda had patients testify to his qualifications as an oncologist. Beveridge and Rivkin, members of the audit team, testified at a time specified but were not allowed to observe the entire hearing. They reported that the patients appeared troubled by the report of fraud. The three professors on the hearing panel knew very little about the case until the hearing. Bezwoda mentioned his letter regarding CAF. The three recognized fraud immediately. The faculty upheld the firing; Bezwoda lost his retirement pension. At the time of his dismissal, there was talk of legal action by Dr. Bezwoda against the university but no legal papers were ever filed. For a time, Bezwoda continued in private practice. In August 2003, the Health Professions Council of South Africa suspended his physician's license for 5 years; this penalty was then suspended for 4.5 years on condition that he not be found guilty of a similar offense within the next 5 years, that he not administer any form of HDC except if based on internationally recognized research, and that he not engage in any form of research on HDC without approval of the relevant authorities (Weiss 2003).

The Second Audit of the First Trial

Weiss had become suspicious of the first South African trial after the audit of the 1999 study. Bezwoda's 1995 study continued to be cited in the United States as evidence of the effectiveness of HDC/ABMT (Bezwoda et al. 1995). It was a randomized study, which everyone had been demanding; it reported positive results with 90 patients; and it was published in the *Journal of Clinical Oncology,* the premier oncology journal, with a favorable accompanying editorial by M. John Kennedy, a transplanter at Johns Hopkins University (Kennedy 1995). Although no one in the United States provided conventional treatment exactly as Bezwoda's control arm specified, the fact that the trial was randomized, reported positive results, and was published in the *Journal of Clinical Oncology,* were persuasive.

When the 1995 study was published, Weiss recalled, "Hoover Dam broke." Transplanters now argued to insurers, "It [HDC/ABMT] is no longer experimental." And, as indicated in chapter 7, Blue Cross Blue Shield Association modified its view. True, the trial had been done in South Africa and little was known about treatment in that first world–third world country. The argument was made that it was unethical to put women in trials in the United States and not offer them HDC/ABMT treatment. Resistance by insurers to offering treatment was regarded as strictly financial. The conclusion was that transplantation works. Why put a patient in a study? Why do a randomized controlled trial? How can this be denied to a 38-year-old mother of two children, aged 2 and 5, who only wishes to see her kids grow up?

After the first audit, Weiss had exchanged e-mail communications with Peter Cleaton-Jones, assistant dean, University of Witwatersrand School of Medicine, who was responsible for inquiry into the Bezwoda affair. Weiss suggested the need to audit the first trial. The university was interested but had no money to finance an audit. "I went to ASCO asking them to finance it, but the executive committee turned down the request on a 9-to-7 vote," Weiss recalled. "NCI, for reasons related to its unwillingness to become involved in the first audit, was not interested" (Weiss 2002b). The University of Witwatersrand wanted an audit in line with international practice to question research done by individuals known to have committed research misconduct.

Weiss assembled an audit team that included himself, Clifford Hudis of Sloan-Kettering, and Lesley Seymour of Queens University, Kingston, Ontario. Roger Dansey, a former colleague of Bezwoda's at Witwatersrand who was then with Peters in Detroit, was asked to be on the team but declined. A South African pharmacist, Geraldine Gill, experienced with drug company trials, was recruited and worked on the audit from September through December 2000. She searched the Hillside Hospital files, the Witwatersrand hospital files, the South African tumor registry files, and all other conceivable sources using the patient names and hospital numbers on the list provided by Bezwoda. She found about 67 of the 90 files. The audit team reviewed the files and concluded that the notes were fabricated, and that this trial was also fraudulent. The Weiss audit team's report was published in the June 1, 2001, issue of the *Journal of Clinical Oncology* (Weiss et al. 2001). In that same issue, the journal would formally retract the Bezwoda paper it had published in 1995 (*Journal of Clinical Oncology* 2001).

News of the second instance of fraud and the retraction would be widely disseminated (NCI 2001). Dr. Larry Norton, in an editorial accompanying the Weiss report and the *Journal of Clinical Oncology* retraction, addressed the dependence of clinical oncology on "the randomized, prospective clinical trial" (Norton 2001, p. 2769). Medicine was just now emerging, he wrote, from "the tyranny of 'expert opinion.'" He added: "Our increasing emphasis on evidence-based medicine will properly replace conjecture with knowledge, tradition with rationality, and subjective experience with objective data" (p. 2769). Weiss and his team had done a "great service," and auditing was "a crucial addition to the scientific method in medicine." He added this caveat: "That the original publication, now being retracted by the Journal, has influenced major thinkers in this field and may have put patients in danger raises the stakes as we consider how we can improve the process to make sure that this never happens again" (p. 2769).

The Data Are Not Yet In

Another response to the 1999 ASCO reports from the transplant community was that the data were preliminary. Karen Antman, who had promoted the HDC/ABMT procedure in the late 1980s and early 1990s as effective treatment on the basis of phase 2 studies, now argued that it was premature to draw conclusions about the procedure's ineffectiveness until the phase 3 trials had run their course. More follow-up data were needed (Antman 2001a, 2001b). Hortobagyi, an early proponent of HDC/ABMT who had then adopted a cautious stance of recommending that the treatment be provided only in clinical trials, also cautioned against premature dismissal of HDC until the data had been reported from the randomized clinical trials.

Dr. Yago Nieto, a member of the University of Colorado Bone Marrow Transplantation Program, a prominent center for HDC/ABMT headed by Roy Jones and Elizabeth Shpall (until she moved to M. D. Anderson), wrote two reviews. In 2000, his abstract read:

> The encouraging results of phase 2 trials suggested a benefit for HDC in high-risk primary breast cancer and some categories of patients with metastatic breast cancer. Some investigators have argued that patient selection might have been a critical factor in those studies. Recently reported randomized trials in patients with chemosensitive metastatic breast cancer have included only small numbers of patients in complete remission and thus have not adequately addressed the relative value of HDC versus maintenance standard-dose chemotherapy in this patient subset. Although initial results of 2 studies have been reported, most randomized phase 3 studies of HDC in high-risk primary breast cancer require longer follow-up before definitive conclusions can be made about its efficacy in this setting. We conclude that the role of HDC for high-risk primary breast cancer or metastatic breast cancer patients has not yet been fully defined. Longer follow-up of the ongoing randomized trials is necessary, and their mature results will help clarify this important question. In the meantime, it is imperative that research continues, to enhance the efficacy of the procedure. (Nieto et al. 2000, p. 476. © 2000. Reprinted with permission from the American Society for Blood and Marrow Transplantation.)

In February 2003, Nieto would publish an article, "The Verdict Is Not In Yet. Analysis of the Randomized Trials of High-Dose Chemotherapy for Breast Cancer" (Nieto 2003). However, the trials reported at the 2003 ASCO meetings would bring the HDC episode much closer to a verdict, and not one supported Nieto, Antman, and the transplant advocates. The 2004 ASCO meeting would not report any reason to question the earlier reports.

The Data Come In Finally

All of the NCI high-priority trials have now reported. Stadtmauer and colleagues reported on the ECOG-Philadelphia trial (E/PBT-01) on metastatic breast cancer, begun in 1990, at the 1999 ASCO meeting and published their final results in the *New England Journal of Medicine* in April 2000 (Stadtmauer et al. 2000). Lippman, one of the signers of the 1990 "Dream Team" document, in an accompanying editorial noted that the phase 2 studies had claimed "rather astounding benefits" compared to historical controls (Lippman 2000, p. 1119), but the "detailed analyses of selection bias" showed the "impossibility of drawing valid conclusions" from such uncontrolled studies. The negative results, he argued, should not diminish enthusiasm for the "prospective evaluation" of other approaches. But such approaches, he continued, "are experimental and should be validated only in appropriately designed trials conducted at centers prepared to analyze and report their results" (p. 1120). He concluded: "We should now acknowledge that, to a reasonable degree of probability, this form of treatment for women with metastatic breast cancer has been proved to be ineffective and should be abandoned in favor of well-justified experimental approaches" (p. 1120).

Martin Tallman and colleagues reported the results of the Intergroup/ECOG trial (INT-0121/E-2190), which began in 1991, at the 2003 ASCO meeting (Tallman et al. 2003a). Those results appeared a month later in a paper in the *New England Journal of Medicine,* which concluded: "The addition of high-dose chemotherapy and autologous hematopoietic stem-cell transplantation to six cycles of adjuvant chemotherapy with CAF may reduce the risk of relapse but does not improve the outcome among patients with primary breast cancer and at least 10 involved axillary lymph nodes" (Tallman et al. 2003b, p. 17).

The CALGB 9082 trial, which began in 1990, had also reported preliminary results at the ASCO 1999 meeting. A manuscript reporting final results was submitted to the *Journal of Clinical Oncology* in September 2003, accepted for publication in August 2004, and published on April 1, 2005 (Peters et al. 2005). Peters was first author and Richard Schilsky, chair of CALGB, the corresponding author. The high-dose regimen of cyclophosphamide, cisplatin, and carmustine (CPB) showed no significant difference compared to the intermediate-dose regimen of the same drugs for the primary endpoint of event-free survival. Overall survival was "identical" for the two arms. Thirty-three patients died of treatment-related causes in the experimental arm compared to none in the control arm. The conclusion: "HD-CPB [the high-dose regimen] with stem-cell support was not superior to ID-CPB [the intermediate dose regimen] for event-free survival or overall survival among all randomized women with high-risk primary breast cancer" (p. 2191).

The SWOG/Intergroup 9623 trial, which had been closed in 2001 due to poor enrollment, presented a final analysis of its results in a poster session at the 2005 ASCO annual meeting. Transplantation did not show superior disease-free or overall survival and actually had poorer outcomes. The abstract concluded: "There is no evidence that adjuvant high dose chemotherapy with AHPCS [autologous hematopoietic progenitor cell support] provides better outcomes for women with ≥4 positive nodes" (Bearman et al. 2005).

In addition to these NCI-sponsored U.S. trials, three other trials would be reported at the 2003 ASCO meeting. Rodenhuis reported further data on the Dutch study, which would also be published in the June 2003 issue of the *New England Journal of Medicine* (Rodenhuis et al. 2003). The Dutch investigators found that "high-dose alkylating therapy improves relapse-free survival among patients with stage II or III breast cancer and 10 or more positive axillary lymph nodes" (p. 7). However, they found "no significant difference" in overall survival. Basser, from Australia, reported on an international trial. In addition, Crown reported on the Anglo-Celtic trial in a poster session. In general, much to the disappointment of the transplanters, these trials reported either no benefit for HDC or marginal benefit for a subset of patients identified only after the fact.

Perspective

In October 1999, Gina Kolata and Kurt Eichenwald, in a front page *New York Times* article, wrote that women had been told "for more than a decade" that HDC/ABMT was "the only treatment that could save their lives" (Kolata and Eichenwald 1999, p. A1). In reality, "no one knew for sure" whether it was better than conventional treatment. Bemoaning this characterization, Dr. Larry Norton, was quoted as saying: "Fifty years from now, we will look at this period with horror and say 'How could this have happened.'" More recently, Dr. John Crown, of St. Vincent's University Hospital, Dublin, would write, "Perhaps no treatment in medical history had as meteoric a rise, or as humiliating a fall from grace" as did HDC/ABMT for breast cancer (Crown 2004, p. 1299). Quite obviously, this story is one that should occasion reflection and effort to draw lessons.

The randomized clinical trials reporting in 1999 showed no significant benefit in overall survival for metastatic or high-risk breast cancer patients treated with HDC/ABMT and those receiving conventional treatment. These results have been confirmed in final reports, which have also failed to identify clearly the subset of women who might benefit from this procedure. More than a full decade was needed to obtain these results in the United States, largely because of the widespread availability of this treatment outside randomized trials. The absence of data of effectiveness of the procedure was not persuasive in the 1990s to patients and physicians. Only clinical trial data showing no effectiveness was persuasive.

The HDC/ABMT story also demonstrates the critical importance of the clinical trial audit. The validation of data is essential to maintaining the trust of patients and the public in the results of clinical trials. The integrity of the data and of the investigators who collect, analyze, and report the data require external scrutiny. Audits, we learn with regret, are essential to data validation. Fortunately, this audit function is well developed in the United States and increasingly used worldwide.

We hope that this account will stimulate reflection within oncology and more broadly within medicine about how such episodes can be avoided in the future. What drove widespread use? "Patient panic," Susan Love would state (Love 2004). Physician "enthusiasm," Gabriel Hortobagyi would say (2004). Money, many others would add. The institutional deficit we discuss in the next chapter allowed a default system of decision making (courts, legislatures, the press) to dominate events of the 1990s and override concern for the careful evaluation of a promising treatment.

Raymond Weiss reflected on his many reviews of contested HDC/ABMT breast cancer cases for the MCOP in the mid-1990s: "Most of the time I said that the evidence of effectiveness came from phase 2, uncontrolled studies, on highly selected patients; that randomized clinical trials were ongoing; that we didn't know if HDC/ABMT, which was still investigational, was better or not" (Weiss 2002a). Regarding the South African trials, especially the initial one, he said: "It was so tragic that Bezwoda contributed to the U.S. controversy in the way he did. I don't think he appreciated what the effect would be. But his 1995 study had a humongous influence. In my work for MCOP, I received medical records for review that many times included both the 1993 Peters paper and the 1995 Bezwoda paper. Bezwoda and Peters had an enormous worldwide impact on the use of this therapy" (Weiss 2002c).

How did women look back on the events of the 1990s? It is impossible to answer this question in any reasonable way without a massive research effort, and then the voices of many whom one would wish to contribute to such a project have been permanently stilled. But, we provide several responses by patients and their advocates that illustrate a range of views and indicate the importance and challenge of listening to patients.

Virginia Hetrick, a southern California resident, was diagnosed in early 1991 with stage III inflammatory breast cancer (Hetrick 2004a).[8] Originally evaluated at the University of California at Los Angeles, she received standard chemotherapy, which reduced her primary tumor by 55% within the next 11 weeks. This receptivity made her a candidate for HDC/ABMT. She was referred to City of Hope and evaluated there in August. Her insurer initially denied coverage but ultimately covered the treatment on threat of litigation and after she arranged for and completed the recommended treatment. "Going in, I was both excited and nervous," she would say; "excited by the prospect that this would be the end of my cancer treatment and I would feel good afterwards, but nervous because it was a [phase 2] clinical trial and I didn't know if [the procedure] it would work" (Hetrick 2004b). Hetrick had no hesitancy about HDC but was told that the hospital was using peripheral blood stem cells and no longer using bone marrow. "No second rate stuff for me," she objected to the oncologist. "I want the real thing." Because bone marrow was no longer a choice, she was persuaded that stem cells were the way to go. Stem cell harvest occurred in the weeks of Christmas and New Year's Day and high-dose treatment began in early January.

Hetrick is a survivor. She described graphically the effects of the treatment: isolation for several weeks; home by early February, with no appetite and mouth sores. But, this determined woman began walking on her street, increasing the distance by 10 house numbers a day, and described herself as "fully functional"

21 months after the transplant. Hetrick is a professional woman, highly oriented to obtaining information about her condition. She attributes her view of the procedure in large measure to her original oncologist at the University of California at Los Angeles, who explained the procedure in detail, gave Hetrick her home phone number, and patiently answered her questions on a weekend call.

Would she do it again? "In a heartbeat," she said, "even though I was about the 50th woman at the City of Hope to have the procedure. Probably the most important thing I learned when I was investigating this [procedure] was that the head of the Bone Marrow Oncology program believed that they would find that the procedure would work well for certain groups of patients and wouldn't work well for others. In the City of Hope studies, inflammatory breast cancer patients tend to turn out particularly well while metastatic patients tend not to have success with this procedure" (V. Hetrick, personal communication to R. A. Rettig, January 25, 2005).

Hetrick is also an original member of You Are Not Alone (YANA), a patient support group to help patients receiving HDC/ABMT for solid tumors. This group provides peer counseling, internships and other training of peer counselors, and stage IV pain management. Strongly oriented to getting information for herself, in the mid-1990s she advised others to investigate and decide for themselves whether to have the procedure and whether to participate in clinical trials. She does not attempt to impose her views on others "trying to make a hard decision" but does provide them information she has derived from the medical literature, City of Hope reports, and other sources. Hetrick supports the use of the procedure, but especially for inflammatory breast cancer.

Alice Philipson was a plaintiff's attorney who successfully fought insurers on behalf of breast cancer patients. She recounted her experience to Shannon Brownlee (Philipson 2000).[9]

> There aren't very many people who do work against insurance companies because there is no money in it. . . . So there aren't that many people who are trained to do it or even willing to do it. I know how to do it. I pretty much do it because of humanitarian and political reasons. You can make a living at it, but you don't get rich. . . . I was a young lawyer out of law school a year when AIDS happened and I joined the gay bar association. [Initially] I was the only one who had sued an insurance company. Now the AIDS referral panel has over 700 lawyers and this huge budget.
>
> My first breast cancer case was 1991. . . . It was the first time someone came to me and said, "I am being denied a life saving treatment." Her name was Ricki. She was 48. She had one child, still in high school. It [her breast cancer] had recurred within 3 years. When I met her, she was stage IV, she had failed the first round of treatment, and it was clearly going to be a fatal illness. It hadn't metastasized, but it was already moving around her body. It had clearly been traveling since the first time. She'd had chemotherapy and a mastectomy. She'd had positive nodes. She had micromets [micrometastases] the first time. . . . She found out about me, she had called around to the regular sources of lawyers. You go to your family lawyer, and they give you a couple of names, and she ended up at these law firms that said "I'll be happy to help, give me $20,000 to start." She knew what she wanted, and she and her husband were going to have to mortgage their house to get it, and she didn't have the money.
>
> She calls me and says "I have stage four breast cancer." What does that mean? "It means I'm going to die. I want this life saving treatment, and my insurance company

won't give it to me." I basically said, there are lots of treatments people want, and I used laetrile as an example. I haven't heard of this [HDC/ABMT], is it laetrile? I told her I had not done a breast cancer case; I'll have to learn the medicine. We made an appointment. I'm pretty strict, you have to bring this, you have to bring that, medical journal articles, hospital records, some money, and the insurance policy. I had to like her and be able to work with her. Ricki came; she had all this stuff, including these articles from Dana-Farber, scientific articles, about this treatment. She had sent her medical records to Dana-Farber, and they suggested she was a good candidate. Antman was on the articles, Bill Peters, Tom Frei. It was the sell job. The local doctor didn't want to do it himself, because he didn't have the expertise or facilities, but the treatment was available at Dana-Farber.

She wanted it done at Dana-Farber or UCSF. I thought it was legitimate, that it was not experimental, that it was cutting edge. And that's the big difference. If it is experimental, truly experimental, there's not much one can do. If it is the standard of care for these kinds of illnesses, it is the only chance this patient has to live. I said OK, we'll try. It [HDC/ABMT] had moved beyond experimental to cutting edge. And, the other factor is they were saying this was a cure, and that's a big deal. If they had said, OK its cutting edge, but we can only buy you a year, I wouldn't have done it. It cost $125,000 at that time, and that's a lot for a few extra month. . . .

I looked for other breast cancer cases, and I didn't find any. . . . I knew that the way you win these cases is only somewhat on whether it is viable; you win [because] the insurance company hasn't done a good job of evaluating it. So part of my approach, when I start to deal with an insurance company, I don't say "give her this treatment or I'm going to sue you." I say, you said no, give me everything you have that leads you to believe this isn't a good treatment. So I started getting all these articles together to persuade them, and because all they had done was send Ricki's file to their medical department, which said uh uh. With the patient, I prepared a giant packet of information, explaining why she was good candidate—she wasn't too old, no other disease—and then the legal argument: this is standard of care. I worked with a PhD who analyzed not the efficacy, but the number of times it had been done, who it had been done for, and whether or not this was standard of care. He looked at journal articles. I don't have to prove it is the best thing since sliced bread.

I sent off the packet. We are working against the clock. If her tumors get too big, she can't do it. We tell them, this is urgent. . . . Every 2 weeks I send them a letter. The insurance company approved it. It took months and months. Things are happening, because you have to have your [bone marrow] harvest when you don't have bone mets. She's getting monitored, and . . . while I'm wrestling with insurance, she has this harvest, and it looks good. She recovers, and everything is go. . . . I don't talk to insurance companies, I write to them. I only do informal conversations. I knew they were doing an inadequate investigation, and I knew I had them dead to rights, because the academic said it was cutting edge treatment.

So Ricki has her transplant. The insurance company said "If you don't tell anybody we approved this, we'll let you do it, but if we decide it isn't a good treatment, we'll bill you for it." But they never bill you. That way they don't go to court and it doesn't become a precedent. She makes it through the transplant. She got it, and of course we never heard boo from the insurance company.

Ricki died within 2 years [of treatment] for a cure. A cure! I was still in contact with her. When she died, I was very sad, because we had become friends, but I have people dying all the time. I think, wow this isn't so great for a cure. I wasn't pleased, but I didn't really approach it as a failure. But boy, that was just the first one. Then the next one died, and the next person. Now I'm starting to both worry about it, and every time I do one of these, I have to get current information. I have to do a Medline search, and the patients have to get it from me. If they can't do it, I don't do the case. So, I am getting stuff, and the cure language is gone. Now it's not a cure anymore. I'm thinking, what's happening here? I have to really have a clean case because I'm going up against the Forces of Evil, and that makes me have to decide what I'm going to spend my energy on. And now the docs aren't saying "it's a cure," [but that] "it buys time." They are not saying, it buys time but you can't raise your head, you are so sick, and it's so horrible and so hard, and you don't have time to say good bye to the people you love. . . . And everybody died. It was a cure that didn't work. Now Dana-Farber and those places stopped saying it was a cure. They were hedging.

Everybody on my caseload [fatally ill people] is going to die, and I have breast cancer, too, so we're all going to die. . . . But had to decide for myself whether I was going to take these cases any more, and I decided not to. HDC/ABMT didn't live up to its promise, it was a horrible treatment, and the outcome didn't match the effort. . . . I decided over time, watching my folks die, and seeing the shift in what was being said by the medical community, that all we were getting was an extension of life at very huge price to the patient in terms of quality of life, and huge financial commitment. And it wasn't worth it. All I was doing was extending the pain. I didn't want to be involved.

Anne Grant is angry. Although she is at peace about her personal decision to undergo HDC, she is angry about a lack of ethics, poor judgment, and greed by the medical and research communities in heavily marketing off-trial HDC without evidence of its superior effectiveness. In the October 19, 1998, issue of *The New Yorker,* Dr. Jerome Groopman wrote about bone marrow transplantation. Groopman, a hematologist-oncologist and frequent contributor to the magazine, described a leukemia patient successfully treated by an allogeneic BMT. He characterized the procedure as "the most powerful weapon in the growing arsenal against cancer." "Nevertheless," he wrote, "I cannot regard it without a measure of horror. It is a treatment of last resort. Even when all goes well, it represents an experience beyond our ordinary imaginings—the ordeal of chemotherapy taken to a near-lethal extreme" (p. 35). Autologous bone marrow transplants, not optimal for leukemias, had been developed for other kinds of cancer. "Suddenly," Groopman wrote, "the prospects for treating cancer changed dramatically: formerly incurable cancer—stubborn metastatic tumors that had resisted normal, survivable diseases of chemotherapy or radiation—might succumb to extraordinary doses" (p. 37). He illustrated this with the case of a friend of his who had been treated for a year for metastatic breast cancer with chemotherapy every 2 or 3 weeks in the second half of 1997. Her condition, evaluated at several leading cancer centers, had been deemed incurable. She and her husband had come to him in Boston to ask about BMT. The three courses explained to her were HDC/ABMT based on "preliminary evidence" suggesting that 20% of women had a 5-year disease-free survival; HDC/ABMT and a "better than even chance that despite a prolonged and harrowing treatment" she would die of cancer; or standard treatment that would "retard the cancer's progression somewhat" and morphine that would ease the pain in the final stages (p. 37). She went forward with the treatment, which "brought [her] as close to death as possible" (p. 37). The treatment effects included "a chemical burn throughout her gastrointestinal tract, from mouth to rectum . . . [and] taking advantage of her lack of immunity, a fungus began to grow in her macerated gut" (p. 37). She survived.

The article prompted a letter to the editor from George Grant, written with his wife, Anne, and published in late 1998 (G. Grant 1998).[10] Anne had received a stem cell transplant for stage II breast cancer in 1995. "We reread my diary from the year of her treatment," the letter read, "and realized that neither one of us could convey the horror of HDC and the years of recovery. What people living with cancer care about is survival and quality of life, and yet the quality of life is dramatically impaired by the possible long-term or even permanent side effects of HDC: chronic fatigue, pain, neuropathy, hearing and memory loss, cognitive impairment, and heart, liver, lung, or kidney damage. The fact is, HDC for breast cancer is experimental, and its efficacy is unproved" (p. 20).

Anne wrote her own account a year later in *MAMM,* a magazine devoted to "women, cancer, and community" (A. Grant 1999). Diagnosed at age 44, and with a mother who had died of breast cancer at age 40, she recounted that "many doctors" recommended HDC as "a new cutting edge treatment." Although little was published on the procedure, she and her husband were told that recovery was 6 to 12 months, that the death rate was "supposed to be less than 3%," and that the procedure would increase her survival chances by 25%. Four rounds of induction treatment caused muscle atrophy and bone and joint pain, created difficulty in walking, and led to frequent falling. She wrote the following:

> By the time I underwent HDC, I felt extremely frail. The 21 days in the hospital were spent sleepless and in unrelenting pain and misery. Friends and family have told me my appearance was frightening. For the next 2 years, nothing felt good and nothing worked quite right. I suffered a clinical depression caused by the chemotherapy drugs and was unable to read, make decisions or handle simple problems. One morning several months after HDC, my husband told me to get dressed so he could take me for a walk. Twenty minutes later he found me sitting on the bed trying to figure out which one of 12 pairs of identical white crew socks to put on. It's 4 years since HDC, and I'm still struggling with long-term, possibly permanent side effects. Pain, balance, memory, neuropathy (nerve pain), cognition (ability to read, comprehend, and remember), stamina and fatigue loom large in my ability to get through the day. One foot has neuropathic damage that requires orthotics, sneakers, and limited walking. (A. Grant 1999, p. 30)

Experience with HDC/ABMT was not limited to the United States. In Sydney, Australia, in 1996 Pam and Rod Baber were faced with a difficult decision (Rod Baber, personal communication to Cynthia Farquhar, September 5, 2003).[11] Pam, in her mid-30s with two young children, had been diagnosed with a recurrence of her breast cancer. She was keen to get the very best that medicine could offer. A discussion with their oncologist lead them to seek the HDC/ABMT procedure. The results from a South African trial, they were told, suggested benefit; therefore, they went ahead with the treatment. Less than 18 months after the treatment finished, Pam had a further recurrence of her disease, which was treated with local radiation therapy. Further recurrences were managed with radiation. Then, in March 1999, a new bombshell hit. Pam was diagnosed with leukemia, possibly the result of the earlier HDC/BMT. More BMTs followed, but finally there was no more that could be done, and Pam died of her leukemia 2 weeks after attending the opening ceremony of the 2000 Sydney Olympics.

Jane Sprague Zones provides a more detached, but not less-engaged view. In late 1995, Zones, a medical sociologist who then chaired the board of directors of the

National Women's Health Network and their breast cancer committee, wrote about the ECRI technology assessment. Its findings were "so disconcerting," she informed readers of the *Breast Cancer Action Newsletter,* that ECRI had formed an advisory committee of breast cancer patient advocates to prepare a consumer-oriented report for widespread dissemination. She reviewed the problems that ECRI's report had revealed: excluding treatment-related deaths that occurred within 30 days after HDC/ABMT, downplaying toxicities, ignoring patient selection bias, and avoiding randomized trials. Zones wrote: "Experimental drugs require regulatory oversight that limits access to treatment only through clinical trials, but experimental medical procedures do not have this requirement" (Zones 1995, p. 2). She also recounted that in the 6 months since the ECRI analysis, she had shared this information with other women, some of whom had been relieved "to be spared a grueling ordeal" and others offended "by the introduction of doubts" about a potentially lifesaving procedure.

In 1998, Zones would write that little had changed in 3 years. A 1995 South African trial had been reported, but the control group had done worse than patients in other conventional treatments, the study was too brief to report long-term outcomes, and the trial involved a small number of patients. In the United States, recruitment to randomized trials was going slowly, due partly to the activity of Response Oncology. A small Dutch trial, however, had found increased risk of cognitive impairment and a greater tendency toward cognitive deficits. She concluded by saying the following:

> HDC raises a common issue in women's health care. The foundation of the women's health movement has been to make accurate information available so that rational decisions about personal and public health care can be made. HDC takes place in a complex social environment that includes providers and insurers with strong opinions and vested interests, affected women and advocates eager for survival choices, and a variety of local settings that provide different treatment options. While we await the outcomes of well-designed randomized clinical trials, we urge women to consider, when possible, entering sound research studies to pursue still experimental treatments. (p. 3)

After the 1999 ASCO meeting, Zones would write of the "little benefit" provided by HDC (Zones 1999). Following the disclosure of fraud in the South African trials, she would write in the May/June 2000 *Breast Cancer Action Newsletter* of the "disappointment and deceit" and "the dismay of women's health advocates around the world" with which the news of fraud was received (Zones 2000). That same newsletter announced that she had been selected as the new board president of Breast Cancer Action (Spector 2000).

We have here two survivors, one highly supportive of the procedure, one highly critical; one woman lost to her family; a plaintiff's lawyer who, after winning several cases, experienced an epiphany and refused to take new ones; and a patient advocate who emphasizes the importance of randomized trials and of truth-telling. All as far as we know are or were aggressive information-seekers. What is owed to such women: hope based on scientific evidence or false hope based on enthusiasm and a willingness to roll the dice? We address this question in the final chapter.

Part IV

The Significance of the Story

10

Values in Conflict

Since 1962, controlled trials have been the common intellectual currency of the drug evaluation process. This did not happen solely because academic scientists believed in the value of such trials, although many did. It happened because Congress, with the advice of academics, imposed the requirement that such trials be the only basis for establishing effectiveness. This has led to a sea change, such that controlled trials are now the accepted standard of evidence for effectiveness for drugs, not just when FDA considers a marketing application, but whenever evidence is discussed in journals or academic environments. Where such trials are not required, however, they are far less often carried out.
—Robert Temple

High-dose chemotherapy with autologous bone marrow transplantation (HDC/ABMT) for breast cancer has historical roots reaching back into the 1970s, if not further, but the events of 1988–1992 basically defined the decade of the 1990s, at least until the 1999 American Society of Clinical Oncology (ASCO) annual meeting. The main features of the HDC/ABMT story as a promising treatment for breast cancer include the emergence of the procedure in the mid- to late 1980s based on small, single-site phase 2 studies, which had either no controls or historical controls. Recognition of the new procedure involved a complex, ill-structured "conversation" between physicians and insurers. As a medical procedure, responsibility for its evaluation fell on the medical profession, health insurers, and the National Cancer Institute (NCI).

By 1990, "a fateful branching" had occurred and subsequent events unfolded along two pathways: widespread and rapid clinical use and limited but slower evaluation by randomized clinical trials. The medical profession, armed with great social legitimacy but divided in its commitment to randomized clinical trials, jumped the gun and sanctioned the procedure as better than conventional treatment. Clinical use was driven by desperate patients, often acting on their physicians' advice; litigation; entrepreneurial oncology; legislative and administrative mandates; and how the media covered the story. We estimate that between 23,000 and 35,000–40,000 women received the HDC/ABMT procedure in the 1989–2002 period.

By contrast, the slower evaluation pathway involved technology assessments and randomized clinical trials. Repeated assessments concluded that existing data did not support claims of the procedure's effectiveness. Interactions among skeptical clinical scientists, health insurers, the NCI, and the cancer cooperative groups led to the initiation of high-priority phase 3 trials in 1990–1991. At the end of the decade, these trials reported that HDC/ABMT provided no significant difference in overall survival between the experimental treatment and conventional therapies. Audits conducted in 2000 of the only two trials reporting benefit judged them fraudulent. Utilization plummeted, and subsequent data have not changed the no benefit conclusion. Of the women who received the procedure, perhaps 1000 were enrolled in randomized clinical trials in the United States.

We draw three primary lessons from our study. First, initial conditions matter. Second, conflicting values permeate the entire experience. Third, no institution existed in the 1990s, or exists today, to manage those conflicting values. From these lessons, we recommend that a new public–private partnership be created under the aegis of the NCI for oncology procedures, as distinct from cancer chemotherapy drugs, and under the relevant National Institutes of Health (NIH) institute for other procedures. This partnership should include the medical profession, health insurers, and patient representatives and have the broad goal of changing the dynamic surrounding the initial conditions so that new untested, costly, and potentially harmful medical procedures do not enter widespread clinical use prematurely. We elaborate the rationale for this recommendation in this chapter. We believe that the lessons we draw apply to procedures involving both public and private health insurers and younger and older patients, and that our recommendation addresses clinical and policy issues that go well beyond the HDC/ABMT experience.

The basic conflict running through the entire HDC/ABMT experience was the need to balance the evaluation of the procedure's effectiveness against making it available to patients before such evidence was firmly established. This conflict can be expected to recur for many future medical innovations. All medical innovations come in distinctive packages: They emerge as specific interventions for particular clinical uses, typically within defined therapeutic areas and often as the property of particular medical specialties. HDC/ABMT focused sharply on breast cancer among solid tumors, first for metastatic and then for high-risk patients, with ownership asserted by bone marrow transplanters.

Medical innovations share many characteristics. What does HDC/ABMT share with other procedures? The variable manifestation of disease and of patient response to treatment is frequent in medicine. The need for evaluation by randomized trials is often essential for determining the effectiveness of many procedures. All life-threatening illnesses are highly charged emotionally. Intense patient demand and physician enthusiasm for the experimental is shared by many new treatments. Political action characterizes many disease entities and treatments.

In early 2005, an important review appeared that compared the effectiveness of new radiation oncology treatments to standard treatments. It analyzed data on 12,734 patients from 57 completed phase 3 randomized trials conducted by the Radiation Therapy Oncology Group from 1968 to 2002. Although innovative treatments were as likely as standard treatments to be successful, they had higher treatment-related mortality. The authors "found no predictable pattern of treatment successes in oncology: sometimes innovative treatments are better than standard ones and vice versa; in most cases there were no substantive differences between experimental and conventional treatments" (Soares et al. 2005, p. 970). They concluded: "The finding that the results in individual trials cannot be predicted in advance indicates that the system and rationale for RCTs [randomized clinical trials] is well preserved and that successful interventions can only be identified after an RCT is completed." The title of an accompanying editorial pungently conveyed the basic message: "The Case for Randomized Trials in Cancer Treatment: New Is Not Always Better" (Grann and Grann 2005).

What is distinctive about medical procedures is that no statutory requirement, no administrative agency exists to serve the function that the Food and Drug Administration (FDA) does for the evaluation of new drugs. Relations among medical researchers, treating physicians, the NIH, and health insurers are not structured systematically. Instead, they are dominated by the relationship between medicine and insurers, which is often characterized by hostility. Consequently, the default decision-making system is decentralized to the courts, entrepreneurs, federal administrative agencies, state legislatures, and media. Demand for the evaluation of procedures may emerge from the weakly organized evaluation system, but it is vulnerable to overrides by the default system.

Numerous examples raise issues similar to those of HDC/ABMT. These include lung volume reduction surgery for bullous emphysema, minimally invasive spinal procedures for discogenic disease such as percutaneous lumbar discectomy and intradiscal electrothermal annuloplasty, HDC with autologous stem cell support for other solid tumors such as ovarian or lung cancer, intravenous immunoglobulin for a variety of autoimmune diseases, and enhanced external counterpulsation for angina pectoris. The health care system confronts a continuing stream of promising new medical technologies today and for the foreseeable future, only some of which will be evaluated by randomized clinical trials. The need for evaluation will not recede but only increase in importance. We suggest one way to respond to this increased need.

Initial Conditions

Our first lesson is that initial conditions matter (Rothman 1977). Why? They drive subsequent events in profound and long-lasting ways. They are as likely to be determined by misplaced enthusiasm as by careful science. What were those conditions? First, HDC/ABMT was seen as promising in clinical and professional terms. Clinically, it had a plausible scientific basis that deserved to be tested. Professionally, it reinforced the identity of the subspecialty of bone marrow transplanters.[1] It would become economically promising for both for-profit and not-for-profit providers, especially as human growth factors and peripheral blood stem cells facilitated a shift from inpatient to outpatient treatment settings.

Second, no regulatory entity existed to require that HDC/ABMT be adequately evaluated before widespread clinical use. The evaluation discussion involved clinicians and clinical scientists, insurers, and the NCI and the cancer cooperative groups. Clinicians and clinician-scientists divided into three groups: skeptics, who believed that randomized trials were necessary to determine whether the new was better than conventional treatment; believers, who "knew" that phase 2 studies justified wider clinical use without such trials; and optimists, who believed that randomized trials were useful but would only confirm the results of phase 2 studies.

Did phase 2 studies of HDC/ABMT generate hypotheses to be tested, or did they justify widespread clinical use without such trials? The latter view required clinicians to overlook or minimize potential patient selection bias resulting from undetected differences between rigorously evaluated phase 2 patients and historical controls. It also dismissed treatment bias that might stem from care given in one center when compared to that provided in a multisite trial.[2] Randomization minimizes both selection and treatment bias. Although oncology has exercised great leadership with respect to the organization and conduct of randomized trials, it remains a persistent fact that only 3%–5% of adult cancer patients are ever enrolled in trials. Jeffrey Abrams, of the NCI, put it this way: "In oncology there is a cadre who believe in clinical trials. There are a lot of oncologists who don't" (Abrams 2002).

This ambivalence highlights the intellectual uncertainty about when a randomized trial is needed and when one can be bypassed. The substantial literature on randomized clinical trials provides little conceptual clarity, and thus little professional guidance to the medical community, on this point. This weakness deserves serious analytical attention by the biostatistical and medical research communities and calls for sustained applied research by the NCI, the FDA, and professional medical societies.

On this issue, the Evidence-Based Discussion Group conducted a survey to identify when randomized trials might be unnecessary (Glasziou 2003). From this survey, the following clinical criteria emerged: A randomized trial might be unnecessary when (1) the all-or-none criterion is satisfied (all patients died before the intervention, but some now survive; or some patients died before the intervention, but none now die); (2) all of the following conditions are met: a bad outcome occurs if the patient is untreated; a dramatic benefit is achieved by treatment; the side effects of treatment are acceptable; no alternative treatment exists; and there is a convincing pathophysiological basis for the treatment; and (3) a randomized trial is *unnecessary* when the treatment effect is dramatic, *inappropriate* when the outcome is rare or occurs far in the future and randomization could reduce effectiveness, *impossible* due to physician refusal to participate or lack of equipoise, and *inadequate* due to low external validity. This survey provides a starting point for the applied research we suggest.

Recognition of a promising new medical procedure becomes crucial under these circumstances, but recognition of a medical procedure is a complex process, often quite contentious, that involves an ill-structured conversation between physicians and health insurers and with a high potential for conflict. No small amount of gamesmanship occurs in this process, involving provider billing and coding practices and preauthorization review and approval by insurers. By contrast, the recognition process for new drugs is quite different. Sponsors of all studies of new drugs in humans must file an Investigational New Drug (IND) application with the FDA before such trials may be started. For new drugs or new indications of use, the transition from phase 2 to phase 3 trials is clearly demarcated and widely reported in the relevant media. Medical procedures require no such pause between emergence from phase 2 studies and introduction into wider clinical use. This phase 2–phase 3 transition is critical because enthusiasm about a new treatment is often intense among researchers at this juncture. But, the need for evaluation is also high, as randomized trials often fail to support a treatment's promise.

Third, oncology legitimated wider clinical use of HDC/ABMT on the basis of phase 2 studies before it had been evaluated in randomized clinical trials. This legitimation by prominent oncologists was perhaps the most influential factor driving events in the 1990s. Indeed, several oncologists became outspoken advocates for the procedure well before phase 3 trials began. Just as randomized trials were being started, HDC/ABMT was represented to patients as a last-best-hope treatment. By the time health insurers, health plans, and other technology assessors asked about data supporting effectiveness, the procedure was being characterized as substantially better than conventional treatment. By the time the first cases were going to court trials, the treatment was being described as standard of care in communities and states across the country. Women were placed at risk of ineffective treatment that many trialists and most technology assessors saw as no better than standard treatment and some saw as worse. This legitimation would severely complicate the ability to recruit women to randomized clinical trials due to the widespread availability of the procedure outside randomized clinical trials.

Gabriel Hortobagyi would later write the following: "Enthusiasm overtook discipline, and well-tested clinical trials methodology was shoved aside by the perception that randomized trials in patients with very poor prognosis were ethically unjustified" (Hortobagyi 2004, p. 2263). Regrettably, patients and others outside medicine do not appreciate the role of enthusiasm among clinicians and clinical scientists for the new, the experimental. Instead, they see a detached commitment to scientific research generating medical breakthroughs and hope for cures of dread diseases. At this transition from phase 2 studies to phase 3 randomized clinical trials, the enthusiasm of experts is most likely to assert itself in ways that are largely hidden to those outside the profession and even to many nonspecialists within medicine. Medical self-regulation is not a guarantor against enthusiasm.

Finally, early clinical use was driven by the dynamic confluence of individual patient demands, physician advice, litigation, financial exploitation, administrative and legislative mandates, and advocacy support, all reinforced by how the media reported the story. Specific decisions involving individual patients were highly decentralized and for the most part uncoordinated. Institutionally, the decentralized and uncoordinated actors defined a "default system" of policymaking and decision making, the net effect of which was a willingness to override the evaluation of the HDC/ABMT procedure by randomized trials. This "default system," which lurched into high gear in the 1988–1992 period, upended and overturned the working assumption of scientists and physicians that the path from clinical research to clinical use proceeds in an orderly and rational way. Not only did no entity require randomized trials, but also the default system was biased toward the experimental, for which the existing evaluation system was unprepared.

Values in Conflict

The second lesson we draw is that conflicting values characterized all participants and permeated all institutions and processes in the HDC/ABMT case. The story's basic conflict pits two legitimate claims against each other. The first is that of individual patient demands for early access to experimental therapy, including insurance coverage and payment. Understood correctly, the claims of individual patients also include access to safe and effective treatment. In the HDC/ABMT case, these claims were usually subordinated to the demand for access to the experimental procedure. The second claim is a collective or societal need to determine if new procedures are better than, comparable to, or worse than standard treatments before wider use and to the corollary need to maintain the integrity of the evaluation process. In short, conflict exists between the expressed needs of the individual and society's need for determining "what works" and controlling costs, especially for unevaluated interventions (Eddy 1996).

The conflict between access and evaluation confronts all parties and all institutions and arises at every stage of the process. Moreover, all parties are conflicted within their frame of reference and in their interactions with others: patients deciding what to do about a diagnosis, physicians advising patients about appropriate therapy, insurers making coverage decisions about new medical technologies, courts adjudicating claims in litigation, executive and legislative bodies mandating benefits, and the media reporting the story. The access-versus-evaluation conflict takes a number of forms: enthusiasm versus discipline, nonrandomized trials versus coin-flip trials, and doctor–patient decision making versus researcher–insurer decision making. However it is resolved in any given instance, this conflict will influence the organization and conduct of clinical trials very strongly, especially in the central task of enrolling patients for randomization.

Acknowledgment that conflicting values characterize HDC/ABMT and other new medical procedures raises the thorny policy question of whether such conflicts can be managed in a rational way. Can we learn from experience, or must we throw up our hands in despair in such situations and let events take their course? Despair is tempting, but if it is to be avoided, we believe that it is both necessary and possible to manage conflicting values better than was done in the HDC/ABMT case. However, no technical solution exists to choosing among conflicting values that is independent of policy, and no sustainable policy is independent of political support. There is no facile win-win solution available by which all parties can be made better off and none worse off. Something must give. Choices must be made, either explicitly or implicitly by inaction. Do these choices involve reasonable and appropriate trades-offs between more of this and less of that? If trade-offs are possible, what are the bases for making them? Or, are the choices between incommensurable values that require an either/or decision? If the choice is between incommensurables—either access or evaluation—are we fated to fight it out in the political realm with the result determined by some Darwinian survival of the fittest?

In the HDC/ABMT case, some parties to the discussion were very good at responding to individual patients: physicians, courts, legislatures, advocates, and the media. Others were much better at responding to the need for population-based data: clinical trialists, the NCI, insurers, and technology assessors. Few were good at responding to both. Yet, only in managing the tension between these conflicting values will effective policy and practice solutions be found. William McGivney described the dilemma by noting that coverage decisions by insurers regarding experimental or investigational procedures are typically go versus no go, whereas individual patients face a risk—benefit choice regarding treatment. Moreover, patient risk–benefit decisions must be made today, whereas opting for evaluation means deferring to some future time the answer to whether the new is better than existing therapy. So, the basic conflict involves individual preferences versus population-based analysis, immediate decisions versus deferred answers. How to respond to this conundrum is a difficult question in the instance and for the entire health care system. Where do we search for common ground that simultaneously allows us to respond to patient demands for access and to maintain the integrity of the evaluation process?

We begin with a rudimentary point: It is essential to listen to patients, especially those with a diagnosis of a terminal or life-threatening disease. Two reasons compel this conclusion. First, patient needs are legitimate. Relief of pain and suffering and avoidance of premature death are highly cherished societal values. Moreover, a society that invests as heavily as does the United States in both public and private financing of medical research generates widespread hope for medical breakthroughs (Brownlee 2003). Such hope may be unrealistic and misleading in many ways, but it would be garish in the extreme to promote it as assiduously as we do and then deny the validity of patient responses to putative breakthroughs. In addition, the country needs a safety valve to accommodate patient demands in ways that do not undermine the systematic evaluation of new medical technologies. In the HDC/ABMT case, the absence of stress-relieving mechanisms for responding to patient demands hampered the management of the basic conflict and slowed evaluation of the procedure.

The critical question is how to respond to patients in the early stages of a new procedure in a way that protects the evaluation process. Listening must be accompanied by articulating the importance of randomized clinical trials at the point when it is genuinely not known whether the experimental treatment is superior to existing therapies. Ways must be found, based on individual values, to respond to the specific needs of identified patients. Ways must also be found, based on community values, to justify and conduct essential clinical trials.

Many interviewees emphasized this lesson. Michael Friedman, formerly head of the NCI Cancer Therapy Evaluation Program, said: "It is important to identify emerging technologies and treatments as early as possible, construct a venue to test these technologies in a formal way, lean more heavily on patient groups and investigators, and use whatever inducements you can to get the best study done, not hastily or clumsily, but as early as you can" (Friedman 2002). John Glick, of the University of Pennsylvania, said: "The need is for trials, to put patients on trials, to not offer treatment outside of trials. We've got to do it right—randomized, prospective, controlled trials, with adequate statistical power to provide answers in a reasonable period of time" (Glick 2002). Hortobagyi said the following:

> This [HDC/ABMT] is a very important episode in oncology, also in medicine. It underlines the critical importance of using the techniques of optimal evaluation, namely, the randomized clinical trials, before getting to societal and insurance angst. It is wrong to come up with uncontrolled studies, not peer reviewed, and to drive clinical practice. A greater degree of discipline is needed by physicians, NIH, NCI, each cancer center. Centers should have been more responsible to this issue—and they were not. When insurers began to pay, the procedure became a cash cow and institutions were less willing to be critical. When the evaluation of patient care is on the basis of income, this is very dangerous. This needs to be recognized as a risk. (Hortobagyi 2002)

In our judgment, it is imperative that society commit itself to the evaluation of new medical innovations. Contrary to popular conceptions, this imperative is not driven solely, or even primarily, by financial considerations, although resources are important. Rather, it is primarily a matter of ensuring that clinical benefits outweigh risks for any given intervention.

The Institutional Deficit

Our third lesson is that an institutional deficit exists, very apparent in the HDC/ABMT case, to manage the basic conflict between access and evaluation of medical procedures. The de facto or default system of decision making (courts, entre-preneurs, federal agencies, state legislatures, and the media) responded well to individual patients, even if the response was not always in a patient's interest. They responded much less well to the societal need for population-based data generated by randomized trials. Indeed, they dominated the more deliberate and orderly evaluation system. Changes in the policies, procedures, and behaviors of these institutions can certainly be suggested, but they are apt to be either modest or so sweeping as to require decades for realization. In general, we are pessimistic that such changes might lead these institutions to deal with the access-versus-evaluation conflict much differently from the way they do now. It is also essential to challenge these institutions regarding their frequent and often uncritical support of the technological imperative that drives much of modern medicine. A need exists for a socially responsible way to evaluate new technology that does not take benefit for granted and that does not exclude cost from consideration. We examine this institutional deficit as reflected in the default decision-making system, after which we propose a remedy.

Lawyers, Judges, and Juries

Courtroom trials constitute one venue in which patients' voices are heard. Lawyers, judges, and juries are well suited to listening to individual patients and taking their demands into account. In theory and practice, courts are designed to protect individuals against arbitrary governmental and nongovernmental actions. Since a woman initiates HDC/ABMT litigation for herself alone (and not for a larger class of patients), the judicial forum ensures attention to her individual claims. Moreover, courts often defer to the treating physician and do not necessarily consider the effects of their rulings on patient populations. Both of these realities tend to favor the individual patient.

Courts do much less well in protecting the integrity of the scientific evaluation process. To do so would work against patients. Had the courts deferred to the statistical uncertainties of clinical science, patients would have won far fewer claims. In contrast to clinical trials, courts are poorly suited for considering populations of patients. Just as important, courtroom trials demonstrate the difficulty of litigating controversial medical procedures that require weighing the competing claims of clinical science. Conflicting claims of scientific validity, such as with silicone breast implants, have long confounded the judicial process. HDC/ABMT offers no exception to the historical record. Despite these advantages, patients did not always win in court. In fact, our results indicate that patients won about 50% of the time, an outcome that was unaffected by the punitive damage award in *Fox v. HealthNet* (No. 219692, Superior Court of California [1993]). What *Fox* changed was the greater willingness of insurers to settle cases afterward than before.

Lawyers and the courts present an inviting target for criticism, but blaming them for the HDC/ABMT fiasco obscures the need to develop better mechanisms for evaluating and controlling new medical procedures and technologies before their widespread diffusion. An important policy lesson from this study is that once a procedure diffuses into practice, it is unlikely that the courts will intervene to check diffusion on scientific grounds. Perhaps the most accurate assessment of our interviews with the attorneys is that both the law and the science failed. As one attorney put it, we were "all sold a bill of goods." Some have speculated that many HDC/ABMT case outcomes resulted from judicial (or juror) sympathy for the dying patient and a concomitant unwillingness to deny a potentially lifesaving treatment (Morreim 2001).[3] Ironically, while many of the decisions favoring the plaintiff may have been motivated by sympathy, only those favoring the insurer expressed that sympathy explicitly.

The Business of Oncology

Oncology is big business. We have highlighted Response Technologies due to the easy availability of information about publicly traded corporations, but many not-for-profit cancer centers, including those in major academic medical centers, also found BMT very profitable. Are entrepreneurial oncologists villains in this story? At one level, the answer is of course. Financial incentives drove both for-profit and not-for-profit entities to promote the widespread use and rapid diffusion of the HDC/ABMT procedure. Entrepreneurs, in both for-profit and not-for-profit institutions, responded to the financial incentives created when prominent oncologists legitimated the procedure in the late 1980s and early 1990s. That legitimation provided the justification for making money from sophisticated oncology services, notwithstanding the absence of adequate evaluation.

On the other hand, entrepreneurial oncologists did little consciously to protect and defend the evaluation process, preferring rather to exploit economic opportunities offered by the slimmest scientific evidence. Although Response Technologies characterized its provision of HDC/ABMT as under clinical trial protocols, these were uncontrolled phase 2 studies, and women were not randomized to any control arm. Moreover, Response declined to participate in trials when Blue Cross plans were paying for patient care costs at a rate below that obtainable from other health insurers. Academic entrepreneurs, though less visible, may have offered women opportunity to participate in phase 3 trials but often did not hesitate to make HDC/ABMT readily available either on a phase 2 protocol or without reference to any trial. Indeed, entrepreneurial oncologists in both for-profit and not-for-profit centers responded to breast cancer patients as businesspeople respond to a market. They supplied a product in response to consumer demand, but they did little to advance the evaluation of that product's effectiveness.

Federal Health Administrators and State Legislators

Legislators listen to constituents, and few have more compelling stories than women with breast cancer. In August 1994, the House of Representatives Post Office and Civil Service Committee challenged the exclusion of HDC/ABMT for women with breast cancer from the policies of health plans participating in the Federal Employees Health Benefits Program administered by the Office of Personnel Management (OPM). This exclusion was interpreted as a feminist cause, not one involving the absence of evidence of effectiveness. Health insurers were depicted as denying benefits to women for financial reasons. Randomized trials were derided as coin-flip trials. In response to the hearing, extensive political pressure, and a weak defense of randomized trials by the NCI, OPM capitulated and required that all 300-plus health plans participating in the Federal Employees Health Benefits Program provide HDC/ABMT as a covered benefit for breast cancer patients. This action, which undermined the evaluation process, argues for inclusion of OPM among the insurers in the public–private partnership we recommend.

Not surprisingly, many states adopted legislative mandates in the mid-1990s requiring that all health plans in their jurisdictions provide HDC/ABMT for breast cancer as a covered benefit. These statutes often responded to the personal situation of a member of the legislature. In Minnesota, for example, the wife of the speaker of the House of Representatives was diagnosed with breast cancer and became the personification of the prospective beneficiary. A lawyer, Mike Hatch, now the attorney general, championed the HDC/ABMT cause and later campaigned unsuccessfully for governor on this basis.

Although a Congressional committee and state legislatures listened to women, they seldom listened to skeptics of the procedure and did nothing to support the evaluation process. Although the Minnesota Blue Cross Blue Shield Association (BCBSA) introduced the ECRI technology assessment into the legislative debate, the report had no effect on the ultimate outcome. The episode suggests that a major audience for the assessments of new medical procedures that are not evaluated by the FDA is, or should be, state legislative bodies. Information from the entity we propose might well temper legislative enthusiasms and contribute to legislative deliberations.

Newspapers and Television Journalists

The media played a critical role in promoting HDC/ABMT to breast cancer patients, and persuading legislators to force insurers to pay for the procedure. Beginning with the first newspaper story about Bill Peters and experimental treatment, journalists told the HDC/ABMT story in heroic terms, with patients playing the tragic victims, insurers and breast cancer the villains, and bold doctors the saviors. Reporters chose to write about the most tragic victims of all, young mothers with breast cancer. They were not intentionally hyping the treatment, but that was certainly the end result. The vast majority of the hundreds of articles that appeared in print about HDC and the dozens of television segments left readers and viewers with three principal conclusions. First, HDC made sense; if a little bit of chemotherapy could cure early cancers, then obviously higher doses were needed for more advanced cases. Second, HDC was an advanced breast cancer patient's only hope. Third, the only thing standing between a patient and the potential cure was money, which insurers did not want to spend.

There were exceptions, of course. In 1993, *60 Minutes* ran a segment suggesting that HDC/ABMT was actually killing or disabling women, not curing them (Kroft 1993). (This story was particularly unusual in that the producer had watched first-hand as his wife died during her own HDC/ABMT treatment.) Even so, the critical stories that appeared before 1999, when the results of four randomized clinical trials showed that HDC was no better than standard-dose chemotherapy, were too few to erase the general impression that HDC/ABMT represented a major advance in the treatment of breast cancer.

Why did reporters get the story wrong? Many medical journalists would argue that they could hardly be expected to have questioned HDC when the medical establishment, including prominent oncologists and bone marrow transplanters, were all telling them the treatment worked. But there were many dissenters, and most reporters dutifully represented the critics' views about HDC, adding a line or two, maybe a paragraph, about the experimental nature of the treatment and its dangers. Even so, most stories left an overall impression that discounted the caveats of the very critics that reporters quoted.

There were many reasons that reporters failed to get the story right, most of them having to do with the culture of journalism and changes in the wider society. Medical journalists (and their editors) are often in the thrall of both prominent doctors and new technologies. Richard Horton, MD, the editor of the British medical journal *The Lancet,* wrote: "Medicine pays almost exclusive homage to the shock of the new" (Horton 1997, p. 872). In fact, so do medical journalists. Going back to the 1930s and 1940s, when the *New York Times* fawned over Walter Freeman, MD, and his then seemingly miraculous new surgery, frontal lobotomy, the media have traditionally embraced new treatments, especially when put forward by charismatic doctors holding prestigious positions in the medical establishment. This is understandable, to a degree; because of their general lack of medical training, journalists must rely on "experts" in medicine. Consequently, reporters found the combination of an authoritative doctor or medical institution presenting a new—potentially lifesaving—treatment almost irresistible. In the case of HDC, reporters accepted without question reports from institutions like ASCO and Duke University, as well as from doctors publicizing the treatment.

This deference to medical authority was glaringly obvious in the stories that appeared after Peters described insurers' HDC/ABMT coverage decisions as "arbitrary and capricious." Stories in newspapers across the nation simply quoted Peters or the press release, some without even asking insurers for comment. Only one or two reporters thought to wonder if the article was not at least a little self-serving in that Duke stood to make money whenever insurers agreed to pay for the procedure.

Reporters were also responding to wider changes in the perception of breast cancer and women's health. By the late 1980s, women were well established in the once all-male bastion of the newsroom, finding themselves for the first time in the position of being able to report and edit stories of their choosing. Women's health was a fresh and vitally interesting topic to both female reporters and readers. When insurers refused to pay for HDC, women reporters often regarded their arguments that the treatment was experimental as merely an excuse for not paying and for ignoring women's health, which was already being sorely neglected by the NIH and Congress.

In the end, reporters found HDC stories compelling to write, and editors wishing to publish, for the simple reason that hope sells. Indeed, the coverage of HDC serves as but one example of the flood of hope-filled stories about medicine that appeared in the second half of the 20th century, and no wonder: Truly miraculous medicine had been pouring out of laboratories and hospitals since shortly after World War II. For the first time in human history, doctors could prevent childhood disease with vaccines, transplant organs, cure once-deadly infection, and even operate on a living heart. By the time HDC came along, medical reporters had gotten used to being the bearers of good news, and their employers knew from their sales figures that while readers were keenly interested in health information, they preferred stories that offered a sense of hope.

Although there are many reasons for the media's failure to cast a critical eye over HDC, there are no easy remedies. The culture of medical reporting does not include the kind of skepticism that political reporters hold for politicians or police reporters for law enforcement officials. Few investigative reporters look critically at medicine, and even fewer media outlets express interest in publishing what they might find. As the media have grown increasingly dependent on advertising by drug companies, they have also become increasingly reluctant to run stories attacking the pharmaceutical industry.

The most effective remedy for uncritical medical science reporting will occur when journalism schools start teaching a different kind of medical journalism. Most medical reporting classes emphasize the gathering of facts and the importance of getting the science right in medical stories. In the case of HDC, the accuracy of the facts should have been secondary to the larger question of evidence in medicine, particularly when the treatment was so expensive and dangerous. While getting the science right is important, journalism schools should also be teaching students to question the motives of doctors and hospitals and to "follow the money," as investigative reporters like to say. Young journalists should learn that medicine is not simply a long string of scientific breakthroughs, of diseases vanquished, but a business, first and foremost, that is often only weakly based on scientific evidence. Like all businesses, medical practitioners have their own self-interests as well as the needs of patients in mind, and good reporters should be always aware of the motives of doctors and medical institutions. Most important, students of journalism should learn from the past and study the mistakes that have been made over the years in the coverage of new and seemingly promising treatments.

An Institutional Remedy

Managing the conflict between access and evaluation requires some agent, some entity, some institution to broker relations among competing interests and conflicting values. But, as indicated, no authoritative, mediating institution exists to manage the conflicts that arise in the evaluation of medical procedures. There is no "FDA equivalent" to insist on evidence of safety and effectiveness and to weigh benefits and risks. Moreover, the default system of decentralized decision making fails to support evaluation and, in the HDC/ABMT instance, promoted wider use of the experimental procedure.

We conclude, therefore, that a new relationship—a public–private partnership—should be established among the institutions primarily responsible for the evaluation of new medical procedures. Who is responsible for evaluating new procedures? Four primary candidates for this authoritative, mediating role are the medical profession, health insurers, the NCI, and patients and their representatives. What roles should these institutions play? What new institutional arrangement is called for?

The Medical Profession

The medical profession is deeply divided regarding how to manage the basic conflict of access versus evaluation for experimental procedures. It manifests no consistency either on how to speak to patients about such procedures or about when randomized clinical trials should be undertaken to test phase 2 hypotheses. Nevertheless, medicine possesses one major asset not available to others, namely, substantial social legitimacy—at the level of the individual physician, the medical specialty, and the clinic or treating institution. This legitimacy, granted in numerous ways, ensures autonomy and shields the profession from the need to grapple with the basic conflict of access versus evaluation when experimental treatments emerge. The medical profession is accountable to no one in failing to deal with this basic conflict, whether at the level of the individual physicians or the profession as a whole.

How does an individual physician inform a woman of a diagnosis of breast cancer and speak to her about options: conventional therapy, experimental therapy, or participation in a randomized clinical trial? A physician's primary obligation is to care for their patients, but different physicians may view existing and new therapies very differently. They may emphasize either the positive features or the inadequacies of conventional treatments. Alternatively, they may emphasize a new treatment's unproven characteristics or its promise. They may recommend strongly a given course of action, or, if genuinely ambivalent, they may recommend participation in a randomized trial or defer to the patient to make her decision.

Framed in this way, it is clear that how a physician presents information will greatly affect what a woman chooses to do. Many studies show just that: How physicians present information is one of the most significant determinants of whether patients agree to participate in randomized clinical trials. The fact that only 3%–5% of adult cancer patients participate in clinical trials suggests, at minimum, tepid physician support for such trials. Whether this weak support results in a bias toward conventional treatment or toward the experimental is an empirical question in any given instance, but the variability of physician advice to patients may promote, intentionally or not, the use of untested procedures that are of no benefit or harmful to patients.

The organized medical profession, as distinct from the individual physician, is central to the evaluation of new medical procedures. It is critical to articulating the justification for randomized clinical trials or suggesting when such trials can be bypassed. It may, however, defer to the individual physician. In the HDC/ABMT case, it deferred to William Peters, who both advocated for and organized critical phase 2 and phase 3 trials while simultaneously advocating for insurance coverage of the procedure as early as 1990. He was tireless in promoting the procedure with large purchasers, state insurance commissions, and others throughout the 1990s. But, he was hardly alone in legitimating the procedure long before it had been evaluated. The American Medical Association lent its support to those seeking coverage. Prominent academic oncologists did the same, attacking insurers for seeking evaluation on the grounds that they were condemning breast cancer patients to certain death. Community oncologists declared the procedure "standard of care" by 1991. Oncology revealed its ambivalent commitment toward randomized clinical trials in many ways. The HDC/ABMT case reveals yet another instance of the weakness of medical self-regulation.

What policies might be suggested to the medical profession regarding the evaluation of new procedures? Exhortation to good behavior is hardly worth considering, but some long-term responses might be considered. For example, oncology and other specialty fellowship and residency programs might develop rigorous training modules that address the conceptual bases both for justifying randomized trials and for bypassing them in certain situations, coupled with detailed case analyses of noteworthy trials. In addition, specialty board certification examinations might devote greater attention to the evaluation of new procedures. Finally, professional societies might redouble their educational efforts related to clinical trials. But, in our view, these responses, although constructive, are rather tepid.

Organizations such as ASCO serve a variety of functions. They organize annual and special meetings for researchers to present the latest results of their investigations. They sponsor journals that publish the results of such research. They provide professional recognition for physicians active in them. They support public policy interventions on behalf of their members before Congress and the executive branch. In the case of ASCO, it has distinguished itself for more than two decades in its advocacy of clinical research, including clinical trials (Krueger 2004). ASCO provided a platform for the presentation of the results of phase 2 studies of HDC/ABMT at successive annual meetings. In 1999, it alerted women in advance of its annual meeting to the forthcoming reports of phase 3 trials that showed no significant difference in overall survival between the experimental procedure and conventional therapy. In 2000, after the documentation of Bezwoda's fraudulent trials, the *Journal of Clinical Oncology* withdrew the 1995 article by the South African and expressed embarrassment at an abstract review process that allowed his 1999 plenary presentation to go unchallenged.

Might ASCO have intervened earlier in the decade, challenging the Dream Team document, for example, as highly premature? Might it have prepared a patient information brochure along the lines of the later ECRI brochure to warn women of the dangers of depending on unconfirmed results of phase 2 studies and citing prior examples of dashed hopes of other "promising" therapies that were later found to be of no benefit? Yes, ASCO might have done all these things, thus satisfying the need both to listen to patients and to protect the integrity of the evaluation process. Should it be prepared to respond in this way in the future, going beyond a passive stance that basically presents the results of any investigator? Again, the answer is yes. Should it do this on its own or in concert with others? We believe it unlikely to act on its own given the weakness of self-regulation in medicine and argue for collaboration with others in the evaluation of new medical procedures.

Insurers

Many health insurers now constitute a major force in pressing for the adequate evaluation of new medical technologies. In general, however, they are divided on how to respond to the basic conflict between access to experimental treatment and adequate evaluation. Should they routinely deny access, should they write their contract language more carefully, should they insist on randomized trials, or should they resist demands for coverage until public pressure requires them to yield for public relations reasons? Most adhere to a position that they are not obligated to finance the evaluation of experimental or investigational treatments from which they are unlikely to benefit financially.

Insurers further argue that the evaluation of new procedures, like research in general, is a public good from which society benefits greatly but for which they, as potential sponsors, cannot capture financial benefits. Therefore, they argue, the evaluation of new medical procedures should be publicly funded. Unlike new drugs and medical devices, for which commercial sponsors assume the cost of evaluation and, if successful, reap financial benefits, medical procedures present a different problem. Their evaluation in randomized trials is expensive. The NIH, never enthusiastic about the costs of large randomized trials, and nonprofit academic institutions face severe budget constraints. Moreover, for-profit sponsors of new procedures cannot establish a proprietary basis for obtaining financial return from the use of procedures, thus eliminating any economic incentive to finance their evaluation.

In response to ongoing efforts by government and academic sources, health insurers and plans have generally resisted financing the evaluation of new procedures. They have developed more flexible approaches to coverage decision making for new treatments for life-threatening or severely disabling conditions; these approaches include technology assessment, limited support of clinical trials, and independent external review. Although technology assessment has matured in methodological and institutional terms in both the public and private sectors, the HDC/ABMT experience reveals several of its limits.

First, the insurance industry is divided in its commitment to technology assessment: Some insurers support superb analytical units, some pay for studies prepared by others, and others exercise the free rider option. Second, even the best assessment organizations can only advise coverage decision makers on the evidence of effectiveness of medical procedures but cannot insulate them from decisions that take external and internal political, economic, legal, and public relations pressures into account. Third, assessments not tied to coverage decision making are not self-executing. ECRI, for example, generates many high-quality reviews of the literature that become advisory to their clients, but clients remain free to do as they wish with this information. Fourth, although registry data were instrumental in persuading BCBSA to modify its position on HDC/ABMT in 1996, such data are not always available, have inherent limitations, and cannot be relied on for evidence of effectiveness or for guidance when phase 2 studies require validation in randomized clinical trials. Fifth, even though some insurers might be committed to generating evidence of clinical effectiveness as a basis for coverage decisions, they lack social legitimacy to speak on behalf of patients or to make the case for rigorous evaluation of experimental procedures. They remain vulnerable to the charge of acting in their financial self-interest.

Finally, although technology assessment had developed in a robust way by the time HDC/ABMT began to diffuse, it did not affect clinical use very strongly. Throughout the 1990s, assessment after assessment concluded that phase 2 studies provided insufficient evidence of treatment effectiveness. But, assessments reporting "no evidence of effectiveness" had virtually no effect on the widespread use of the procedure, as the OPM and Minnesota cases make clear. Decisive assessments depend on randomized trials for data, as do systematic reviews and clinical practice guidelines. Only when the phase 3 trials reported no benefit in 1999 was there any effect on utilization. Data showing ineffectiveness finally trumped the absence of data of effectiveness, reinforcing an old political lesson that you can't fight something with nothing.

What has changed in the past decade in how insurers respond to new medical procedures? Four noteworthy developments stemmed directly from experience with HDC/ABMT. First, US HealthCare financed the Philadelphia trial and did so before the NCI initiated its trials. Regrettably, no other insurers supported this effort. Second, the BCBSA's demonstration project, in which 17 Blue plans participated, was designed to pay for patient care costs of randomized clinical trials without challenging the traditional health insurance business model. Although it was limited in its effect by the relatively few plans that participated and perhaps by a low reimbursement for the procedure, the BCBSA demonstration project deserves consideration as the basis for future use.

Third, independent medical review, pioneered by the Medical Care Ombudsman Program and promoted by Aetna, allowed an insurer to ask an expert panel to review the appropriateness of an investigational procedure for a specific patient. For Aetna, individual coverage disputes between a patient and the health plan medical director would be sent to a panel of three nationally known oncologists. A recommendation by one physician to treat was decisive; a unanimous recommendation not to treat included the willingness of the experts to defend their judgment in court. The mechanism juxtaposes the expert judgment of nationally known oncologists against that of the patient's treating physician, thus potentially offsetting the undue influence of a single local physician as an expert witness in a court trial. Supporters of medical review also supported randomized clinical trials. Over 40 states have since adopted independent medical review. We believe that this represents both conceptual and institutional progress.

Finally, on reflection, it becomes clear that the transition from phase 2 studies to phase 3 randomized clinical trials has become more visible and that phase 3 trials have become very public events. They are no longer the exclusive province of scientific medicine. Public information about new treatments, available to all parties via the Internet and Worldwide Web, becomes very important at this juncture. In this respect, ECRI, not an insurer but a technology assessment organization, led the way. The ECRI patient brochure, prepared with the help of women's health and breast cancer patient advocacy groups, and written for the intelligent and interested patient, highlights the great value of carefully prepared information made available when a patient is considering a treatment decision. The brochure, published in 1996 when HDC/ABMT diffusion was nearing its peak, would have been of greater value had it been available much earlier. It is worth noting that BCBSA has posted the results of its technology assessments on its Web site for the past 2 years. Had this been done in the 1990s, it might have affected the course of events. To be effective, information useful to patients needs to be made available at the time a phase 3 trial is initiated, not after the fact.

The National Cancer Institute

Only the NCI stands close enough to the center of the conflicting values and competing interests surrounding new oncology procedures to ensure that their evaluation is as rigorous as FDA's evaluation of new drugs. NCI currently plays three roles that might be expanded: managing more actively than at present the transition from phase 2 studies to phase 3 randomized clinical trials of procedures; negotiating agreement with insurers on financing patient care costs of clinical trials when a procedure is involved; and engaging in an aggressive patient communication program early in the life of a controversial experimental procedure. Although NCI might act on its own, in the following section we propose a collaborative public–private partnership in which it exercises leadership.

First, the transition from phase 2 studies to phase 3 randomized trials must be recognized as the critical transition for procedures. It is at this stage when active discussion occurs within the scientific community—among clinical researchers, cooperative groups, cancer centers, and the NCI—about whether the hypotheses emerging from phase 2 studies are sufficiently robust to warrant a randomized trial. Ideally, this discussion should follow an orderly process that results in a science-based decision about a phase 3 trial, but it is also at this stage when the danger of jumping the gun is greatest. If premature clinical enthusiasm overrides discipline, control over the timely evaluation of a procedure is lost, and the default system of decision making takes over.

A second expanded role for the NCI involves financing clinical trials of procedures, trials that are not sponsored by pharmaceutical firms. Although it is true that phase 3 trials are expensive and difficult to organize, expense is a fact and not an argument. All processes—whether they involve research and development, production, or marketing—have some segments that are more expensive than others. The expense of phase 3 trials does not justify failure to conduct them. The NCI should abandon the argument advanced more than a decade ago for shifting the costs of all NCI clinical trials to health insurers.[4] That "all or nothing, take it or leave it" argument was little more than a thinly disguised plea for cost shifting to a party with deep pockets. This argument is a quid without a quo. Instead, it should commit itself to seeking common ground with insurers on the issue of financing randomized clinical trials.

Third, the NCI should adopt a more aggressive leadership role in advising prospective patients about experimental and investigational treatments as they emerge. The NCI already provides substantial information on its Web site about clinical research, but much of the social utility of that information depends on when it is provided to patients actively seeking such information. Midway through the HDC/ABMT trials, the NCI's public information office became active in seeking to understand barriers to patient accrual. It also became active in 1999 on the threshold of the ASCO meeting as the NCI learned that four trials would report no benefit, but it provided no advice to patients about HDC/ABMT before that, leaving that task to treating physicians, clinical trialists, cooperative groups, and cancer centers. It is reasonable to expect the NCI to generate and actively disseminate information to patients as new procedures move from phase 2 studies to phase 3 randomized clinical trials. Information should indicate the results and limits of phase 2 studies and the rationale for a phase 3 randomized trial based on the medical literature.

In suggesting an expansion of these three existing NCI roles—managing the phase 2–phase 3 transition, focusing on financing expensive but untested procedures, and communicating aggressively to patients—we believe that responsibility should be shared with the medical profession, health insurers, and patients as discussed in the section on negotiating the new arrangement.

Is there a role for the FDA in the evaluation of medical procedures? We think not, but the issue deserves some discussion. The FDA had already approved the single-agent drugs used in the HDC/ABMT combination chemotherapy regimens. (It would also approve human growth factor in 1991.) For the agency to assert authority over combinations of previously approved drugs would require additional statutory authority and would certainly encounter the opposition of organized medicine. However, the FDA review of not-yet-approved drugs with effectiveness that is manifest only in combination with other agents is very much under discussion (B. Goldman 2003a, 2003b). Consideration might be given to the FDA review of combination drug regimens consisting of single agents previously approved. The counterargument, of course, is that the use of combinations found in HDC/ABMT regimens is, and should remain, the practice of medicine and therefore be off-limits to FDA review. What about dosages that greatly exceed the approved indications for the single-agent drugs used in HDC/ABMT combination regimens? Again, this is a gray area not contemplated by existing statutory or regulatory authority. Is the testing of combination high-dose regimens consisting of single-agent drugs approved for much lower doses simply the practice of medicine? Or, is it an issue that should call forth FDA review? Oncologists are likely to insist on the former. Advocates for patient safety and well-being might well insist on FDA review.

If one views the HDC/ABMT "procedure" as off-label use of FDA-approved drugs, then one might argue for an expanded regulatory role for the agency. The availability of effective chemotherapy agents in cancer is still sufficiently limited for oncologists and patients, to say nothing of legislators in the U.S. Congress, to resist strenuously such expansion. The historic relations between the FDA, the NCI, and oncology have been fractious enough to rule expansion of FDA authority out of the question. The FDA regulation of new drugs for cancer, restricted primarily to single-agent evaluation, coexists alongside tolerance for a good deal of clinical experimentation. The proposal we advocate would restrict this regime of tolerance somewhat without creating a new regulatory entity.

Patients and Their Representatives

Is there a role for patient representatives in the arrangement we propose? We believe the answer is yes. The breast cancer advocacy movement was and is a complex movement at the individual, local, and national levels. It derives its forcefulness primarily from the personal experience of women with breast cancer. The movement was not always very supportive of evaluating HDC/ABMT by randomized trials. Quite often, individual women, advised by their physicians, and breast cancer patient advocates supported access to the procedure independent of randomized clinical trials. Coverage denials of the procedure by health insurers and health plans were seen as depriving women of lifesaving treatment for financial reasons.

Few national organizations actively challenged the merits of the HDC/ABMT procedure. Few, in fact, ever took a formal position on the procedure, at least not until the events of 1999 and 2000. Several refused to be swept along by pressures to endorse the procedure. Out of this emotional cauldron, surprisingly, would come a commitment to evidence-based medicine that has permanently changed the clinical research landscape. The National Breast Cancer Coalition (NBCC), which would discuss HDC/ABMT again and again over several years, would eventually articulate a clear and deep commitment to providing experimental treatments only within the context of randomized clinical trials.

These NBCC discussions led initially to the creation of Project LEAD in 1995 and the Clinical Trials Project in 1996. Project LEAD (for Leadership, Education, and Advocacy Development) is a training program designed to teach breast cancer activists the language and concepts of science; how to read the scientific literature critically; how to remain current on breast cancer research; how to understand breast cancer research decision making; to recognize the wide array of advocacy opportunities; and to "gain confidence to speak up, ask questions and find common ground with scientists" (NBCC 2004b, p. 1). The 3-day training program is held in various cities across the United States several times a year. Its curriculum considers the drug development process, the scientific contributions of phase 2, 3, and 4 breast cancer clinical trials, endpoints of trials, quality of life, research protocols, ethical issues, data safety monitoring boards and interim data analysis, examination of specific trials, and media reporting of cancer. Faculty are drawn from NBCC staff, members of coalition organizations, the NCI, the FDA, and leading cancer research institutions.

The NBCC Clinical Trials Initiative was established "to encourage and improve critical breast cancer clinical trials research, and increase access to high quality clinical trials for all breast cancer patients" (NBCC 2000a, p. 1). This initiative involves partnerships with the scientific community and industry, which are entered if the study is "designed to answer an important, novel question relevant to breast cancer," is well designed; is conducted in an ethical manner; adheres to the guidelines of the International Committee of Medical Journal Editors' "Uniform Requirements for Manuscripts Submitted to Biomedical Journals" (ICMJE 2005) provides a mechanism for payment of patient care costs of trial participants; addresses NBCC's concerns about "the inclusion of a diverse population and inappropriate exclusion of specific populations" (NBCC 2000a, pp. 1–2). This initiative has resulted in NBCC partnerships with Genentech on the HER2 (Herceptin) phase 3 clinical trial; with the Breast Cancer International Research Group and Aventis Oncology on a phase 3 trial of a new use of Herceptin; with Genentech on a phase 3 trial of Avastin, a potentially new antiangiogenic therapy; and with Biomira, Inc., in a phase 3 trial of Theratope vaccine. These two initiatives demonstrate that patient advocates can confront the issues of new treatments realistically and affirm the importance of adequate evaluation.

Negotiating a New Institutional Arrangement

We believe that the institutional deficit described must be remedied. The evaluation of new medical procedures, whether in breast cancer, more broadly in oncology, or in medicine in general, deserves more attention than it has received. The conflict between access and evaluation requires effective management of conflicting values to avoid jumping the gun before experimental procedures have been adequately evaluated. The alternative can be very costly—in human lives, in the burden of toxicities, in financial costs, and in the elusive commodity of trust in the health care system.

We propose a new arrangement among and between the medical profession, health insurers, the NCI for oncology and the other NIH institutes for other disease entities, and patients. Does this imply a new regulatory entity? No. In our view, a new regulatory regime appears neither politically feasible nor clearly desirable. Ruling out a new regulatory regime does not imply simply strengthening existing institutions without changing the relationships among them. Although in this chapter we have suggested modest steps that the major parties might take on their own to improve the evaluation process, reliance solely on the current institutional arrangements offers no assurance that an HDC/ABMT experience will be avoided in the future. We believe that a new collaborative relationship is needed among the primary parties to the evaluation of medical procedures.

We recommend that a public–private partnership be created under the aegis of the NCI for oncology procedures and under the relevant NIH institute for other procedures, which includes the medical profession, health insurers, and patient representatives. The broad goal of this partnership would be to change the dynamic surrounding the initial conditions associated with the emergence of a new medical procedure. The explicit purpose would be to see that new unevaluated, costly, and potentially harmful medical procedures do not enter widespread clinical use prematurely. The factor that would trigger action by this partnership is the transition of a procedure from phase 2 studies to phase 3 randomized clinical trials. A determination regarding the expense of patient care costs of the procedure compared to conventional therapies would inform deliberations.

We expect that this partnership would generate summary information about a given medical procedure (the hypotheses generated by phase 2 studies and the "equipoise rationale" for undertaking a phase 3 randomized clinical trial) that would be disseminated widely to patients, physicians, insurers, and the general public.[5] Information generated by the partnership should be made an obligatory part of local and central institutional review board (IRB) deliberations and should be incorporated into the individual patient informed consent process.

The heart of the partnership proposal is the expectation that health insurers would finance patient care costs for expensive but promising new procedures identified as ripe for NCI-sponsored phase 3 randomized clinical trials. In return, they would be parties to an authoritative statement from the partnership that articulated the clinical rationale for a randomized trial of a new treatment and provided them protection from legal demands to cover it outside such trials.

In the absence of an existing agency for the evaluation of procedures, it is appropriate to ask under whose authority might this entity be established? Congress could clearly direct the NCI to convene a group to negotiate such a partnership. Existing NCI authority, we believe, is adequate to convene a meeting to discuss this proposal. In all likelihood, the convening of a work group on this proposal would require prior deliberations by the principal institutions involved and a "champion" to insist that the general interest of patients and the broader public interest in the evaluation of medical procedures should override institutional self-interest.

What incentives might lead the parties to enter into such a nonregulatory, voluntary partnership? The lesson that conflicting values need to be managed is hardly self-executing. Essentially, the parties involved would have to recognize that their self-interest would be better served in this way than by existing arrangements. The factors that might motivate the major parties to come together include reducing the delay in determining whether an experimental procedure is better than conventional treatment, increasing support for enrolling patients in randomized trials, clarifying the risks to patients of treatments that have not yet been evaluated, and damping of the costs of litigation and payment for experimental treatments. That the general public might be better served as well provides a potential, but weaker, reason for action.

A further incentive that might encourage the creation of such an arrangement would be the recognition that sweeping proposals for change (e.g., that insurers should finance patient care costs of all NCI-sponsored clinical trials or that insurers should be taxed on their premiums to support clinical research) are demonstrated nonstarters of the past decade. Starting with a narrowly focused area of agreement might establish the venue for discussions about larger possibilities. We would expect that the NCI and medical professional societies would actively support this partnership if health insurers would agree to finance patient care costs of randomized trials. We would expect insurers to support this partnership if they were shielded from litigation related to medical procedures that had yet to be evaluated. If the partnership encouraged "free riders" among health insurers and health plans, the U.S. Congress should consider establishing this partnership by statute.

What benefits might accrue from such a partnership? It would remedy the institutional deficit where it is weakest, at the front end, where the transition from phase 2 studies to phase 3 randomized trials occurs, where zealots for new procedures currently have an advantage based on enthusiasm and not always on data. It would frame the access-versus-evaluation conflict in terms of the hypotheses generated by phase 2 studies, the data supporting such studies, the rationale for a randomized trial, and the plan for generating the needed information.

Information from such a partnership would be authoritative, involving all primary parties to the discussion. This would contrast with current arrangements by which none of the major parties are clearly responsible for anything, and power flows to the actors in the default system. Information would be provided to and for individual patients, individual physicians, and all those actively engaged in patient decision making, as well as for those with institutional responsibilities. Such information would justify restricting the availability of the procedure in question to randomized trials. This information should be widely available in many forms (on the Web, as a brochure, as an announcement in professional journals, etc.) for reaching multiple audiences. Including such information in deliberations of local and central IRBs should be obligatory, thus reducing the variability to which IRBs are vulnerable on scientific matters, leaving them to focus on the ethical issues of informed consent. The statement should be made part of the individual patient informed consent process. Such a partnership would put timely information in the hands of information-seeking patients as they confront their treatment options, one of which would be a randomized trial. The ECRI patient brochure could serve as a model, but such a partnership might also stimulate much needed attention to patient communication.

An authoritative statement from the partnership would also serve as a benchmark for those lacking medical expertise (courts, legislatures, administrative agencies, and the media) regarding the scientific status of a putative breakthrough treatment. It would remove the presumption of expertise currently granted to local treating physicians in court cases and anchor it in a national authoritative entity. It would invert the current situation in which the absence of an authoritative entity, in effect, cedes authority on a decentralized basis to the default system of courts, legislatures, administrative agencies lacking expertise, and the media.

Independent medical review should be a corollary to all of the above actions. It now exists in over 40 states. This innovation allows national experts to consider the appropriateness of a given experimental procedure for a specific individual patient, thus reducing the expert status of the ordinary community physician. It provides a way to listen to the individual patient, constitutes a societal safety valve for troublesome cases, and allows the evaluation process to move forward.

What obstacles exist to this proposal being considered, let alone adopted? The absence of a convening authority may be the biggest obstacle. Inertia also militates against change. A judgment, correct or not, that an HDC/ABMT case is unlikely to recur would provide another reason for inaction. A conclusion that the costs of change are greater than the benefits would deter adoption. Finally, whatever the benefits to other parties and the general public, a judgment by any of the major parties that their independence was being constrained in an unacceptable way would stop this proposal in its tracks.

A major obstacle involves the financing of clinical trials. Public financing of oncology clinical trials has been established in interagency agreements between the NCI and the Department of Defense (DoD) and the NCI and the Department of Veterans Affairs (DoD/NCI 1996; Department of Veterans Affairs/NCI 1997). An Institute of Medicine report in 2000 said that 206 patients had participated in the DoD program by April 1999; of more than 11,000 eligible patients; more than half had breast cancer, and about two thirds were in phase 2 trials and one third in phase

3 trials. The DoD benefit was apparently seen as a way to obtain HDC/ABMT. As most patients were in phase 2 trials, they would have avoided randomization (Aaron et al. 2000). The Veterans Affairs was not tracking the number of patients enrolled in trials under this agreement. In response to this Institute of Medicine report, President Clinton issued an executive memorandum that required Medicare to cover patient care costs for beneficiaries enrolled in clinical trials, including cancer trials (Aaron et al. 2000). These arrangements reflect policy decisions by federal government agencies and constitute significant developments of the past decade, but they do not bind private health insurers and health plans, for whom such arrangements require economic incentives responsive to their financial situation.

The historic NCI position articulated by Wittes, and extended to the NIH, argued that the NIH budgetary constraints limited its ability to finance phase 3 trials, and that insurers should finance such trials for the greater social good. Its scope included all NCI-sponsored clinical trials, with no role for insurers in determining priorities. This view amounts to little more than an expressed preference for someone else's money. It is not a negotiating position but a statement of self-interest. It should be abandoned for a strategy that provides incentives for both parties. We believe that our proposal is at least a first step toward such a strategy.

Similarly, ASCO adopted a policy statement "Reimbursement and Coverage Implications of Clinical Trials in Treatment of Cancer" more than a decade ago (ASCO 1992). It criticizes insurers for excluding coverage of experimental or investigational treatments on the grounds that such a policy increasingly "is used to deny coverage for high quality therapy associated with clinical trials" (p. 1). It urges insurers to adopt policies "that enhance a cancer patient's access to medically appropriate treatment options" (p. 1), which include phases 1 through 4 clinical trials. The rationale for this policy, like that of the NCI, leans heavily on patient benefit, implicitly on benefit to the research enterprise, but offers nothing in return to insurers. It is time to acknowledge that proposals that have gone nowhere in over a decade either lack the political support that would result in federal legislation or the financial or legal incentives that would bring insurers to the table.

A growing body of research done in the past decade has shown than the patient care costs of most oncology clinical trials are modest, not much higher than the comparable costs of conventional treatment, and potentially easily absorbed by insurers (Chirikos et al. 2001; Fireman et al. 2000; Wagner et al. 1999). Goldman and colleagues have shown that the incremental patient care costs of oncology clinical trials are modest for most trials, on average 6.5% higher for nonpediatric clinical trial participants than for nonenrollees. They suggest—without recommending—that such costs can be absorbed by insurers with relative ease (D. P. Goldman et al. 2003). We suggest that insurers should routinely cover patient care costs of experimental treatments when they fall in a normal cost range. Indeed, there is reason to believe that insurers absorb the costs of many trials because they go unrecognized. The patient care costs of HDC/ABMT trials were not modest but were some multiple of those of conventional treatment. The financial beneficiaries were hospitals, clinics, and physicians, at the expense of insurers. The economic incentive to health insurers to finance trials under such circumstances is weak indeed. The entity we propose here need not be invoked for trials with marginal incremental patient care costs. Our proposal applies mainly to expensive new procedures for which clinical evidence of effectiveness is absent and for which only a randomized trial can generate decisive data.

Our proposal is hardly a magic bullet. Conflicting values existed at every stage of the HDC/ABMT experience, as we have indicated. They guarantee that conflict would accompany efforts to create this kind of partnership. This proposal is consistent with other recent and prior proposals that indicate genuine frustration at the inadequacy of existing relationships among the key institutional actors. In 2004, Dr. Mark McClellan, administrator of the Centers for Medicare and Medicaid Services and formerly commissioner of Food and Drugs, indicated at the ASCO annual meeting that Medicare was developing a Memorandum of Understanding with the NCI regarding how those agencies could cooperate to improve coverage decision making for cancer therapeutics and diagnostics (Goldberg 2004). McClellan was quoted as saying the following:

> One of the goals is to make sure that we are developing reimbursement frameworks that are appropriate for the new kinds of treatments that are coming along for cancer care. We want to make sure that our procedures for paying for these treatments and getting the *effective* [emphasis added] treatments to patients are effective and timely, and informed by the best science and clinical experience. We are also going to be working hard to increase the body of knowledge that clinicians and patients can use to guide decisions about how to use these new technologies effectively. (p. 2)

The Memorandum of Understanding would involve the joint CMS [Centers for Medicare and Medicaid Services]-NCI identification of "high-priority clinical questions," a "systematic process for consultations," devising "more efficient methods of collecting clinical evidence" on new cancer treatments, development of a process for "the prospective identification and evaluation of emerging technologies," and "sharing data and resources" for improving the quality of care (Goldberg 2004, p. 3). The CMS plan also involves reportedly cooperative efforts to "identify and initiate high-priority clinical trials in areas where clinicians and patients have said that they need more and better clinical information to guide their decision making about new or competing treatment regimens" (p. 3). William McGivney, formerly at Aetna, now chief executive officer of the National Comprehensive Cancer Network, welcomed the news: "It's an excellent idea. There needs to be a meeting of minds on the process for making clinical treatment decisions and the process for making coverage policy" (p. 2).

Current proposals also echo several made a decade ago that highlighted the need for systematic evaluation of new medical technologies. In 1994, the Physician Payment Review Commission proposed an entity to evaluate new medical procedures (Physician Payment Review Commission 1994). The following year, the BCBSA proposed an "urgent care" approach to evaluating high-priority procedures (Gleeson 1998). In 1999, the New Jersey Association of Health Plans, representing nine health insurers in the state, entered into a "voluntary agreement" to finance the routine costs of patient care for individuals participating in phase 1, 2, and 3 cancer clinical trials (New Jersey Association of Health Plans 2000). These costs would include "physician fees, laboratory expenses, administration of treatment, and continuing evaluation of the health of the patient" (p. 1), according to the association. The *New York Times* would report the following:

> The insurers are acting partly out of frustration. Currently, many researchers cannot find enough patients to volunteer for studies that determine whether treatments work. With their new initiatives, the insurers hope to funnel more patients into scientifically valid studies so that the effectiveness of a treatment can be determined more quickly. (Kolata and Eichenwald 1999, p. C1)

The evaluation of medical and surgical procedures, as distinct from new therapeutic agents, has also received recent attention from two surgeons. Strasberg and Ludbrook (2003) examined procedures that are "permitted entry into ordinary use after much more limited evaluation, or even after no evaluation" (p. 938). They listed as recent examples of "harm or potential harm" laparoscopic cholecystectomy, radiofrequency ablation of metastatic colorectal tumors in the liver, and live donor right hemiliver transplantation. Their review of "current safeguards" for protection of patients receiving innovative therapies ("both novel and unvalidated") focused on weaknesses of the human subjects' informed consent process. Strasberg and Ludbrook suggested four potential steps toward solution of the issue of evaluating procedures. These include clarifying the meaning of significant innovation; triggering a patient protection process for procedures so identified; determining which agencies should have responsibility for overseeing and monitoring evaluation of the procedure; and finding a funding mechanism for evaluation.

Our proposal addresses these issues by avoiding the semantic jungle of defining and listing significant innovations and by restricting the triggering process to procedures identified as sufficiently promising to warrant randomized clinical trials and sufficiently costly to require attention to the patient care costs of such trials. Oversight would be provided by a public–private partnership that involves clinical researchers, insurers, patients' representatives, and the NCI or the relevant NIH institute. Finally, financing the patient care costs of randomized clinical trials would be assumed by health insurers in return for a front-end authoritative statement that the effectiveness of the procedure in question was unknown, and that a randomized trial was required to determine its benefit. Such a statement, we believe, grants insurers protection against providing the experimental treatment outside clinical trials.

Slouching toward Evidence-Based Medicine

Modern medicine is clearly moving toward greater reliance on evidence-based clinical practice (Guyatt et al. 2002). The reasons are clear. At root, this movement results from the recognition that the individual physician is overwhelmed by the flood of new scientific and clinical information that appears in the journal literature on a weekly, if not daily, basis. This flood of new information creates the need for methods of synthesis, such as clinical practice guidelines, that go beyond the traditional review article. The result is a gradual restriction of idiosyncratic physician autonomy in favor of a more systematic collective means of relating clinical science to clinical practice. In addition, the country has demonstrated a decreasing tolerance for clinical practice that fails to provide effective clinical care. The phenomenon of jumping the gun manifest in the HDC/ABMT story is less and less defensible over time.

Although a regulatory system for evaluating new drugs has been in place for four decades, no such system exists for the evaluation of medical procedures. We propose, not a regulatory scheme, but a voluntary coming together of medical scientists, health insurers, the NIH (as represented by its constituent institutes), and representatives of the patient community. The basis for this coming together is the recognition that the existing system does not work. Subjecting 23,000–40,000 women to a difficult, highly toxic experimental procedure, as in the HDC/ABMT case, while providing the procedure to only 1000 women through randomized trials and waiting a decade for answers to how the experimental compares to conventional treatment is an experiment not worth repeating.

We do not advocate a new regulatory regime supported by congressional legislation. Neither do we argue for continued reliance on the current institutional arrangement. Some might suggest that "the system worked" in the HDC/ABMT case, that at the end of the day randomized clinical trials decisively resolved the issue of the procedure's effectiveness or lack thereof, both for metastatic and high-risk breast cancer. Some might also argue that a decade is substantially shorter than the 80 years it took to challenge the Halstad mastectomy procedure. This is cold comfort. The argument that the system worked draws solace from the avoidance of major institutional breakdown, which is hardly an endorsement for a well-ordered system. The challenge of evaluating new medical procedures deserves a collaborative approach involving all relevant parties, including the general public.

Medical procedures deserve careful evaluation before they have diffused widely to determine if the new therapy is comparable to or better than existing treatment. An explosion of new therapies is occurring throughout medicine, and by all reports, we can expect this to continue and probably increase. The effectiveness of these new treatments is often unclear, and some that proclaim major benefits may only provide marginal advances; some may actually deliver harms. Moreover, the effects of new treatments on health care costs cannot be avoided forever. It is economically, if not morally, untenable to expect that patients be provided with continuous access to new, untested therapy and that automatic payment by insurers be accepted as the societal norm.

Information should be generated at the transition to phase 3 trials about what is known, what is not known, and why randomized trials are essential. This information should be available to patients considering decisions about the appropriate course of treatment, physicians telling patients about their choices, IRBs evaluating phase 3 protocols for informed consent, and insurers evaluating coverage. In return for information that supports testing experimental procedures only in randomized trials, insurers should finance patient care costs of the appropriate publicly sponsored phase 3 trials. This will speed the acquisition of data about effectiveness.

Finally, we believe that the arrangement proposed for medicine, insurers, the NCI, and patients and their representatives would stand the current relations with the default system institutions upside down. Rather than yield de facto control to the decentralized courts, entrepreneurs, legislatures, administrators, and media, a centralized defense of randomized clinical trials would encourage a more balanced view of the access-versus-evaluation issue. It would establish a benchmark that would require these other institutions to justify a different course. It would temper the enthusiasm that physicians bring to new medical procedures before their adequate evaluation. It would diminish the vulnerability of courts to their limited capacity to evaluate scientific medicine. It would dampen the effects of the popular media in highlighting the promise and minimizing the risk of untested procedures.

Epilogue

What is hope? Hope is both a verb and a noun, an act of looking forward, a visualization of a future event or state, an attitude by which an individual confronts a difficult but not impossible situation, such as a diagnosis of breast cancer with varying treatment options. Hope comes with expectations for rescue, relief, restoration, or cure, while understanding the great uncertainty about the prospects for restoring health. Dictionaries often define hope in circular ways (e.g., one definition of the noun is "something hoped for"). More helpful is this discussion of synonyms: "Expect, hope, look mean to await some occurrence or outcome. *Expect* implies a high degree of certainty and usually involves the idea of preparing or envisioning. *Hope* implies little certainty but suggests confidence or assurance in the possibility that what one desires or longs for will happen. *Look to* implies assurance that expectations will be fulfilled; *look for* implies less assurance and suggests an attitude of expectancy and watchfulness" (Merriam-Webster's Collegiate Dictionary, 10th edition, 1997, p. 408).

In contrast to false hope, a central element in hope is the general understanding that expectations are realistic. Realism is based in part on biology, in part on the human spirit, in part on the dynamic interaction of patient and physician. Jerome Groopman, in *The Anatomy of Hope,* in a chapter entitled "False Hope, True Hope," recounts his vacillation in encounters with several patients early in his medical career. "I had swung wildly," he writes, "between matter-of-factly revealing shattering statistics and hiding salient facts behind euphemistic evasions, unable in each case to locate a middle ground" (pp. 50–51). For a subsequent patient, he found that "Richard had come closer to the middle ground where both truth and hope could reside. I had seen that it was possible" (p. 57).

Realistic expectations are also based on the kind of individuals involved. Joan Didion, in *The Year of Magical Thinking,* writes the following:

> One thing I noticed . . . was that many people I knew, whether in New York or California or in other places, share a habit of mind usually credited to the very successful. They believed absolutely in their own management skills. They believed absolutely in the power of the telephone numbers they had at their fingertips, the right doctor, the major donor, the person who could facilitate a favor at State or Justice. The management skills of these people were in fact prodigious. The power of their telephone numbers was in fact unmatched. I had myself for most of my life shared the same core belief in my ability to control events. . . . Yet I had always at some level apprehended, because I was born fearful, that some events in life would remain beyond my ability to control or manage them. Some events would just happen. (p. 98)

Marjorie Williams, in *The Woman at the National Zoo*, a book of her essays edited by Timothy Noah, her husband, displays the behaviors of which Didion writes. Diagnosed with liver cancer, Williams recorded much of the final three and one-half years of her life in compelling terms. During that time she consulted numerous physicians in Washington and New York. Her husband inquired about compassionate use of a new drug still in the clinical trial stage, but to no avail. Her experience reflects one dynamic of hope driving behavior of newly diagnosed cancer patients. When a diagnosis of cancer is presumed to be terminal, such individuals may drive events along the path of unrealistic expectations, reasoning that they are willing to try anything.

False hope is based on a set of unrealistic expectations, encouraged through incomplete or faulty information or by a patient's unwillingness to acknowledge the limits of medicine. For HDC/ABMT for breast cancer, false hope was the genuine promise of a treatment that deserved careful evaluation, but around which exaggerated and unrealistic expectations were created about its benefit. Careful evaluation of HDC/ABMT was required because of the biological nature of breast cancer and the high toxicity of the treatment. Although there was no deliberate effort to deceive women, the combined effect of salesmanship by physicians, lawyers, legislators, entrepreneurs, and the press led one of our respondents to say, "We were all sold a bill of goods."

Can we identify in advance those medical procedures that offer false hope because they are based on unrealistic expectations? For breast cancer, the answer is yes. Unrealistic expectations derive from early studies of few patients that lack adequate controls, studies with promise that constitutes a valid hypothesis to be tested but that provide no justifiable basis for physician enthusiasm or exaggeration by others.

For breast cancer, realism about new procedures requires that expectations be validated by essential randomized clinical trials. True hope, therefore, requires patience and the willingness to wait for credible scientific evidence of benefit generated by randomized trials. (Interestingly, the Spanish verb *esperar* means both to hope and to wait.) Patience, in turn, requires mechanisms to protect the integrity of the evaluation process and ensure against widespread premature clinical use of untested innovations. Hence, we have the abiding tension with which we all must contend: how to counsel patience and advocate for thorough evaluation of new treatments when individuals see such treatments as their best hope for life. We must engage in the search for where biology and hope reside. This search must provide a mechanism for access to clinical trials for promising new treatments. There is no escape from this challenge.

Appendix

Evidence-Based Reviews of Clinical Trials

Evidence-based reviews of clinical trials have become common in the medical literature in the past two decades. The Oxford Group, the Cochrane Collaboration, and the Evidence-based Practice Centers sponsored by the Agency for Healthcare Research and Quality all support such reviews. In brief, these systematic reviews constitute an activity committed to summarizing the evidentiary basis of medical practice. This development reflects a sea change in views of the 1980s—away from emphasis on expert consensus and toward systematic reviews of scientific evidence. Both institutions and processes now exist to review data from randomized trials.

In this appendix we present a summary of two Cochrane Collaboration systematic reviews by Farquhar and Basser of all the available randomized trials as of March 2005, both in the United States and internationally (1,2). One review addresses high-risk breast cancer trials, the other metastatic breast cancer trials. Their conclusions are presented here.

High-Risk Breast Cancer

For women with high-risk breast cancer (nonmetastatic disease), 20 potential studies were found. Two were excluded: One did not compare high-dose chemotherapy with a conventional regimen, and the other was invalidated by scientific misconduct (3,4). Of the remaining 18 trials, 5 were ongoing (5–9), and 13 were included in the review (10–22). Only 5 of them have been published so far.

The 13 trials randomized 5111 women, of whom 99% were included in intention-to-treat analyses. Of the studies, 9 used acceptable methods of randomization and allocation concealment; details were unavailable for the other four (10,12,15,22). Eleven studies described using risk stratification to balance the groups with respect to baseline prognostic factors such as the number of positive nodes, hormone receptor status, and menopausal status (11–15,17–22). The prescribed minimum number of involved lymph nodes required by the inclusion criteria ranged from 4 to 10. Eleven of the trials delivered an initial course of conventional dose chemotherapy to all participants, with the high-dose arm proceeding to a myeloablative regimen. In the other two trials, the experimental arm had a combination of high-dose chemotherapy drugs in sequence, with no prior conventional-dose chemotherapy (16,17). In all cases, high-dose therapy was supported by stem cells or bone marrow harvested during the initial stages. The proportion of women randomized to high-dose treatment who did not actually receive it varied from 4% to 31% in the eight trials that supplied this information.

Among women with high-risk breast cancer, statistically significant benefit in event-free survival for the high-dose group was found at 3 years (relative risk [RR] 1.12, 95% confidence interval [CI] 1.02–1.46) and at 4 years (RR 1.34, 95% CI 1.17–1.53). This benefit was no longer evident at 5 years (RR 1.03, 95% CI 0.97–1.09). Regarding overall survival rates, there was no statistically significant difference between the treatments at any stage of follow-up (measured at 3, 4, 5, and 6 years). These results are presented in figures A.1 and A.2.

Several of the trials involving women with high-risk breast cancer reported quality-of-life outcomes. Results varied, but although the high-dose arms reported significantly worse quality-of-life scores around the time of treatment, in general there was little difference between the arms at 6–12 months (11–13). However, in one study women in the high-dose arm still scored significantly lower on physical and functional measures at 1 year. In another study, 20% of women on each arm reported fatigue, sore muscles, decreased sexual interest, and sweating as adverse effects of therapy at 4 years (22). In the Dutch trials (13,14), cognitive function tests administered to a subset of women at a median of 2 years after treatment showed an elevated risk of cognitive impairment in the high-dose group compared with a control group who had not had any chemotherapy ($P = .006$). However, at 4 years the tests were repeated, and the results suggested that cognitive dysfunction after chemotherapy may be transient, although there was a high attrition rate of initially cognitively impaired women in the high-dose arm.

Metastatic Breast Cancer

For women with metastatic breast cancer, 11 potentially suitable studies were found. Three were excluded: two did not make the comparison of interest, and one was invalidated by scientific misconduct (23–25). Of the remainder, two trials were ongoing at the time of this review (26, 33), and six were included in the review (27–32). Only three of them have been published as this review was conducted.

Three of the six trials concerning metastatic disease described satisfactory methods of randomization and allocation concealment (27,28,32); the other trials were unclear. The six trials randomized 866 women, of whom 98% were analyzed by intention to treat. The proportion of women randomized to high-dose treatment who did not actually receive it varied from 6% to 21% in the five trials that supplied this information. Although only three trials described used risk stratification (27,29,31), all reported that baseline prognostic factors were well balanced between the groups, with the exception of one study, which had more women with central nervous system and pulmonary metastases on the high-dose arm (31). All these studies required the participants to have had no prior chemotherapy for metastatic disease. All but one delivered an initial course of conventional chemotherapy to all women, with the experimental arm proceeding to high-dose treatment. In one trial, the experimental arm had a combination of high-dose chemotherapy drugs in sequence, without prior conventional chemotherapy (32).

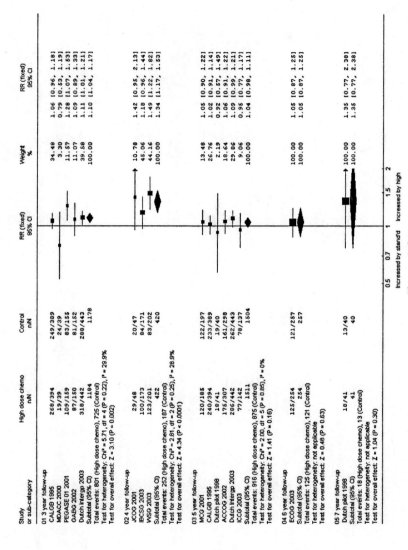

Figure A.1

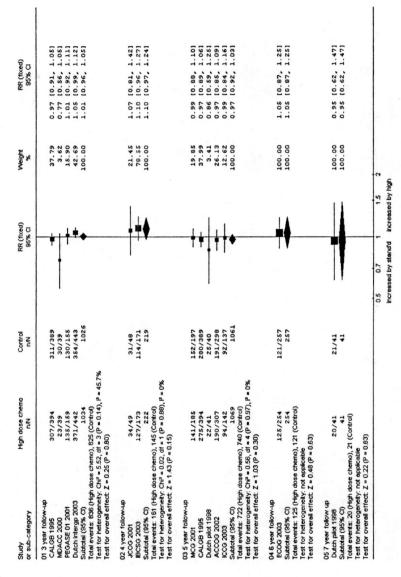

Study or sub-category	High dose chemo n/N	Control n/N	RR (fixed) 95% CI	Weight %	RR (fixed) 95% CI
01 3 year follow-up					
CALGB 1995	307/394	311/389		37.79	0.97 [0.91, 1.05]
MDACC 2000	23/39	30/39		3.62	0.77 [0.56, 1.05]
PEGASE 01 2001	135/159	130/155		15.90	1.01 [0.92, 1.11]
Dutch Intergp 2003	371/442	354/443		42.69	1.05 [0.99, 1.12]
Subtotal (95% CI)	1034	1026		100.00	1.01 [0.96, 1.05]
Total events: 836 (High dose chemo), 825 (Control)					
Test for heterogeneity: Chi² = 5.52, df = 3 (P = 0.14), I² = 45.7%					
Test for overall effect: Z = 0.25 (P = 0.80)					
02 4 year follow-up					
JCOG 2001	34/49	31/48		21.45	1.07 [0.81, 1.42]
IBCSG 2003	127/173	114/171		78.55	1.10 [0.96, 1.27]
Subtotal (95% CI)	222	219		100.00	1.10 [0.97, 1.24]
Total events: 161 (High dose chemo), 145 (Control)					
Test for heterogeneity: Chi² = 0.02, df = 1 (P = 0.88), I² = 0%					
Test for overall effect: Z = 1.43 (P = 0.15)					
03 5 year follow-up					
MCG 2001	141/185	152/197		19.85	0.99 [0.88, 1.10]
CALGB 1995	275/394	280/389		37.99	0.97 [0.89, 1.06]
Dutch pilot 1998	22/41	25/40		3.41	0.86 [0.59, 1.25]
ACCOG 2002	190/307	191/298		26.13	0.97 [0.85, 1.09]
ICCG 2003	94/142	92/137		12.62	0.99 [0.84, 1.16]
Subtotal (95% CI)	1069	1061		100.00	0.97 [0.92, 1.03]
Total events: 722 (High dose chemo), 740 (Control)					
Test for heterogeneity: Chi² = 0.56, df = 4 (P = 0.97), I² = 0%					
Test for overall effect: Z = 1.03 (P = 0.30)					
04 6 year follow-up					
ECOG 2003	125/254	121/257		100.00	1.05 [0.87, 1.25]
Subtotal (95% CI)	254	257		100.00	1.05 [0.87, 1.25]
Total events: 125 (High dose chemo), 121 (Control)					
Test for heterogeneity: not applicable					
Test for overall effect: Z = 0.48 (P = 0.63)					
05 7 year follow-up					
Dutch pilot 1998	20/41	21/41		100.00	0.95 [0.62, 1.47]
Subtotal (95% CI)	41	41		100.00	0.95 [0.62, 1.47]
Total events: 20 (High dose chemo), 21 (Control)					
Test for heterogeneity: not applicable					
Test for overall effect: Z = 0.22 (P = 0.83)					

0.5 0.7 1 1.5 2

Increased by stand'd   Increased by high

Figure A.2

Among women with metastatic disease, a significant benefit in event-free survival for the high-dose group was found at 1- and 2-year follow-up (RR 1.79, 95% CI 1.4–2.24; RR 1.96, 95% CI 1.32–2.90, respectively), and one study showed the high-dose arm still benefiting at 3-year follow-up, although this study was the smallest in the review, with only 61 women (31). Again, no benefit was evident at 5-year follow-up. These results must be interpreted with caution because much of the data is immature, and the results at 3-years were statistically heterogeneous. When overall survival was considered, there was no statistically significant difference between the treatments at any stage of follow-up (which was measured at 1, 3, and 5 years). These results are presented in figures A.3 and A.4.

All the studies of women with metastatic disease reported on median time to tumor progression and median overall survival time; however, as no individual data were available, it was not possible to combine results. Three studies found a significant difference between the two arms in time to tumor progression, and one found a difference of borderline significance, all favoring the high-dose arm. However, the study with the longest follow-up, which had followed 184 women for a median of 57 months, found no significant difference between the groups for this outcome. None of the trials found a significant difference between the two arms in median overall survival time.

Only one of the studies involving women with metastatic disease reported quality-of-life outcomes (27): at 6 months, total mood disturbance was significantly worse in the high-dose arm than in the control arm.

Adverse Events

Treatment-related mortality was significantly higher in the high-dose chemotherapy arms for both groups of women (high-risk breast cancer group: RR 8.48, 95% CI 4.08–17.61; metastatic group: RR 4.07, 95% CI 1.39–11.88). In the high-dose arms, 64 women with high-risk breast cancer and 15 women with metastatic disease died from treatment-related toxicity, while in the control arms there were 4 and 2 deaths, respectively. These results are presented in figures A.5 and A.6.

Adverse effects were more frequent and severe in the high-dose groups. Toxicities included neutropenia (low white blood cell count) and acute effects such as fatigue; vomiting; inflammation of the mucous membranes, especially the oral cavity; and diarrhea, along with organ toxicities. Long-term adverse effects included avascular necrosis, peripheral neuropathy, hearing loss, congestive heart failure, and pulmonary fibrosis. There was no statistically significant difference between the groups in the frequency of occurrence of secondary malignancies, although one trialist reported that it was as yet too early to evaluate this risk.

Sensitivity Analyses

In the review of trials for women with high-risk breast cancer, trials were excluded (in turn) that were not explicit about randomization and allocation methods, did not analyze by intention to treat, or did not report balanced prognostic factors in the two

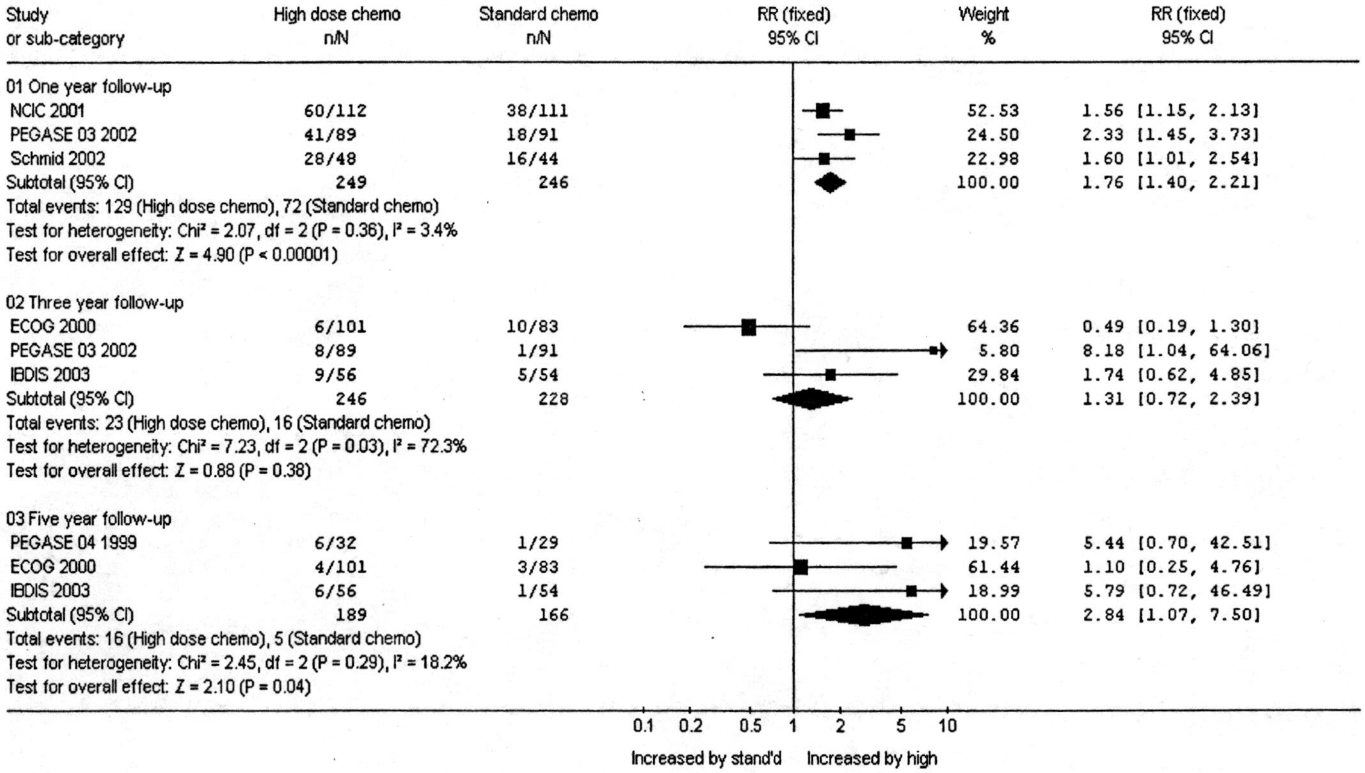

Study or sub-category	High dose chemo n/N	Standard chemo n/N	RR (fixed) 95% CI	Weight %	RR (fixed) 95% CI
01 One year follow-up					
NCIC 2001	60/112	38/111		52.53	1.56 [1.15, 2.13]
PEGASE 03 2002	41/89	18/91		24.50	2.33 [1.45, 3.73]
Schmid 2002	28/48	16/44		22.98	1.60 [1.01, 2.54]
Subtotal (95% CI)	249	246		100.00	1.76 [1.40, 2.21]

Total events: 129 (High dose chemo), 72 (Standard chemo)
Test for heterogeneity: Chi² = 2.07, df = 2 (P = 0.36), I² = 3.4%
Test for overall effect: Z = 4.90 (P < 0.00001)

02 Three year follow-up					
ECOG 2000	6/101	10/83		64.36	0.49 [0.19, 1.30]
PEGASE 03 2002	8/89	1/91		5.80	8.18 [1.04, 64.06]
IBDIS 2003	9/56	5/54		29.84	1.74 [0.62, 4.85]
Subtotal (95% CI)	246	228		100.00	1.31 [0.72, 2.39]

Total events: 23 (High dose chemo), 16 (Standard chemo)
Test for heterogeneity: Chi² = 7.23, df = 2 (P = 0.03), I² = 72.3%
Test for overall effect: Z = 0.88 (P = 0.38)

03 Five year follow-up					
PEGASE 04 1999	6/32	1/29		19.57	5.44 [0.70, 42.51]
ECOG 2000	4/101	3/83		61.44	1.10 [0.25, 4.76]
IBDIS 2003	6/56	1/54		18.99	5.79 [0.72, 46.49]
Subtotal (95% CI)	189	166		100.00	2.84 [1.07, 7.50]

Total events: 16 (High dose chemo), 5 (Standard chemo)
Test for heterogeneity: Chi² = 2.45, df = 2 (P = 0.29), I² = 18.2%
Test for overall effect: Z = 2.10 (P = 0.04)

0.1 0.2 0.5 1 2 5 10

Increased by stand'd   Increased by high

Figure A.3

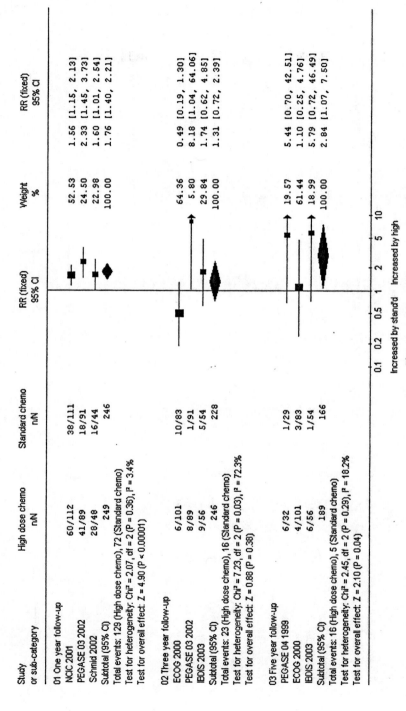

Study or sub-category	High dose chemo n/N	Standard chemo n/N	RR (fixed) 95% CI	Weight %	RR (fixed) 95% CI
01 One year follow-up					
NCIC 2001	60/112	38/111		52.53	1.56 [1.15, 2.13]
PEGASE 03 2002	41/89	18/91		24.50	2.33 [1.45, 3.73]
Schmid 2002	28/48	16/44		22.98	1.60 [1.01, 2.54]
Subtotal (95% CI)	249	246		100.00	1.76 [1.40, 2.21]
Total events: 129 (High dose chemo), 72 (Standard chemo)					
Test for heterogeneity: Chi² = 2.07, df = 2 (P = 0.36), I² = 3.4%					
Test for overall effect: Z = 4.90 (P < 0.00001)					
02 Three year follow-up					
ECOG 2000	6/101	10/83		64.36	0.49 [0.19, 1.30]
PEGASE 03 2002	8/89	1/91		5.80	8.18 [1.04, 64.06]
IBDIS 2003	9/56	5/54		29.84	1.74 [0.62, 4.85]
Subtotal (95% CI)	246	228		100.00	1.31 [0.72, 2.39]
Total events: 23 (High dose chemo), 16 (Standard chemo)					
Test for heterogeneity: Chi² = 7.23, df = 2 (P = 0.03), I² = 72.3%					
Test for overall effect: Z = 0.88 (P = 0.38)					
03 Five year follow-up					
PEGASE 04 1999	6/32	1/29		19.57	5.44 [0.70, 42.51]
ECOG 2000	4/101	3/83		61.44	1.10 [0.25, 4.76]
IBDIS 2003	6/56	1/54		18.99	5.79 [0.72, 46.49]
Subtotal (95% CI)	189	166		100.00	2.84 [1.07, 7.50]
Total events: 16 (High dose chemo), 5 (Standard chemo)					
Test for heterogeneity: Chi² = 2.45, df = 2 (P = 0.29), I² = 18.2%					
Test for overall effect: Z = 2.10 (P = 0.04)					

0.1 0.2 0.5 1 2 5 10

Increased by stand'd   Increased by high

Figure A.4

Study or sub-category	High dose chemo n/N	Standard chemo n/N	RR (fixed) 95% CI	Weight %	RR (fixed) 95% CI
MCG 2001	1/185	0/197		6.04	3.19 [0.13, 77.90]
CALGB 1995	32/394	0/389		6.27	64.18 [3.94, 1044.39]
Dutch pilot 1998	0/41	0/40			Not estimable
MDACC 2000	1/39	0/39		6.23	3.00 [0.13, 71.46]
JCOG 2001	0/48	0/47			Not estimable
PEGASE 01 2001	1/159	0/155		6.31	2.93 [0.12, 71.26]
ACCOG 2002	5/307	0/298		6.32	10.68 [0.59, 192.27]
GABG 2002	3/150	2/152		24.76	1.52 [0.26, 8.97]
Dutch Intergp 2003	5/442	0/443		6.22	11.02 [0.61, 198.78]
ECOG 2003	9/254	0/257		6.20	19.22 [1.12, 328.55]
IBCSG 2003	4/173	0/171		6.27	8.90 [0.48, 163.99]
ICCG 2003	3/142	2/137		25.37	1.45 [0.25, 8.53]
WSG 2003	0/201	0/202			Not estimable
Total (95% CI)	2535	2527		100.00	8.44 [4.06, 17.54]

Total events: 64 (High dose chemo), 4 (Standard chemo)
Test for heterogeneity: Chi² = 10.98, df = 9 (P = 0.28), I² = 18.1%
Test for overall effect: Z = 5.72 (P < 0.00001)

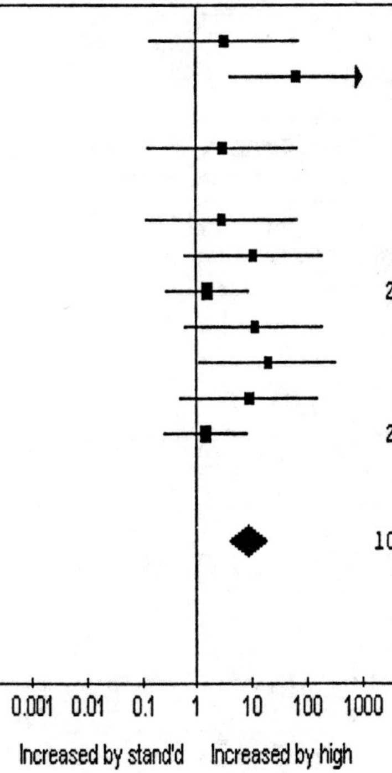

0.001 0.01 0.1 1 10 100 1000

Increased by stand'd   Increased by high

Figure A.5

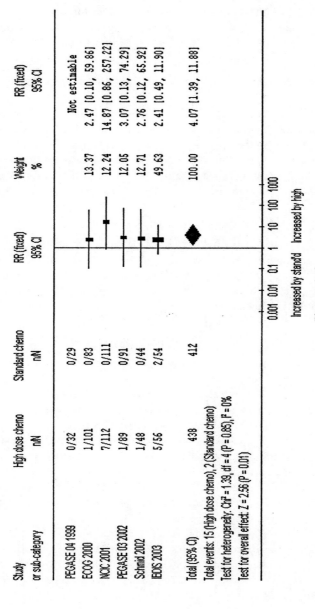

Study or sub-category	High dose chemo n/N	Standard chemo n/N	RR (fixed) 95% CI	Weight %	RR (fixed) 95% CI
PEGASE 04 1999	0/32	0/29			Not estimable
ECOG 2000	1/101	0/83		13.37	2.47 [0.10, 59.86]
NCIC 2001	7/112	0/111		12.24	14.87 [0.86, 257.22]
PEGASE 03 2002	1/89	0/91		12.05	3.07 [0.13, 74.29]
Schmid 2002	1/48	0/44		12.71	2.76 [0.12, 65.92]
IBDIS 2003	5/56	2/54		49.63	2.41 [0.49, 11.90]
Total (95% CI)	438	412		100.00	4.07 [1.39, 11.88]

Total events: 15 (High dose chemo), 2 (Standard chemo)
Test for heterogenity: Chi² = 1.39, df = 4 (P = 0.85), I² = 0%
Test for overall effect: Z = 2.56 (P = 0.01)

0.001 0.01 0.1 1 10 100 1000

Increased by stand'd   Increased by high

Figure A.6

arms. This did not affect the statistical significance of the results; the exclusion of the trial that used carmustine (BCNU) in the high-dose regimen also had no effect, and it accounted for over 60% of treatment-related deaths in the review. The exclusion of studies that included women with four to nine positive nodes resulted in a pooled risk ratio of 1.08 (95% CI 0.99–1.19) in event-free survival for women in the high-dose arm at 3 years. There were insufficient trials reporting each outcome to allow any sensitivity analysis in the review involving women with metastatic disease.

Conclusions

Although there is statistically significant evidence that high-dose chemotherapy with autologous bone marrow transplantation improves event-free survival compared to conventional-dose chemotherapy, there is no statistically significant evidence of benefit in overall survival for women with either high-risk or metastatic breast cancer. High-dose chemotherapy with bone marrow or stem cell transplantation should not be given to women with high-risk or metastatic breast cancer outside clinical trials.

Comment

Only the published studies had mature data on survival rates, while the others gave estimates based on their results to date. The systematic reviews in the Cochrane Library will be updated as more data become available. A full report of both reviews is available on the Cochrane Library (www.cochrane.org).

References

1. Farquhar C, Basser R, Marjoribanks J, Lethaby A. High dose chemotherapy and autologous bone marrow or stem cell transplantation versus conventional chemotherapy for women with early poor prognosis breast cancer. *The Cochrane Database of Systematic Reviews* 2003, Issue 1. Art. No.: CD003139. DOI: 10.1002/14651858.CD003139.
2. Farquhar C, Basser R, Hetrick S, Lethaby A, Marjoribanks J. High dose chemotherapy and autologous bone marrow or stem cell transplantation versus conventional chemotherapy for women with metastatic breast cancer. *The Cochrane Database of Systematic Reviews* 2002, Issue 4. Art. No.: CD003142. DOI: 10.1002/14651858.CD003142.
3. Bergh J, Wiklund T, Erikstein B, et al. Tailored fluorouracil, epirubicin and cyclophosphamide compared with marrow-supported high-dose chemotherapy as adjuvant treatment for high-risk breast cancer: a randomized trial. *Lancet* 2000; 356:1384–91.
4. Bezwoda W. Randomized, controlled trial of high dose chemotherapy (HD-CNVp) versus standard dose (CAF) chemotherapy for high-risk, surgically treated, primary breast cancer. 1999. Available at: http://www.asco.org. Accessed August 29, 2002.
5. Isaacs RE, Adkins DR, Spitzer G, Freeman S, Pecora AL, Weaver C. A phase III multi-institution randomized study comparing standard adjuvant chemotherapy to intensification with high-dose chemotherapy (HDC) and autologous peripheral blood progenitor cell (PBPC) rescue in patients with stage II/IIIA breast cancer with 4–9 involved axillary lymph nodes. 1999. Available at: http://www.asco.org. Accessed July 24, 2002.

6. Nieto Y, Champlin RE, Wingard JR, et al. Status of high-dose chemotherapy for breast cancer: a review. *Biol Blood Marrow Transplant* [serial online] 2000; 6: 476–85. Available at: http://bloodline.net. Accessed July 10, 2003.

7. A multicenter phase III randomized trial comparing docetaxel in combination with doxorubicin and cyclophosphamide (TAC) with TAC followed by high dose chemotherapy with mitoxantrone, cyclophosphamide and vinorelbine (HDCT) with autologous peripheral stem cell transplantation and G-CSF in adjuvant treatment of operable breast cancer with 4 or more positive axillary nodes. Available at: http://www.bcirg.org. Accessed June 25, 2002.

8. Randomized multicentric exploratory study phase III evaluating the contribution of the therapeutic intensification with autotransplantation of hematopoietic cells in non metastatic breast cancer with ganglionic invasion. 2002. Available at: http://www.fnclcc.fr. Accessed August 20, 2002.

9. NCI high priority trial: phase III randomized study of intensive sequential doxorubicin, paclitaxel and cyclophosphamide versus doxorubicin and cyclophosphamide followed by STAMP I and STAMP V combination chemotherapy with autologous stem cell rescue in women with primary breast cancer and at least 4 involved axillary lymph nodes. 2001. Available at: http://www.cancer.gov/clinical_trials. Accessed June 21, 2002.

10. Nitz UA, Frick M, Mohrmann S, et al. Tandem high-dose chemotherapy versus dose-dense conventional chemotherapy for patients with high-risk breast cancer: interim results from a multicenter phase III trial Available at: http://www.asco.org. Accessed July 31, 2003.

11. Crown J, Lind M, Gould A, et al. High-dose chemotherapy (HDC) with autograft (PBP) support is not superior to cyclophosphamide (CPA), methotrexate and 5-FU (CMF) following doxorubicin (D) induction in patients (pts) with breast cancer (BC) and 4 or more involved axillary lymph nodes (4+LN): the Anglo-Celtic I study. 2002. Available at: http://www.asco.org. Accessed June 28, 2002.

12. Peters WP, Rosner G, Vredenburgh J, et al. Updated results of a prospective, randomized comparison of two doses of combination alkylating agents (AA) as consolidation after CAF in high-risk primary breast cancer involving ten or more axillary lymph nodes (LN): CALGB 9082/SWOG 9114/NCIC Ma-13. 2001. Available at: http://www.asco.org. Accessed June 28, 2002.

13. Rodenhuis S, Bontenbal M, Beex LVAM, et al. High-dose chemotherapy with hematopoietic stem-cell rescue for high-risk breast cancer. *N Engl J Med* 2003; 349:7–15.

14. Schrama JG, Faneyte IF, Schornagel JH, et al. Randomized trial of high dose chemotherapy and hematopoietic progenitor-cell support in operable breast cancer with extensive lymph node involvement: final analysis with 7 years of follow-up. *Ann Oncol* 2002; 13:689–98.

15. Tallman M, Gray R, Robert N, Phase III study of conventional adjuvant chemotherapy with or without high-dose chemotherapy and autologous stem cell transplantation in patients with stage II and III breast cancer at high-risk of recurrence (INT 0121). 2003. Available at: http://www.asco.org. Accessed June 10, 2003.

16. Zander AR, Kruger W, Kroger N, et al. High-dose chemotherapy with autologous hematopoietic stem-cell support (HSCS) versus standard-dose chemotherapy in breast cancer patients with 10 or more positive lymph nodes: first results of a randomized trial. 2002. Available at: http://www.asco.org. Accessed April 16, 2002.

17. Basser R, O'Neill A, Martinelli G, et al. Randomized trial comparing up-front, multi-cycle dose-intensive chemotherapy (CT) versus standard dose CT in women with

high-risk stage 2 or 3 breast cancer (BC): first results from IBCSG Trial 15–95. 2003. Available at: http://www.asco.org. Accessed June 5, 2003.

18. Bliss JM, Vigushin D, Kanfer E, et al. Randomized trial of high dose therapy using cyclophosphamide, thiotepa and carboplatin in primary breast cancer patients with four or more histologically involved positive nodes (ISRCTN: 52623943). 2003. Available at: http://www.asco.org. Accessed June 11, 2003.

19. Tokuda Y, Tajima T, Narabayashi M, et al. Randomized phase III study of high-dose chemotherapy (HDC) with autologous stem cell support as consolidation in high-risk postoperative breast cancer: Japan Clinical Oncology Group (JCOG9208). 2001. Available at: http://www.asco.org. Accessed July 24, 2002.

20. Gianni A, Bonadonna G. Five-year results of the randomized clinical trial comparing standard versus high-dose myeloablative chemotherapy in the adjuvant treatment of breast cancer with >3 positive nodes (LN+). 2001. Available at: http://www.asco.org. Accessed June 27, 2002.

21. Hortobagyi GN, Buzdar AU, Theriault RL, et al. Randomized trial of high-dose chemotherapy and blood cell autografts for high-risk primary breast carcinoma. *J Natl Cancer Inst* 2000; 92:225–33.

22. Roche H, Viens P, Biron P, Lotz JP, Asselain B. High-dose chemotherapy for breast cancer: the French PEGASE experience. *Cancer Control* 2003; 10:42–7.

23. Madan B, Broadwater G, Rubin P, et al. Improved survival with consolidation high-dose cyclophosphamide, cisplatin and carmustine (Hd-Cpb) compared with observation in women with metastatic breast cancer (Mbc) and only bone metastases treated with induction adriamycin, 5-fluorouracil and methotrexate. 2000. Available at: http://www.asco.org. Accessed July 10, 2003.

24. Peters WP, Jones RB, Vredenburgh J, et al. A large, prospective, randomized trial of high-dose combination alkylating agents (CPB) with autologous cellular support (ABMS) as consolidation for patients with metastatic breast cancer achieving complete remission after intensive doxorubicin-based induction therapy (AFM). 1991. Available at: http://www.asco.org. Accessed June 15, 2002.

25. Bezwoda W. High dose chemotherapy with hematopoietic rescue as primary treatment for metastatic breast cancer: a randomized trial. *J Clin Oncol* 1995; 13:2483–9.

26. Rosti G, Ferrante P, Prosper F, Crown J, Dazzi C, Marangolo M. High dose chemotherapy in breast cancer in Europe: EBMT database and ongoing trials. In: Dicke KA, Keating A, eds. *Autologous Blood and Marrow Transplantation X: Proceedings of the Tenth International Symposium 2001.* Available at: http://www.bloodline.net. Accessed July 10, 2003.

27. Stadtmauer EA, O'Neill A, Goldstein LJ, et al. and the Philadelphia Bone Marrow Transplant Group. Conventional-dose chemotherapy compared with high-dose chemotherapy plus autologous hematopoietic stem-cell transplantation for metastatic breast cancer. *N Engl J Med* 2000; 342:1069–76.

28. Crown J, Perey L, Lind M, et al. Integrity of tandem high-dose chemotherapy (HDC) versus optimized conventionally-dosed chemotherapy (CDC) in patients (pts) with metastatic breast cancer (MBC): the International Randomized Breast Cancer Dose Intensity Study (IBDIS I). 2003. Available at: http://www.asco.org. Accessed June 11, 2003.

29. Crump M, Gluck S, Stewart D, et al. A randomized trial of high-dose chemotherapy (HDC) with autologous peripheral blood stem cell support (ASCT) compared to standard therapy

in women with metastatic breast cancer: a National Cancer Institute of Canada Clinical Trials Group Study. 2001. Available at: http://www.asco.org. Accessed July 25, 2002.

30. Biron P, Durand M, Roche H, et al. High dose thiotepa, cyclophosphamide (CPM) and stem cell transplantation after 4 FEC 100 compared with 4 FEC alone allowed better disease survival but the same overall survival in first line chemotherapy for metastatic breast cancer: results of the PEGASE 03 French Protocols. 2002. Available at: http://www.asco. org. Accessed April 16, 2002.

31. Roche H, Viens P, Biron P, Lotz JP, Asselain B. High-dose chemotherapy for breast cancer: the French PEGASE experience. *Cancer Control* 2003; 10:42–7.

32. Schmid P, Samonigg H, Nitsch T, et al. Randomized trial of up front tandem high-dose chemotherapy (HD) compared to standard chemotherapy with doxorubicin and paclitaxel (AT) in metastatic breast cancer (MBC). 2002. Available at: http://www.asco.org. Accessed April 16, 2002.

33. Kroger N, Kruger W, Zander AR. High dose chemotherapy in breast cancer: current status of ongoing German trials. In: Dicke, KA, Keating, A, eds., *Autologous Blood and Marrow Transplantation X: Proceedings of the Tenth International Symposium 2001.* Available at http://www.bloodline.net/. Accessed July 2003.

Notes

Chapter 1

1. Doxorubicin is a cytotoxic antibiotic, also known by its commercial name, Adriamycin. *Neoadjuvant chemotherapy* refers to chemotherapy administered before surgery.

2. Kidney, heart, and liver transplantation are the most frequently performed whole organ procedures worldwide, followed at some distance by pancreas and lung transplantation. The 1990 Nobel Prize in Medicine and Physiology was awarded to Dr. Joseph E. Murray for his work in whole organ transplantation and to Dr. E. Donnal Thomas for his pioneering work in bone marrow transplantation.

3. The statements of these three consensus conferences are found on the NIH Web site at http://consensus.nih.gov/1980/1980AdjuvantTherapyBreastCancer024.html.htm, http://consensus.nih.gov/1985/1985AdjuvantChemoBreastCancer052html.htm, and http://consensus. nih.gov/1990/1990EarlyStageBreastCancer081html.htm. Both the 1980 and 1985 statements indicate that they are "no longer viewed by NIH as guidance for current medical practice." The 1990 statement "reflects the panel's assessment of medical knowledge available at the time," thus providing "a snapshot in time" of new knowledge that is "inevitably accumulating through medical research." The most recent statement, Adjuvant Chemotherapy for Breast Cancer, NIH Consensus Statement Online 2000 November 1–3; 17(4):1–23, is found at http://consensus.nih.gov/2000/2000AdjuvantTherapyBreastCancer114.html.htm, accessed February 17, 2006.

4. Amgen's G-CSF is known as Filgrastin; the Immunex/Berlex GM-CSF, a yeast-derived molecule, is known as Sargramostim. Several other forms of GM-CSF include Molgramostim, a molecule based on *Escherichia coli* and tested but not marketed in the United States, and Regramostim, derived from Chinese hamster eggs.

5. This list was taken from "Locations That Are Doing Clinical Trials of Autologous Bone Marrow Transplants for Breast Cancer as of September 15, 1989." A copy was obtained from the files of the National Alliance of Breast Cancer Organizations and is retained in the project files.

Chapter 2

1. Meta-analysis is a statistical technique used to summarize the results of several clinical studies in a single weighted estimate of outcomes in which more weight is given to the results of studies with more events and sometimes to studies of higher quality.

2. The organizations were the American Medical Association, American Society of Clinical Oncology, Association of American Cancer Institutes, Association of Community

Cancer Centers, Candlelighters Childhood Cancer Foundation, Memorial Sloan-Kettering Cancer Center, National Cancer Institute, and National Institute of Allergy and Infectious Diseases. The statement was published as a letter from Mary McCabe and Michael Friedman, reflecting the "coordination" that had been provided by NCI.

3. Aubry, a coauthor of this book, was Senior Vice President and Medical Director of Blue Shield of California (1989–1995) and chaired the Medical Advisory Panel of the Technology Evaluation Center of Blue Cross Blue Shield Association (1993–1999). In these capacities, he participated in a number of events described here. Early in the project, he prepared a summary of his experience for the benefit of our entire research team (Aubry 2002).

4. A trial "powered" to determine that a 20% improvement in some specified outcome (e.g., overall survival) compared to placebo or standard treatment is not a chance occurrence will require a sample of patients of a certain size. If the objective is to detect a 10% improvement, then more patients will be required. The cost of a clinical trial is related directly to the number of patients needed and enrolled.

5. Complete response indicates tumor volume has regressed to the point at which it is no longer detectable; partial response means that the tumor has regressed by at least 50%.

6. Medicare was essentially unaffected by HDC/ABMT as patients were typically younger women in their 40s and 50s, not women over 65 years of age.

7. Eddy's review, published in the *Journal of Clinical Oncology* in April 1992, had been submitted in February 1991, revised in response to reviewer's comments, and updated through October 1991; it was accepted by the journal on November 18, 1991.

8. The document was entered into evidence in *Harris v. Mutual of Omaha Companies*, 1992, WL 421489 (S.D. Ind. 1992) (see Rose 2002, p. 308).

9. Copies of these letters are in the files of this project. Some were addressed to Ms. Michele Coad of Culp, Guterson and Drader, One Union Square, 600 University Street, Seattle, Washington 98101–3143. Others were addressed simply To Whom it May Concern.

10. The project conducted a Nexis-Lexis search of all newspaper, wire service, and television reports on HDC/ABMT for the period 1988 through 2001 and compiled three large notebooks in the process, which are in the project files.

Chapter 3

1. *Fox v. HealthNet*, No. 219692, Superior Court of California (1993).

2. This section is adapted from Jacobson (2002).

3. Modern products liability law introduced the concept of no-fault liability, by which the manufacturer of a mass-produced good can be held liable for injuries even if it was not at fault.

4. The preponderance of the evidence standard means that it is more likely than not (even if 50.1% to 49.9%) that the facts favor the plaintiff.

5. In certain circumstances, courts may rule that industry custom is inadequate and impose liability for not investing enough in accident prevention. See, for example, *United States v. Carroll Towing Company, Inc.*, 159 F.2d 169 (2d Cir. 1947), and *The T. J. Hooper*, 60 F.2d 737 (2d Cir. 1932).

6. *Lauro v. The Travelers Insurance Co.*, 261 S0.2d 261, 266 (La. 1972).

7. In some cases, courts have determined that resource constraints on hospitals or physicians are relevant in determining the standard of care. See, for example, *Hall v. Hilbun*, 466 S0.2d 856 (Miss. 1985); *Lauro v. The Travelers Insurance Co.*, 261 S0.2d 261 (La. 1972).

8. *Hall v. Hilbun*, 466 S0.2d 856 (Miss. 1985).

9. *Gala v. Hamilton*, 715 A.2d 1108 (Pa. 1998).

10. During the past 20 years, numerous states have enacted tort reforms, such as limitations on damage awards, to address what some scholars believe is an out-of-control tort system. Most of the legislative reforms have been pro-defendant, partly in response to loosening of procedural rules that were perceived to be pro-plaintiff (Jacobson 1989).

11. The Court established a gatekeeper model in which the trial judge would be expected to determine the soundness of the scientific evidence, such as whether it had appeared in peer-reviewed journals. See *Daubert v. Merrell Dow Pharmaceuticals*, 509 U.S. 579 (1993); *General Electric Co. v. Joiner*, 522 U.S. 136 (1997); and *Kumho Tire Co. v. Carmichael*, 526 U.S. 137 (1999). Note that these new federal evidentiary standards were established after the initial wave of contested HDC/ABMT litigation had taken place. Even under the previous standard, *Frye v. United States*, 293 F. 1013 (D.C. Cir. 1923), however, the defense was unable to prevent physicians from testifying for plaintiffs. Under the Frye standard, expert testimony was admissible if generally accepted by the scientific community. Under that malleable standard, the quality of the science was rarely examined, and experts were rarely blocked from testifying. For reasons discussed in this chapter, the plaintiffs' expert witnesses easily satisfied either standard. For a thorough review of this issue, see Shuman (2001). See also *Adams v. Blue Cross/Blue Shield of Maryland, Inc.*, 757 F. Supp. 661, 668 (D.Md. 1991), ruling that the Frye standard did not apply to "the practical evaluation of a medical treatment to decide whether it is accepted." Neither our interviews nor our review of the cases indicated any pre-post Daubert differences in witness testimony.

12. Legislative history of the Employee Retirement Income Security Act of 1974, at p. 3456 (1976). The Employee Retirement Income Security Act of 1974, 29 U.S.C. § 1001 et seq.

13. 29 U.S.C. Art. 1021–1031.

14. 29 U.S.C. Art. 1051–1061.

15. 29 U.S.C. Art. 1081–1086.

16. 29 U.S.C. Art. 1101–1114.

17. See Jacobson (2002) for a more detailed discussion.

18. *Firestone Tire and Rubber Co. v. Bruch*, 489 U.S. 101, 108 (1989).

19. *Citizens to Preserve Overton Park, Inc., v. Volpe*, 401 U.S. 402 (1971).

20. *Pirozzi v. Blue Cross–Blue Shield of Virginia*, 741 F. Supp. 586 (E.D. Va. 1990).

21. See *Pirozzi*, 741 F. Supp. at 589.

22. In some instances, employees may only see a summary plan description not the actual contract itself.

23. *Healthcare America Plans, Inc., v. Bossmeyer*, 1998 U.S. App. LEXIS 31323 (10th Cir. 1998).

24. If an ERISA-covered plan is involved, courts will usually defer to the plan's interpretation.

25. *McEvoy v. Group Health Cooperative of Eau Claire*, 570 N.W.2d 397 (Wis. 1997).

26. Id.

27. Our interviews (described in chapter 4) suggest that settlement activity increased markedly after the decision in *Fox v. HealthNet*.

28. See *Killian v. Healthsource Provident Administrators, Inc.*, 152 F.3d 514, 516 (6th Cir. 1998) ("To guard against [the risk of illness from infection], HDC patients frequently undergo either autologous bone marrow transplant, or as in this case, peripheral stem cell rescue."). See also *Smith v. CHAMPUS*, 97 F.3d 950, 957 n.8 (7th Cir. 1996) ("[I]t is our understanding that HDC/ABMT and HDC/PSCR—which both fall under the broader label HDC/ASCR or 'HDC with stem cell rescue'—are essentially the same in the treatment of breast cancer."); *Mattive v. Healthsource of Savannah, Inc.*, 893 F. Supp. 1559, 1572 (S.D. Ga. 1995) ("The [c]ourt recognizes that the ABMT and the PSCR accomplish the same thing when used in conjunction with HDC in treating cancer patients . . . but the procedures for removing the stem cells are different.").

29. *Sweeney v. Gerber Products Co. Medical Benefits Plan,* 728 F. Supp. 594 (D. Neb. 1989); *Thomas v. Gulf Health Plan, Inc.,* 688 F. Supp. 590 (S.D. Ala. 1988).

30. *Thomas v. Gulf Health Plan, Inc.,* 688 F. Supp. 590 (S.D. Ala. 1988).

31. Id. at 593.

32. Id. at 596.

33. Id. at 595.

34. *Sweeney,* 728 F. Supp. at 597.

35. *Pirozzi v. Blue Cross–Blue Shield of Virginia,* 741 F. Supp. 586 (E.D. Va. 1990).

36. Id. at 592.

37. Id. at 592.

38. Id. at 588.

39. Id. at 594.

40. *White v. Caterpillar, Inc.,* 765 F. Supp 1418 (W.D. Mo. 1991).

41. Id. at 1423.

42. *Kulakowski v. Rochester Hospital Services Corp.,* 779 F. Supp. 710 (W.D.N.Y. 1991).

43. Id. at 715.

44. *Jenkins v. Blue Cross Blue Shield of Michigan,* 1994 WL 901184 (N.D. Ohio, May 9, 1994).

45. Id. at 11.

46. *Smith v. CHAMPUS,* 97 F.3d 950 (7th Cir. 1996).

47. Id. at 958 n.12.

48. *Holder v. Prudential Insurance Co.,* 951 F.2d 89 (5th Cir. 1992).

49. Id. at 91.

50. *Adams v. Blue Cross/Blue Shield of Maryland, Inc.,* 757 F. Supp. 661, 675 (D. Md. 1991).

51. Id. at 663.

52. *Nichols v. Trustmark Insurance Co.,* 1 F. Supp. 2d 689, 699 (N.D. Ohio 1997).

53. Id. at 700.

54. *Pirozzi v. Blue Cross–Blue Shield of Virginia,* 741 F. Supp. 586, 591 (E.D. Va. 1990).

55. *Adams v. Blue Cross/Blue Shield of Maryland, Inc.,* 757 F. Supp. 661 (D. Md. 1991).

56. Id. at 671.

57. *CompreCare Insurance Co. v. Snow,* no. 92-CV-8087, 1993 WL 330929 (Colo. Dist. Ct. February 12, 1993).

58. *Healthcare America Plans, Inc., v. Bossemeyer,* 953 F. Supp 1176 (D. Kan. 1996).

59. Id. at 1191.

60. *Caudill v. Blue Cross and Blue Shield of North Carolina, Inc.,* 999 F.2d 74, 80 (4th Cir. 1993).

61. Id.

62. *Harris v. Mutual of Omaha Cos.,* 992 F.2d 706 (7th Cir. 1993).

63. *Bechtold v. Physician's Health Plan of Northern Indiana, Inc.,* 19 F.3d 322 (7th Cir. 1993).

64. *Fuja v. Benefit Trust Life Insurance Co.,* 18 F.3d 1405, 1408 (7th Cir. 1994).

65. Id. at 1411.

66. Id. at 1412.

67. As an interesting side note to *Fuja,* following the Seventh Circuit's reversal of the district court's holding that the insurer was obligated to cover Ms. Fuja's HDC/ABMT treatment, the insurance company sued the hospital to recover the payments it had already made. The trial court held that the insurer was not required to pay for treatments that did not qualify as medically necessary, and that the hospital must return the payments, *Trustmark Insurance Company v. University of Chicago Hospitals,* No. 94 C 4692, 1997 WL 610294 (N.D. Ill. September 29, 1997), but the Seventh Circuit overturned that ruling as well, holding that the

insurer's promise to pay for the treatment induced action on the part of the hospital and did not place any conditions or qualifications (such as the decision being affirmed on appeal) on the payments, *Trustmark Insurance Company v. University of Chicago Hospitals,* 207 F.3d 876 (7th Cir. 1997).

68. 29 U.S.C. § 1001 (1994).

69. See also *Van Boxel v. Journal Co. Employee's Pension Trust,* 836 F.2d 1048, 1049 (1987).

70. *Firestone Tire Rubber Co. v. Bruch,* 489 U.S. 101, 108 (1989).

71. *Scalamandre v. Oxford Health Plans, Inc.,* 823 F. Supp. 1050 (E.D. N.Y. 1993).

72. 229 F.3d 729 (9th Cir. 2000).

73. *Scalamandre,* 823 F. Supp. at 1062.

74. *Holder v. Prudential Insurance Co.,* 951 F.2d 89, 90 (5th Cir. 1992).

75. *Ulrich v. Caterpillar,* No. 93 C 5271, 1993 WL 478990 (N.D. Ill. November 18, 1993).

76. *Bechtold v. Physicians Health Plan of Northern Indiana,* 19 F.3d 322 (7th Cir. 1994).

77. *Bossemeyer,* 953 F. Supp. at 1192.

78. *Bucci v. Blue Cross–Blue Shield of Connecticut,* 764 F. Supp. 728 (D. Conn. 1991).

79. *Kulakowski v. Rochester Hospital Service,* 779 F. Supp. 710, 716 (W.D. N.Y. 1991).

80. *White v. Caterpillar,* 765 F. Supp. 1418 (W.D. Mo. 1991).

81. *Bucci,* 764 F. Supp. at 732.

82. *Killian v. Healthsource Provident Administrators,* 152 F.3d 514 (6th Cir. 1998).

83. 5 U.S.C. §§ 8901–8914 (1988).

84. 10 U.S.C. §§ 1071–1106 (1988 and Supp. V 1993).

85. *See* 32 C.F.R. 199.17.

86. *Caudill v. Blue Cross & Blue Shield of North Carolina,* 999 F.2d 74, 80 (4th Cir. 1993).

87. *Harris v. Mutual of Omaha Cos.,* 992 F.2d 712 (7th Cir. 1993).

88. Administrative Procedure Act, 5 U.S.C. § 706(2)(A) (1994).

89. 32 C.F.R § 199.4(g)(15). Interestingly, in *Hawkins v. Mail Handlers Benefit Plan,* the court found that, due to the differences in the wording of the policies, CHAMPUS had acted arbitrarily and capriciously, but OPM had not. *Hawkins v. Mail Handlers Benefit Plan,* no. 1:94CV6, 1994 WL 214262 (W.D. N.C. January 28, 1994).

90. *Bishop v. CHAMPUS,* 917 F. Supp 1469, 1478 (E.D. Wash. 1996).

91. *Mashburn v. Mail Handlers Benefit Plan,* no. 3:94–0549, 1994 WL 715962 (M.D. Tenn. August 4, 1994). Both Mail Handlers and CHAMPUS were initially named as defendants, but the complaint against Mail Handlers was dismissed, leaving only CHAMPUS's denial at issue.

92. 97 F.3d 950 (7th Cir. 1996).

93. Id. at 959.

94. *Taylor v. Blue Cross/Blue Shield of Michigan,* 517 N.W. 2d 864 (Mich. Ct. App. 1994).

95. *Tepe v. Rocky Mountain Hospital and Medical Services,* 893 P. 2d. 1323 (Colo. Ct. App. 1994).

96. Although the procedural history of many of these cases is not clear, the most common reason for removal to federal court (other than the fact that the claim involved ERISA) was diversity jurisdiction. The U.S. Constitution grants the federal courts the authority to hear cases based on the diversity of the litigants, such as cases between citizens of different states or between a citizen of the United States and a citizen of a foreign country. U.S. CONST., art. 1, § 2. Diversity jurisdiction requires that the amount in controversy be greater than $75,000. 28 U.S.C. § 1332(a) (1993).

97. *Dahl-Eimers v. Mutual of Omaha Life Insurance Co.,* 986 F.2d 1379 (11th Cir. 1993).

98. *Nichols v. Trustmark Insurance Co. (Mutual),* 1 F. Supp.2d 689 (N.D. Ohio 1997).

99. *Frendreis v. Blue Cross Blue Shield of Michigan,* 873 F. Supp. 1153 (N.D. Ill. 1995).

100. *O'Rourke v. Access Health, Inc.,* 668 N.E.2d 214 (Ill. Ct. App. 1996).

101. *Wolfe v. Prudential Insurance Co.,* 50 F.3d 793 (10th Cir. 1995).

102. 29 U.S.C. § 1144(a).

103. *Bast v. Prudential Insurance Co.,* 150 F.3d 1003 (9th Cir. 1998).

104. Id. at 1011.

105. *Reger v. Espy,* 836 F. Supp. 869 (N.D. Ga. 1993).

106. Id. at 872.

107. Id. at 872–873.

108. 29 U.S.C. §§ 701–797b (1988); 42 U.S.C. §§ 12101–12213 (1993); *Dodd v. Blue Cross & Blue Shield Association,* 835 F. Supp. 888 (E.D. Va. 1993).

109. *Dodd,* 835 F. Supp. at 891.

110. *Henderson v. Bodine Aluminum, Inc.,* 70 F.3d 958 (8th Cir. 1995).

111. *Reed v. Wal-Mart Stores, Inc.,* 197 F. Supp. 2d 883 (E.D. Mich. 2002).

112. Id. at 886.

113. *Whitney v. Empire Blue Cross & Blue Shield,* 920 F. Supp. 477 (S.D. N.Y. 1996), *vacated,* 106 F.3d 475 (2d. Cir. 1997).

114. *Taylor v. Blue Cross/Blue Shield of Michigan,* 517 N.W.2d 644 (Mich. App. Ct. 1994).

115. *Frendreis v. Blue Cross Blue Shield of Michigan,* 873 F. Supp. 1153, 1157 (N.D. Ill. 1995).

116. Id. at 1158.

117. *Simkins v. NevadaCare, Inc.,* 299 F.3d 729, 735 (9th Cir. 2000).

118. *Healthcare America Plans, Inc., v. Bossemeyer,* 953 F. Supp 1176, 1176, 1188 (D. Kan. 1996).

119. Id. at 1188.

120. *Caudill v. Blue Cross and Blue Shield of North Carolina,* 999 F.2d 74 (4th Cir. 1993); *Lowey v. HealthChicago,* No. 92 C 7657, 1994 WL 194265 (N.D. Ill. May 16, 1994); *Roseberry v. Blue Cross and Blue Shield of Nebraska,* 821 F. Supp. 1313 (D. Neb. 1992).

121. See, for example, *Bechtold v. Physicians Health Plan of Northern Indiana, Inc.,* No. F 92–239, 1993 WL 625573, 8 (N.D. Ill. Mar. 19, 1993).

122. *Dahl-Eimers v. Mutual of Omaha Life Insurance Co.,* 812 F. Supp. 1193. 1195, *rev'd* 986 F.2d 1379 (11th Cir. 1993).

123. *Dahl-Eimers,* 812 F. Supp. at 1197.

124. *Dahl-Eimers,* 986 F.2d at 1382–1383.

125. *Sluiter v. Blue Cross and Blue Shield of Michigan,* 979 F. Supp. 1131 (E.D. Mich. 1997).

126. *Whitehead v. Federal Express Corp.,* 878 F. Supp. 1066 (W.D. Tenn. 1994).

127. *Tepe v. Rocky Mountain Hosp. and Medical Services,* 893 P. 2d. 1323, 1328 (Colo. Ct. App. 1994).

128. *Duckwitz v. General American Life Ins. Co.,* 812 F. Supp. 864 (N.D. Ill. 1993).

129. *Caudill v. Blue Cross–Blue Shield of North Carolina,* No. 92-94-CIV-7-F, 1992 WL 486661 (E.D. N.C. August 24, 1992), *affm'd* 999 F.2d 74, 80 (4th Cir. 1993).

130. *Hasty v. Central States, Southeast & Southwest Areas Health & Welfare Fund,* 851 F. Supp. 1250, 1260 (N.D. Ind. 1994).

131. *Wilson v. Group Hospital and Medical Services, Inc.,* 791 F. Supp. 309, 314 (D. D.C. 1992).

132. See Morreim (2001, p. 413), "Such desperation- or sympathy-guided rulings are not merely expensive. They set a terrible legal precedent if we want empirical judgments to be guided by empirical evidence."

133. *Harris v. Mutual of Omaha Co.,* IP 92–1089-C, 1992 WL 421489, *1 (S.D. Ind. August 26, 1992).

134. *Hill v. Trustmark Insurance Co.,* No. 6:96 CV 50, 1996 WL 170117 (E.D. Tex. Jan. 31, 1996).

Chapter 4

1. One anticipated strategy—conflict of interest based on financial incentives—was only peripherally raised. Most cases did not directly address this issue. It was widely reported that the issue was directly presented during the *Fox v. HealthNet* testimony but dropped before the jury ruled on it. After the trial, jurors expressed bewilderment regarding why such testimony was presented but then not presented to the jury for deliberation. See, for example, Grinfeld (1999) and Larson (1996).

2. *Adams v. Blue Cross/Blue Shield of Maryland, Inc.*, 757 F. Supp. 661, 666 (D.Md. 1991).

3. A defense attorney maintained that this comment was made in jest and largely taken out of context. Regardless of how it was intended, it reinforced the prevailing anti–managed care sentiment. Although the comment was not entered into evidence, plaintiff's counsel quoted it in the closing argument. The defense attorney's objection that it was not in evidence was overruled.

4. One respondent said that the defense victories were flukes.

5. In *Pirozzi v. Blue Cross–Blue Shield of Virginia*, 741 F. Upp. 586 (E.D. Va. 1990), for instance, the court noted that "Blue Cross relies heavily on the absence of phase II studies relating to the efficacy of HDCT-ABMT. This reliance is misplaced. To begin with, nothing in the Plan requires that a treatment be the subject of completed phase III studies to escape the experimental exclusion."

6. This language invited disputes over prevailing clinical practices.

7. See also Newcomer (1990). "Listing coverages and exclusions creates a natural tension between the marketing department and the medical and actuarial departments of commercial third-party payers" (p. 1702). One respondent characterized this tension as a dance between attorneys and markets and then a business decision for the plan based on risk exposure.

8. This is quoted directly from the official court transcript. A respondent termed this a bait-and-switch strategy, knowing that most patients will not challenge the denial.

9. Pertinent to the plaintiffs' contractual ambiguity arguments, the witness admitted that the contract did not define the general medical community. This left the witness open to cross-examination regarding differing ways of defining the community.

10. Previously, the witness had qualified this statement by noting that "There is no evidence from phase III medical literature that such treatments significantly change the outcome of the primary disease process."

11. For a vivid example of how this dynamic played out in court, see *Smith v. Office of Civilian Health and Medical Program of the Uniformed Services*, 97 F.3d 950 (7th Cir. 1996). In that case, the majority focused on the lack of RCTs proving the scientific efficacy, while the dissent focused on the procedure's diffusion among community oncologists.

12. *Sarchette v. Blue Shield of California*, 223 Cal.Rptr. 76 (Cal. 1987), footnote 1.

13. The ability of plaintiffs to demonstrate inconsistency creates some long-term coverage concerns for insurers. If a company makes a decision to pay for one subscriber, then how will it look later? How can one decision be presented so that it does not create a binding precedent? A defense attorney suggested that external review would minimize subsequent risk. A similar issue the plaintiff exploited in the *Fox* case (again, widely reported) was that the defendant's outside consultant said that HDC/ABMT was widely adopted in the community. Aubry noted that insurers were also concerned about potential health plan liability for approving a harmful, toxic, and ineffective procedure. This concern did not emerge during our interviews, perhaps because defense counsel did not want to pursue inconsistent theories of the case between this concern and informed consent. If the defense focused on the patient's informed consent, then it would be hard to argue that despite informed consent, the plan could be liable for nonetheless approving a harmful procedure.

Of course, attorneys are free to pursue conflicting theories (and often do). Given the fact that the defense's informed consent theories were ineffective, pursuit of this alternative strategy might have been preferable.

14. This is quoted directly from the plaintiff's trial brief. The insurer argued that because these concerns were biologically different (due partly to dissimilar relapse/remission patterns), they demanded a different response from the insurer. In short, the plaintiff's contentions "compared apples to oranges."

15. In several transcripts, plaintiffs' attorneys introduced evidence that the insurer telephoned the treating physician to argue against the HDC/ABMT recommendation. In some instances, the calls were perceived as threatening continued referrals. At least one physician testified that he changed the treatment recommendation in response.

16. An issue not raised in our interviews, but important for context, is that the economics favored using HDC/ABMT at community hospitals. The procedure was profitable for both the hospital and the oncologist.

17. *DeMeurs v. HealthNet,* No. 239338, Riverside County Superior Court (December 13, 1995).

18. Several respondents, including both plaintiffs' and defense attorneys, characterized medical directors' testimony as frequently arrogant and cocky.

19. Careful reading of the available transcripts confirms this observation. In several transcripts, the defense's cross-examination either allowed the plaintiff's expert to reiterate how widespread the procedure was by the early 1990s or failed to nail down the scientific reasons why the procedure should have been considered experimental. For example, one defense attorney asked the expert the following question: "Isn't it true that the weight of peer-review articles as of the middle of 1992 at least came to the conclusion that high-dose chemotherapy for stage IV breast cancer is promising or was promising?" From subsequent questioning, the defense meant to show that the articles concluded that further clinical trials were needed. In my view, however, this allowed the witness to state again how widespread the procedure's use was at that time.

20. One defense counsel said that *Fox* put the "fear of God" in us. Based on this, one defense attorney advised the client to cover doubtful cases for which the patient had a potential argument. "If I cover everything, I won't lose my job through a huge verdict."

21. In support, one plaintiffs' attorney cited an August 15, 1990, letter from Elizabeth F. Brown, MD, director of the Department of Technology Assessment at the AMA, stating that "Constant refinement and investigation move the practice of medicine forward. Nowhere is this more true than in the field of oncology where new combinations and doses of drugs and radiation therapy are always under study. Thus, a rigid interpretation of the term investigational is particularly problematic for terminally ill patients who may have very limited treatment options."

22. This is why, for instance, insurers balked at covering alternative medicine.

23. This is a statement from the closing argument reported in a trial transcript.

24. At least one of our defense attorneys was unabashedly critical of Peters's study, calling it "political, manipulated, and deliberately misleading with fabricated numbers."

25. *Adams v. Blue Cross/Blue Shield of Maryland, Inc.*, 657 F. Supp. 661, 671 (D.Md. 1991).

26. This respondent derisively parodied an opening statement: "I begin with a prayer that the Lord will give me the eloquence to award this woman's child damages to live a reasonable life."

27. On the other hand, a plaintiffs' attorney noted that a "showy" client alienated the jury.

28. The respondent said, "Once the litigation started, plans retrenched and overreacted. They circled the wagons when attacked."

29. At least in concept, plans are designed to think about patient populations. What seems to have gotten lost in the HDC/ABMT case is the balance between individuals and the patient population.

30. He added that depositions were no more revealing: "I want to see my children grow. What else can I do?"

31. For a comprehensive discussion of the managed care backlash, see the articles in the *Journal of Health Politics, Policy and Law* 1999;24:873–1218. To our knowledge, no one has quantified, or attempted to quantify, the extent to which any particular factor contributed to the backlash.

32. According to Morreim (2001): "If any conclusion is obvious, it is that throughout much of medicine no particular practices 'prevail.' There is no such thing as 'the' standard of care" (p. 30).

33. Compare *Adams v. Blue Cross/Blue Shield of Maryland, Inc.,* 757 F. Supp. 661 (D. Md. 1991), holding that widespread HDC/ABMT use among community oncologists met the standard of care, with *Healthcare America Plans, Inc., v. Bossemeyer,* 953 F. Supp. 1176 (D. Kan. 1996) holding just the opposite.

34. *Bossemeyer,* 953 F. Supp. at 1183 (D. Kan. 1996). This case was largely decided based on ERISA's narrow arbitrary and capricious standard, which sets a very high bar for a plaintiff to meet. Nonetheless, the appellate court noted that "The very fact that significant controversy existed as to the status of the procedure in treating stage II breast cancer seems to suggest it had not yet won general acceptance in the medical community." *Healthcare America Plans, Inc., v. Bossemeyer,* 166 F.3d 347, 5 (10th Cir. 1998) (unpublished table decision).

35. For an insightful look at the inherent problems in determining the standard of care, see the symposium articles in the *Wake Forest Law Review* 2002;37:663–955.

36. For different reasons, Professor Haavi Morreim shares this conclusion (2001, p. 30).

37. *Glauser-Nagy v. Medical Mutual of Ohio,* 987 F. Supp. 1002, 1016 (N.D. Ohio 1996).

38. *Smith v. CHAMPUS,* 97 F. 3d 950, 956–957 (7th Cir. 1996), cited approvingly in *Glauser-Nagy,* 987 F. Supp. at 1016.

39. For an extended discussion of this issue, see Jacobson (2002, pp. 189–193). Compare, for example, the *Adams* and *Glauser-Nagy* cases. In *Adams,* the court relied almost entirely on community oncologists' testimony to rule that HDC/ABMT met the standard of care, but in *Glauser-Nagy,* the court relied almost entirely on the scientific literature showing a lack of long-term superiority for HDC/ABMT. See also *Smith v. CHAMPUS,* 97 F. 3d 950, 956–957 (7th Cir. 1996) and *Glauser-Nagy,* 987 F. Supp. at 1016.

40. When we read some of the contract language, we clearly understand what the insurer intended. At the same time, the language would be very difficult for most patients to understand, even if brought to their attention, and the contracts can be quite misleading.

41. For two reasons, this is a dubious assertion. First, recent issues of scientific fraud and perennial questions about the ability of peer review to identify serious problems suggest that a science court would not be a panacea. Second, it is not clear that a science court is more effective in this regard than cross-examination in open court.

42. As a cautionary note, the respondent referred to the recent attempt in California to gather stakeholders to define medical necessity. According to the respondent: "It was easy to get agreement on the definition, including a cost-effectiveness provision. But the discomfort was that 'everyone felt that the definition would be used against them.'" See also Singer and Bergthold (2001).

43. In response, a plaintiff's attorney argued that this advantage would dissipate if external review became merely a rubber stamp for denial of care. It could then be attacked as not being implemented in good faith. For an analogous situation in which a managed care plan

misused the contractual arbitration provision, see *Engalla v. The Permanente Medical Group, Inc.*, 938 P.2d 903 (Cal. 1997).

Chapter 5

1. The registry data presented here are preliminary and were obtained from the Statistical Center of the International Bone Marrow Transplant Registry and Autologous Blood and Marrow Transplant Registry. The analysis has not been reviewed or approved by the Advisory or Scientific Committees of the International Bone Marrow Transplant Registry and ABMTR.

2. In mid-2004, the Medical College of Wisconsin created the Center for International Blood and Marrow Transplant Research, a partnership that includes the ABMTR, the International Bone Marrow Transplant Registry, and the National Marrow Donor Program (http://www.ibmtr.org).

3. Diagnoses other than breast cancer were grouped using Clinical Classification Software, a tool developed at the Agency for Healthcare Research and Quality that is used for clustering patient diagnoses into a manageable number of clinically meaningful categories.

4. The registry data presented here are preliminary and were obtained from the Statistical Center of the International Bone Marrow Transplant Registry and ABMTR. The analysis has not been reviewed or approved by the Advisory or Scientific Committees of the International Bone Marrow Transplant Registry and ABMTR.

5. Chemotherapy, although not strictly a diagnosis, has an assigned *ICD* diagnostic code.

6. In 1995, Salick sold half of the stock in his firm to Zeneca Group, PLC, a U.K. pharmaceutical firm, which completed the purchase in 1997.

7. Response Technologies changed its name to Response Oncology on October 23, 1995, executed a reverse stock split, and began trading on the NASDAQ National Market under the symbol ROIX.

8. This is from an undated Response Technologies, Inc., document that is clearly an internal Response-generated document, probably used with hospitals and prospective cancer centers in discussions about affiliation. Its six sections are "Profile of RTI"; "Delivery System"; "Reasonable and Appropriate Therapy"; "Costs"; "Breast Cancer"; and "Appendices."

Chapter 6

1. In a September 3, 2004, interview, Smith recalled events this way. "NIH said this was experimental. The NIH guy rolled on me. Not in the testimony. My recollection is that he gave Norton room to go beyond experimental."

2. Jones attached the June 6, 1994, letter supporting his testimony and signed by him, William Peters, Stephanie Williams of the University of Chicago, Gary Spitzer of St. Louis University, Richard Champlin of the M. D. Anderson Cancer Center, and Nancy Davidson of Johns Hopkins University.

3. The conditions for which the treatment was already considered standard were acute lymphocytic or nonlymphocytic leukemia, advanced Hodgkin's lymphoma, advanced non-Hodgkin's lymphoma, advanced neuroblastoma, and testicular, mediastinal, retroperitoneal, and ovarian germ cell tumors.

4. Our interviews suggest that all of the debate took place in the House of Representatives. The Senate followed the lead once the House passed the mandate.

5. Some opponents were less than charitable in describing this involvement.

6. According to respondents from the insurance industry, the woman was not covered because she would have fared well under conventional therapy "and was lucky to get through ABMT," even though her survival was attributed to ABMT. Indeed, these respondents considered it ethically wrong to place her in a clinical trial because her cancer was stage II. Nonetheless, she had name recognition and was a highly effective spokesperson for the mandate effort.

7. This assertion seems dubious given the amount of money involved for physicians and hospitals. It was strongly challenged by insurer respondents, who talked about financial incentives to the treating physicians and oncologists.

8. It does not appear that the industry offered to pay for the clinical trials.

9. Some respondents suggested that "the legislature did not care about the clinical trials." Others indicated that the issue was raised, although they also agreed that the trials played a minor role in the debate. Keep in mind that legislators are likely to be very happy to use scientific evidence to support whatever legislation is being proposed.

10. More than one observer noted that HTAC was set up as something of a consolation prize to Republicans and business interests when Democrats controlled both houses of the state government.

11. ECRI was sufficiently concerned about how its work was being presented in the media that the organization's president wrote an op-ed piece trying to explain why ECRI's research did not support a mandate. To the best of our knowledge, this piece was not published, although an op-ed article written by Arthur Caplan supporting ECRI's position was published in *St. Paul Pioneer Press,* April 12, 1995. The episode confirms the insurance industry's frustration about not being able to present its version through the media.

12. Although apparently not raised directly at the hearings, opponents of repeal argued that the insurance industry overstated the costs of the mandate and the effects on premium costs. To support these accusations, opponents of repeal noted that the insurers covered everything for prostate cancer and covered Viagra but not female contraceptives. One of the plaintiffs' attorneys we interviewed raised a similar point during the litigation regarding coverage for treatment costs for males when the clinical evidence was ambiguous but not for HDC/ABMT.

13. These observations were offered in reviewing a book by Marcia Angell (1996)

Chapter 7

1. These functions have been continued in the successors to the National Center for Health Services Research: the Agency for Health Care Policy and Research (1989–1995) and the Agency for Healthcare Research and Quality (1995–present).

2. The BCBSA provides centralized services to but does not control the individual Blue Cross Blue Shield health plans. Its technology assessments are advisory only.

3. This committee met regularly three times a year to consider coverage requests for new procedures, review the relevant literature, and make recommendations to the medical director.

4. In 1971, Monaco had organized a candlelight demonstration around the home of Representative Paul Rogers (D, Fla.), the chairman of the Subcommittee on Health of the House Commerce Committee, when he appeared reluctant to support legislation to increase cancer research funds.

5. The MCOP would later become a major activity of the Medical Care Management Corporation.

6. The HMO Group consists of group and staff model health maintenance organizations.

7. This was formerly the Emergency Care Research Institute, now simply ECRI.

Chapter 8

1. In this period, the NCI designated a clinical trial as high priority in the hope that this would assist patient recruitment. No additional funds resulted from priority status. The designation was discontinued in 1997.

2. It might be argued that equipoise required comparison of the conventional versus the experimental treatment. Henderson saw dosage as the issue, and that it was unknown whether a high or intermediate dose was more effective.

3. Illustrating trial complexity, the ECOG protocol for INT 0121 (ECOG 2190) (revised in January 1995) noted that "Memorial Sloan-Kettering is only a CALGB member for the Intergroup Breast Cancer Studies and is usually not included in the CALGB roster" (p. vi). The protocol EST 2190 is 64 pages long; its main categories are background; objectives; selection of patients; randomization/registration procedures; treatment plan; measurement of effect; study parameters; drug formulation and procurement; statistical considerations; records to be kept; patient consent and peer judgment; and references (of which there were 92).

4. Henderson suggests that the fact that both arms were experimental made randomization easier. Abrams notes that many trial participants were recruited by Peters from the large Duke transplant program.

5. Attendees included Klausner, Robert Wittes, Mary McCabe, and Jeff Abrams for the NCI; Robert Comis, the chair of ECOG; Richard Schilsky, chair of CALGB; Allen Lichter, then president of ASCO; Amy Langer of the National Alliance of Breast Cancer Organizations; Wade Aubry, BCBSA; and others.

Chapter 9

1. Anthony Elias, who had become the breast cancer transplanter at Dana-Farber after the departures of Peters and Antman, went to tandem transplants. In Milan, Gianni reported a nonrandomized study of tandem transplants.

2. This section is based on three lengthy interviews with Weiss on May 14, May 18, and October 10, 2002.

3. The NCI had required all cooperative groups to audit clinical trials in response to congressional concerns over scientific misconduct in the late 1970s.

4. Peters had tried to recruit Bezwoda to the Barbara Ann Karmanos Cancer Institute in Detroit at one point and later recruited Dansey, Bezwoda's colleague.

5. South Africa classified individuals as white, black, colored, or Indian at that time.

6. Amgen and Immunex paid for the trip through US Oncology; members were reimbursed expenses and received a fee.

7. Nurses are called Sister in South Africa, as they are in many British Commonwealth countries.

8. This discussion used by permission of Virginia Hetrick.

9. This discussion used by permission of Alice Philipson and Shannon Brownlee.

10. *The New Yorker* restricts letters to one signature.

11. This discussion used by permission of Rod Baber.

Chapter 10

1. Procedures often define subspecialties. High-dose chemotherapy compares in this respect to dialysis and nephrology, transurethral resection and urology, and heart catheterization and interventional cardiology.

2. Furthermore, the staging of a disease, which is critical to establishing comparability between experimental and historical populations, typically changes, becoming more precise over time. As staging changes, it often results in some reclassification of patients from one stage to another, further confounding the interpretation of study results.

3. "Such desperation- or sympathy-guided rulings are not merely expensive. They set a terrible legal precedent if we want empirical judgments to be guided by empirical evidence" (Morreim 2001, p. 413).

4. This argument became and remains the de facto position of the NIH, advanced in the mid-1990s in negotiations between the NIH and the then so-named American Association of Health Plans.

5. The Agency for Healthcare Research and Quality has established such a partnership with private institutions, designated as Evidence-based Practice Centers, for conducting technology assessments.

References

Introduction

Chamberlin TC. The method of multiple working hypotheses. *Science* 1965; 148:754–9.

Flyvbjerg B. *Making Social Science Matter: Why Social Inquiry Fails and How It Can Succeed Again.* Cambridge, UK: Cambridge University Press, 2001.

Chapter 1

American Cancer Society. *Cancer Facts & Figures 2003–2004.* Atlanta, GA, 2004. Available at http://www.cancer.org/downloads/STT/CAFF2003BrFPWSecured.pdf. Accessed December 28, 2004.

American Cancer Society. *Breast Cancer Facts & Figures 2005–2006.* Atlanta, GA, 2005. Available at http://www.cancer.org/downloads/STT/CAFF2005BrF.pdf. Accessed July 20, 2006.

Antman K, Eder JP, Elias A, et al. High-dose combination alkylating agent preparative regimen with autologous bone marrow support: the Dana-Farber Cancer Institute/Beth Israel Hospital experience. *Cancer Treat Rep* 1987; 71:119–25.

Brandt SJ, Peters WP, Atwater SK, et al. Effect of recombinant human granulocyte-macrophage colony-stimulating factor on hematopoietic reconstitution after high-dose chemotherapy and autologous bone marrow transplantation. *N Engl J Med* 1988; 318:869–76.

Canales MA, Arrieta R, Hernandez-Garcia MC, et al. Factors influencing collection and engraftment of CD34+ cells in patients with breast cancer following high-dose chemotherapy and autologous peripheral blood progenitor cell transplantation. *J Hematother Stem Cell Res* 2000; 9:103–9.

Canellos GP. Bone marrow transplantation as salvage therapy in advanced Hodgkin's disease: allogeneic or autologous. *J Clin Oncol* 1985; 3:1451–4.

Dana-Farber Cancer Institute. Emil Frei III, MD, honored for his role in developing first treatment leading to complete cure for childhood leukemia. Available at http://www.dana-farber.org/abo/news/press/040704.asp. Accessed on November 16, 2004.

DeVita VT. Dose-response is alive and well. *J Clin Oncol* 1986; 4:1157–9.

DeVita VT, Schein PS. The use of drugs in combination for the treatment of cancer: rationale and results. *N Engl J Med* 1973; 288:998–1006.

Eder JP, Antman K, Peters W, et al. High-dose combination alkylating agent chemotherapy with autologous bone marrow support for metastatic breast cancer. *J Clin Oncol* 1986; 4:1592–7.

Food and Drug Administration. G-CSF approved to protect cancer chemo patients. Press release, P91–6. Rockville, MD: Food and Drug Administration, 02/21/1991.

Frei E 3rd, Canellos GP. Dose: a critical factor in cancer chemotherapy. *Am J Med* 1980; 69:585–94.

Gelman RS, Henderson IC. A reanalysis of dose intensity for adjuvant chemotherapy trials in stage II breast cancer. *SAKK Bull* 1987; 4:10–2.

Gentry C. Insurance companies balk at breast-cancer treatment. *St. Petersburg Times,* September 4, 1990:1A.

Goodman E. A health-research bias. Op-Ed. *Boston Globe,* June 21, 1990:15.

Handelsman H. *Reassessment of autologous bone marrow transplantation* (SuDoc HE 20.6512/7:988/3). Health Technology Assessment Reports, 1988. Rockville, MD: National Center for Health Services Research and Health Care Technology Assessment, Public Health Service, U.S. Dept. of Health and Human Services, 1988.

Hansen JA, Anasetti C, Beatty PG, Martin PJ, Thomas ED. Allogeneic marrow transplantation: the Seattle experience. In: Teraski PI, ed. *Clinical Transplants 1989.* Los Angeles: UCLA Tissue Typing Lab, 1989:105–14.

Henderson C. Interview by RA Rettig. May 17, 2002a.

Henderson C. E-mail to RA Rettig, forwarded by F Jordan, June 12, 2002b.

Henderson IC. Adjuvant chemotherapy of breast cancer: a promising experiment or standard practice? *J Clin Oncol* 1985; 3:140–3.

Henderson IC, Canellos GP. Cancer of the breast: the past decade (first of two parts). *N Engl J Med* 1980a; 302:17–30.

Henderson IC, Canellos GP. Cancer of the breast: the past decade (second of two parts). *N Engl J Med* 1980b; 302:78–90.

Henderson IC, Hayes DF, Gelman R. Dose-response in the treatment of breast cancer: a critical review. *J Clin Oncol* 1988; 6:1501–15.

Hernon P. Dying of cancer, woman battles insurance firm. *St. Louis Post-Dispatch,* July 12, 1992:1A.

Hortobagyi GN. Developments in chemotherapy of breast cancer. *Cancer* 2000; 88:3073–9.

Howe RF. Maryland patient wins coverage for treatment. *Washington Post,* April 19, 1990:C1.

Hryniuk W, Bush H. The importance of dose intensity in chemotherapy of metastatic breast cancer. *J Clin Oncol* 1984; 2:1281–8.

Hryniuk W, Levine MN. Analysis of dose intensity for adjuvant chemotherapy trials in stage II breast cancer. *J Clin Oncol* 1986; 4:1162–70.

Hudis CA, Munster PN. High-dose therapy for breast cancer. *Semin Oncol* 1999; 26:35–47.

Larson E. The soul of an HMO. *Time,* January 22, 1996; 147:44–52.

Leff L. Cancer patient has no regrets over win that came too late. *Washington Post,* December 17, 1990a:D3.

Leff L. Maryland mother's chance at life hinges on trial; patient sues insurers for cancer treatment cost. *Washington Post,* April 17, 1990b:B1.

Lerner BH. *The Breast Cancer Wars: Hope, Fear, and the Pursuit of a Cure in 20th-Century America.* New York: Oxford University Press, 2001.

National Institutes of Health. Adjuvant chemotherapy for breast cancer. *NIH Consensus Statement Online July* 14–16, 1980; 3:1–4. Available at http://consensus.nih.gov/1980/ 1980AdjuvantTherapyBreastCancer024html.htm. Accessed July 18, 2002.

National Institutes of Health. Adjuvant chemotherapy for breast cancer. *NIH Consensus Statement Online* September 9–11, 1985; 5:1–19. Available at http://consensus.nih.gov/1985/1985AdjuvantChemoBreastCancer052html.htm. Accessed January 7, 2005.

National Institutes of Health. Treatment of early-stage breast cancer. *NIH Consensus Statement Online* June 18–21, 1990; 8:1–19. Available at http://consensus.nih.gov/1990/1990EarlyStageBreastCancer081html.htm. Accessed July 18, 2002.

National Institutes of Health. Consensus Conference. Treatment of early-stage breast cancer. *JAMA* 1991; 265:391–5.

Peters WP. The rationale for high-dose chemotherapy with autologous bone marrow support in the treatment of breast cancer. In: Dicke KA, Spitzer G, Zander AR, eds. *Autologous Bone Marrow Transplantation: Proceedings of the First International Symposium.* Houston, TX: University of Texas M. D. Anderson Hospital and Tumor Institute, 1985:189–95.

Peters WP. The effect of recombinant human colony-stimulating factors on hematopoietic reconstitution following autologous bone marrow transplantation. *Semin Hematol* 1989; 26:18–23.

Peters WP, Eder JP, Henner WD, et al. High-dose combination alkylating agents with autologous bone marrow support: a phase 1 trial. *J Clin Oncol* 1986; 4:646–54.

Peters WP, Ross M, Vredenburgh JJ, et al. High-dose chemotherapy and autologous bone marrow support as consolidation after standard-dose adjuvant therapy for high-risk primary breast cancer. *J Clin Oncol* 1993; 11:1132–43.

Peters WP, Shpall EJ, Jones RB, et al. High-dose combination alkylating agents with bone marrow support as initial treatment for metastatic breast cancer. *J Clin Oncol* 1988; 6:1368–76.

Rettig RA. *Cancer Crusade : The Story of the National Cancer Act of 1971.* Princeton, NJ: Princeton University Press, 1977; republished by Authors Choice Press, New York, 2005.

Rodenhuis S. The status of high-dose chemotherapy in breast cancer. *Oncologist* 2000; 5:369–75.

Tobias JS, Weiner RS, Griffiths CT, Richman CM, Parker LM, Yankee RA. Experience with cryopreserved autologous marrow infusion following high dose chemotherapy. *Eur J Cancer* 1977; 13:269–77.

Williams SF, Mick R, Desser R, Golick J, Beschorner J, Bitran JD. High-dose consolidation therapy with autologous stem cell rescue in stage IV breast cancer. *J Clin Oncol* 1989; 7:1824–30.

Williams SF, Gilewski T, Mick R, Bitran JD. High-dose consolidation therapy with autologous stem cell rescue in stage IV breast cancer: follow-up report. *J Clin Oncol* 1992; 10:17443–7.

Chapter 2

Ahmed T. Professor of Medicine, Director of Bone Marrow Transplantation Services, New York Medical College, Valhalla, New York. Letter to M Coad, Culp, Guterson & Drader, May 6, 1992.

American Medical Association. Diagnostic and therapeutic technology assessment. Autologous bone marrow transplantation—reassessment. *JAMA* 1990; 263:881–7.

American Society of Clinical Oncology. Policy Statement: Reimbursement for Cancer Treatment: Coverage of Unlabeled Drug Indications. Approved 1990, revised 1993. Alexandria, VA: American Society of Clinical Oncology. Available at http://www.asco.org/prof/pp/html/m_unlab.htm. Accessed September 6, 2000.

American Society of Clinical Oncology. Bone marrow transplants increase survival for breast cancer patients. American Society of Clinical Oncology. Press release. May 19,1992.

Antman K, Schnipper LE, Frei E 3rd. The crisis in clinical cancer research. Third-party insurance and investigational therapy. *N Engl J Med* 1988; 319:46–8.

Antoine F. Are health insurers denying patients quality care? *J Natl Cancer Inst* 1989; 81:1766–8.

Aronson N. Interview by RA Rettig, PD Jacobson, and WM Aubry, March 14, 2002.

Artig T. Bone Marrow Transplant Program Coordinator, University of Utah Medical Center, Salt Lake City, Utah. Letter To Whom It May Concern. May 7, 1992.

Ascensao JL. Professor of Medicine, Director, Bone Marrow Transplant Program, University of Nevada-Reno, Reno, Nevada. Letter to M Coad, Culp, Guterson & Drader, May 29, 1992.

Aubry WM. Summary presentation prepared for RA Rettig, CM Farquhar, and PD Jacobson, March 5, 2002.

Bazell R. Topic of cancer. *The New Republic* 1990; 203:9–12.

Bazell R. Interview by S Brownlee, September 16, 2004.

Belanger D, Moore M, Tannock I. How American oncologists treat breast cancer: an assessment of the influence of clinical trials. *J Clin Oncol* 1991; 9:7–16.

Bergthold LA. Medical necessity: do we need it? *Health Aff* 1995; 14:180–90.

Blum D. What patients want to know. *Forum on Emerging Treatments for Breast Cancer.* Bethesda, MD: National Cancer Institute, Health Improvement Institute, Candlelighters Childhood Cancer Foundation, 1991, 101–5.

Boodman SG. Advocates of breast cancer research come of age: politics of an illness. *The Times Union* April 24, 1994:E1.

Boston Women's Health Book Collective. *Our Bodies, Ourselves.* New York: Simon and Schuster, 1973.

Boston Women's Health Book Collective. Our bodies ourselves, 2004. Available at: http://www.ourbodiesourselves.org/bwhbc.htm. Accessed December 28, 2004.

Brown E. Autologous bone marrow transplantation. Letter To Whom It May Concern, on behalf of the American Medical Association, Chicago, IL, August 14, 1990a.

Brown E. Use of the term investigational. Letter To Whom It May Concern, on behalf of the American Medical Association, Chicago, IL, August 15, 1990b.

Brownlee S. Bad science and breast cancer. *Discover* 2002; 23:73–8.

Brownlee S. Interview by RA Rettig, September 14, 2004.

Cancer Letter. Funding for cooperative research threatened. *Cancer Lett* November 3, 1989; 15:1.

Cancer Letter. Clinical cooperative groups asked to develop tamoxifen prevention trial: CGOPs to participate. *Cancer Lett* July 6, 1990a; 16:1–4; Group chairmen propose four more trials for high priority status, 16:5–6.

Cancer Letter. Lasagna Committee report advocates faster drug approval, insurance coverage for investigational drugs, ancillary costs. *Cancer Lett* September 7, 1990b; 16:2.

Chalmers TC, van den Noort S, Lockshin MD, Waksman BH. Summary of a workshop on the role of third-party payers in clinical trials of new agents. *N Engl J Med* 1983; 309:1334–6.

Ciobanu N., Associate Professor of Medicine, Director, Bone Marrow Transplant Program, Albert Einstein Cancer Center, Bronx, New York. Letter to M Coad, Culp, Guterson & Grader. June 2, 1992.

Clark WF, Garg AX, Blake PG, Rock GA, Heidenheim AP, Sackett DL. Effect of awareness of a randomized controlled trial on use of experimental therapy. *JAMA* 2003; 290:1351–5.

Davidson NE. Out of the courtroom and into the clinic. *J Clin Oncol* 1992; 10:517–9.

Doctors Group. Women and Their Bodies. Boston: New England Free Press, 1970.

Eddy DM. High-dose chemotherapy with autologous bone marrow transplantation for the treatment of metastatic breast cancer. *J Clin Oncol* 1992; 10:657–70.

Eddy DM. Interview by RA Rettig. October 29, 2003.

Elfenbein GJ, Professor of Internal Medicine, Director, Division of Bone Marrow Transplantation, Chief, Bone Marrow Transplant Service, H. Lee Moffitt Cancer Center & Research Institute, University of South Florida, Tampa, Florida. Letter To Whom It May Concern. April 30, 1992.

Epstein S. *Impure Science: AIDS, Activism, and the Politics of Knowledge.* Berkeley: University of California Press, 1996.

Forum on Emerging Treatments for Breast Cancer. Bethesda, MD: Co-sponsored by National Cancer Institute, Health Improvement Institute, and Candlighters Childhood Cancer Foundation, June 11, 1991.

Gelband H, U.S. Congress, Office of Technology Assessment. *The Impact of Randomized Clinical Trials on Health Policy and Medical Practice: Background Paper.* Washington, DC: Congress of the United States, 1983.

Gentry C. Insurance companies balk at breast-cancer treatment. *St. Petersburg Times* September 4, 1990: p. 1A.

Gleeson S. Interview by RA Rettig, October 19, 2002.

Glick J. Interview by RA Rettig, March 25, 2002.

Haney DQ. Study shows blood growth factor useful in cancer treatment. *Associated Press,* Boston, April 6 and 7, 1988.

Henderson C. Interview by RA Rettig, May 17, 2002.

Herzig RH. Marion F. Beard Professor, Director, Bone Marrow Transplant Program, University of Louisville, Louisville, Kentucky. Letter To Whom It May Concern. May 27, 1992.

Institute of Medicine. *Assessing Medical Technologies.* Washington, DC: National Academy Press, 1985.

Institute of Medicine. *Medical Technology Assessment Directory.* Washington, DC: National Academy Press, 1988.

Kadar AG. The sex-bias myth in medicine. *The Atlantic* August 1994, 274:66.

Kiernan LA. NH women sue to get coverage of cancer. *Boston Globe* October 6, 1991:31.

Kolata G. Interview by S Brownlee, September 28, 2004.

Kushner R. *Breast Cancer: A Personal History and Investigative Report.* New York: Harcourt, Brace, Jovanovich,1975.

Kushner R. *Why Me: What Every Woman Should Know about Breast Cancer to Save Her Life.* New York: New American Library, 1977.

Langer A. Interview by RA Rettig, April 2, 2004.

Lazarus H. Director, Bone Marrow Transplant Program, Ireland Cancer Center, University Hospitals of Cleveland, Case Western Reserve University, Cleveland, Ohio. Letter To Whom It May Concern. May 8, 1992.

Leff L. Maryland mother's chance at life hinges on trial; patient sues insurers for cancer treatment cost. *Washington Post* April 17, 1990:B1.

Lerner BH. *The Breast Cancer Wars: Hope, Fear, and the Pursuit of a Cure in 20th-Century America.* New York: Oxford University Press, 2001.

Loupe D. 'Self-transplants' prolong some lives. *Atlanta Journal and Constitution* October 22, 1991:A1.

Love SM, Lindsey K. *Dr. Susan Love's Breast Book.* New York: Addison-Wesley, 1991.

Love SM, Lindsey K. *Dr. Susan Love's Breast Book.* 3rd ed. New York: HarperCollins, 2000.

Marks HM. *The Progress of Experiment : Science and Therapeutic Reform in the United States, 1900–1990.* Cambridge, UK: Cambridge University Press, 1997.

Marshall E. The politics of breast cancer. *Science* 1993; 259:616–7.

McCabe M, Friedman MA. Impact of third-party reimbursement on cancer clinical investigation: a consensus statement coordinated by the National Cancer Institute. *J Natl Cancer Inst* 1989; 81:1585–6.

McGlave P. Professor of Medicine, Director, Adult Bone Marrow Transplantation Program, University of Minnesota Medical School, Minneapolis, Minnesota. Letter to M. Coad, Culp, Guterson & Grader. May 5, 1992.

McGrory B. Courts overruling insurers reluctant to cover breast cancer therapy. *Boston Globe* May 6, 1990: p. 44.

McMillan R. Director, Weingart Center for Bone Marrow Transplantation, Scripps Clinic and Research Foundation, LaJolla, California. Letter To Whom It May Concern. April 27, 1992.

Michigan Society of Hematology and Oncology. Position on ABMT for Breast Cancer. Ann Arbor, Michigan, n.d.

National Alliance of Breast Cancer Organizations. *Autologous Bone Marrow Transplantation: Facing the Challenge* [videotape]. New York: National Alliance of Breast Cancer Organizations, 1992.

National Institutes of Health. History of congressional appropriations, 1980–1989. Available at http://officeofbudget.od.nih.gov/PDF/appic3806%20-%20transposed%20%2080%20-%2089.pdf.

National Women's Health Network. About NWHN: Our Mission. Available at http://www.womenshealthnetwork.org/about/overview.php. Accessed March 25, 2004.

Newcomer LN. Defining experimental therapy: a third-party payer's dilemma. *N Engl J Med* 1990; 323:1702–4.

Newhouse JP. Medical care costs: how much welfare loss? *J Econ Perspect* 1992; 6:3–21.

Peters WP, Lipman ME, Bonadonna G, DeVita VT, Holland JF, Rosner GL. High dose chemotherapy and autologous bone marrow support for breast cancer: a technology assessment. Confidential draft, July 1990.

Peters WP, Rogers MC. Variation in approval by insurance companies of coverage for autologous bone marrow transplantation for breast cancer. *N Engl J Med* 1994; 330:473–7.

President's Cancer Panel. *Final Report of the National Committee to Review Current Procedures for Approval of New Drugs for Cancer and AIDS.* Washington, DC: National Cancer Institute, August 15,1990: i–xi, 1–15.

Reed EC. Assistant Professor of Medicine, Clinical Director, Bone Marrow Transplant Unit, University of Nebrask Medical Center, Omaha, Nebraska. Letter To Whom It May Concern. April 28, 1992.

Rettig RA. Technology assessment: an update. *Invest Radiol* 1991; 26:165–73.

Rettig RA. *Health Care in Transition: Technology Assessment in the Private Sector.* Santa Monica, CA: RAND, 1997.

Rose LJ. Autologous bone marrow transplants. *Health Aff* 2002; 21:308.

Rosenthal E. Patient's marrow emerges as key cancer tool. *New York Times* March 27, 1990:C1.

Silver SM. Director, Adult Bone Marrow Transplant Program, University of Michigan Medical Center, Ann Arbor, Michigan. Letter to M Coad, Culp, Guterson & Grader. April 28, 1992.

Stabiner, Karen. Women warriors. *Los Angeles Times Magazine,* November 5, 1995, p. 10.

Stadtmauer E. Interview by RA Rettig, May 20, 2002.

Tobias JS, Weiner RS, Griffiths CT, Richman CM, Parker LM, Yankee RA. Experience with cryopreserved autologous marrow infusion following high dose chemotherapy. *Eur J Cancer* 1977; 13:269–77.

Tutschka PJ. Professor of Medicine and Pathology, Division of Bone Marrow Transplantation, James Cancer Center and Research Institute, The Ohio State University, Columbus, Ohio. Letter to Culp, Guterson & Grader, To Whom It May Concern. May 29, 1992.

Ungerleider R Friedman M. Sex, trials and data tapes. *J Natl Cancer Inst* 1991; 83:16–17.

Vogler WR. Professor of Medicine, Department of Medicine, Division of Hematology/Oncology, Emory University School of Medicine, Atlanta, Georgia. Letter To Whom It May Concern. April 27, 1992.

Weisbrod B. The health care quadrilemma: an essay on technological change, insurance, quality of care, and cost containment. *J Econ Lit* June 1991; 523–552.

Wittes RE. Paying for patient care in treatment research—who is responsible? *Cancer Treat Rep* 1987; 71:107–13.

Chapter 3

Abraham KS. Judge-made law and judge-made insurance: honoring the reasonable expectations of the insured. *Virginia Law Review.* 1981; 67:1151–91.

Antman K, Gale RP. Advanced breast cancer: high-dose chemotherapy and bone marrow autotransplants. *Ann Intern Med* 1988; 108:570–4.

Brostron JC. The conflict of interest standard in ERISA cases: can it be avoided in the denial of high dose chemotherapy treatment for breast cancer? *DePaul J Health Care Law* 1999; 1:6.

Cramm T, Hartz AJ, Green MD. Ascertaining customary care in malpractice cases: asking those who know. *Wake Forest Law Rev* 2002; 37:699–755.

ERISA Litigation Reporter. Courts continue to struggle with the exclusion in medical plans for experimental procedures: a review of the circuit court cases concerning high dose chemotherapy as a treatment for cancer in connection with autologous bone marrow transplant or peripheral stem cell rescue. *ERISA Litigation Rep* 1996; 4:6.

Giese W. Adjudication of third party payment for high dose chemotherapy and bone marrow rescue in the treatment of breast cancer. *DePaul J Health Care Law* 1996; 1:205–42.

Jacobson PD. Medical malpractice and the tort system. *JAMA* 1989; 262:3320–7.

Jacobson PD. *Strangers in the Night: Law and Medicine in the Managed Care Era.* New York: Oxford University Press, 2002.

Jacobson PD, Rosenquist CJ. The diffusion of low-osmolar contrast agents: technological change and defensive medicine. *J Health Politics, Policy and Law* 1996; 21:243–66.

Kennedy KJ. The perilous and ever-changing procedural rules of pursuing an ERISA claims case. *Univ Missouri at Kansas City Law Rev* 2001; 70:329–84.

Lauro v. The Travelers Insurance Co., 261 S0.2d 261, 266 (La. 1972).

Lippman ME. High-dose chemotherapy plus autologous bone marrow transplantation for metastatic breast cancer. *N Engl J Med* 2000; 342:1119–20.

Mayer M. From access to evidence: an advocate's journey. *J Clin Oncol* 2003; 21:3881–4.

Mello MM, Brennan TA. The controversy over high-dose chemotherapy with autologous bone marrow transplant for breast cancer. *Health Aff* 2001; 20:101–17.

Morreim EH. From the clinics to the courts: the role evidence should play in litigating medical care. *J Health Polit Policy Law* 2001; 26:409–27.

Shuman DW. Expertise in law, medicine, and health care. *J Health Polit Policy Law* 2001; 26:267–90.

Stadtmauer EA, O'Neill A, Goldstein LJ, et al. Conventional dose chemotherapy compared with high-dose chemotherapy plus autologous hematopoietic stem-cell transplantation for metastatic breast cancer. *N Engl J Med* 2000; 342:1069–76.

Thomas v. Gulf Health Plan, Inc., 688 F. Supp. 590 (S.D. Ala. 1988).

Chapter 4

Ader M. Investigational treatments: a legal perspective. *Technologica* July 1995: 1, 3, 5–6.

American Medical Association Diagnostic and Therapeutic Technology Assessment. Autologous bone marrow transplantation: reassessment. *JAMA* 1990; 263:881–7.

Bovbjerg RJ. The medical malpractice standard of care: HMOs and customary practice. *Duke Law J* 1975: 1375–1409.

Brown E. Use of the term investigational. Letter To Whom It May Concern, on behalf of the American Medical Association, Chicago, IL. August 15, 1990.

Eddy DM. High-dose chemotherapy with autologous bone marrow transplantation for the treatment of metastatic breast cancer. *J Clin Oncol* 1992; 10:657–70.

Glaspy JA. Interview by RA Rettig, October 23, 2002.

Grinfeld MJ. How does Hiepler do it? What a family law firm did to become managed care's biggest headache. *California Lawyer* 1999; 19:44–8.

Jacobson PD. *Strangers in the Night: Law and Medicine in the Managed Care Era.* New York: Oxford University Press, 2002.

Jacobson PD, Rosenquist CJ. The diffusion of low-osmolar contrast agents: technological change and defensive medicine. *J Health Polit Policy Law* 1996; 21:243–66.

Journal of Health Politics, Policy and Law 1999; 24:873–1218.

Larson E. The soul of an HMO. *Time,* January 22, 1996; 147:44–52.

Morreim EH. *Holding Health Care Accountable: Law and the New Medical Marketplace.* New York: Oxford University Press, 2001.

Newcomer LN. Defining experimental therapy: a third-party payer's dilemma. *N Engl J Med* 1990; 323:1702–4.

Rose LJ. Autologous bone marrow transplants. *Health Aff* 2002; 21:308.

Singer SJ, Bergthold LA. Prospects for improved decisionmaking about medical necessity. *Health Aff* 2001; 20:200–6.

Wake Forest Law Review 2002; 37:663–955.

Weiss RB. Breast cancer litigation: another aspect of the story. 2001. Available at: http://www.afip.org/Departments/legalmed/legmed2001/breast.htm. Accessed Jan. 13, 2005.

Chapter 5

Agency for Healthcare Research and Quality, HCUP Databases. Healthcare Cost and Utilization Project (HCUP). 2004. Available at http://www.hcup-us.ahrq.gov/nisoverview.jsp. Accessed January 1, 2005.

Banchik D. *Basic Report: Response Technologies, Inc.* Irvine, CA: LH Friend, Weinross & Frankson, June 9, 1991.

Birch, Robert. Interview by RA Rettig, January 30, 2004.

Dexheimer E. Courting disaster. Part 2 of 2. *Westword,* November 2, 1994. Available at http://www.westword.com/issues/1994-11-02/feature2_print.html. Accessed January 18, 2005.

ECRI. *High-Dose Chemotherapy with Autologous Bone Marrow Transplantation and/or Blood Cell Transplantation for the Treatment of Metastatic Breast Cancer.* Plymouth Meeting, PA: ECRI, 1995.

Gale RP, Park RE, Dubois R, et al. Delphi-panel analysis of appropriateness of high-dose chemotherapy and blood cell or bone marrow autotransplants in women with breast cancer. *Clin Transplant* 2000; 14:32–41.

Hortobagyi GN. Chemotherapy of breast cancer: a historical perspective. *Semin Oncol* 1997; 24:S171–4.

Hudis CA, Munster PN. High-dose therapy for breast cancer. *Semin Oncol* 1999; 26:35–47.

Hurd DD, Peters WP. Randomized, comparative study of high-dose (with autologous bone marrow support) versus low-dose cyclophosphamide, cisplatin, and carmustine as consolidation to adjuvant cyclophosphamide, doxorubicin, and fluorouracil for patients with operable stage II or III breast cancer involving 10 or more axillary lymph nodes (CALGB Protocol 9082). Cancer and Leukemia Group B. *J Natl Cancer Inst Monogr* 1995; 19:41–4.

Imrie K, Esmail R, Meyer RM. The role of high-dose chemotherapy and stem-cell transplantation in patients with multiple myeloma: a practice guideline of the Cancer Care Ontario Practice Guidelines Initiative. *Ann Intern Med* 2002; 136:619–29.

Kroft S. The most promising treatment? Is bone marrow transplant really the answer to curing breast cancer? *60 Minutes* September 26, 1993.

Lagnado L. Planned New York center sends shivers through competitors. *Wall Street Journal* August 12, 1996a:B1.

Lagnado L. Famed cancer center gives in to managed care. *Wall Street Journal* October 25, 1996b:B1.

Lagnado L. Sloan-Kettering Cancer Center seeks to keep rival Salick out of New York. *Wall Street Journal* December 6, 1996c:B5.

Leff R, Spinolo J, Feinberg B. Letter. *Wall Street Journal* March 29, 1993:A13.

Love SM. Interview by RA Rettig, September 1, 2004.

Mighion K, Gesme DH, Rifkin RM, Bennett CL. Growth of oncology physician practice management companies. *Cancer Invest* 1999; 17:362–70.

Olmos DR. Cancer clinics, managed-care firm team up. *Los Angeles Times* May 11, 1994a:D1.

Olmos DR. Salick breaks new ground in deal with Florida HMO. *Los Angeles Times* July 14, 1994b:D3.

Paris E. A personal affair (Bernard Salick and his Salick Health Care Inc.). *Forbes* June 2, 1986:98.

Peters WP, Eder JP, Henner WD, et al. High-dose combination alkylating agents with autologous bone marrow support: a phase 1 trial. *J Clin Oncol* 1986; 4:646–54.

Peters WP, Rosner G, Vredenburgh J, et al. Updated results of a prospective, randomized comparison of two doses of combination alkylating agents (AA) as consolidation after CAF in high-risk primary breast cancer involving 10 or more axillary lymph nodes (LN): CALGB 9082/SWOG 9114/NCIC Ma-13, 2001. Available at http://www.asco.org/asco/publications/abstract_print_view/1,1148,_12–002643–00_18–0010–00_19–0081,00.html. Accessed January 5, 2005.

Raeburn P. Maverick researcher's approach to developing cancer drugs is faltering. *Associated Press,* Franklin, TN, December 19, 1988.

Rebello K. Salick plans 24-hour cancer clinics. *Money* 1987:3B.

Response Technologies, Inc. Internal report. N.d.:1–35.

Rodenhuis S, Richel DJ, van der Wall E, et al. Randomised trial of high-dose chemotherapy and haemopoietic progenitor-cell support in operable breast cancer with extensive axillary lymph-node involvement. *Lancet* 1998; 352:515–21.

Salick B. Interview by RA Rettig, October 24, 2002.

Salick B. Interview by RA Rettig, February 11 and 12, 2003.

Stadtmauer EA, O'Neill A, Goldstein LJ, et al. Conventional-dose chemotherapy compared with high-dose chemotherapy plus autologous hematopoietic stem-cell transplantation for metastatic breast cancer. Philadelphia Bone Marrow Transplant Group. *N Engl J Med* 2000; 342:1069–76.

Stadtmauer EA, O'Neill A, Goldstein LJ, et al. Conventional-dose chemotherapy compared with high-dose chemotherapy (HDC) plus autologous stem-cell transplantation (SCT) for metastatic breast cancer: 5-year update of the "Philadelphia Trial" (PBT-1). 2002. Available at http://www.asco.org/ac/1,1003,_12–002643–00_18–0016–00_19–00169,00.asp. Accessed January 5, 2005.

Steiner C, Elixhauser A, Schnaier J. The healthcare cost and utilization project: an overview. *Eff Clin Pract* 2002; 5:143–51.

U.S. Department of Health and Human Services, Public Health Service, Centers for Disease Control and Prevention, National Center for Health Statistics. *National Hospital Discharge Survey for 1990 and 1991.* Hyattsville, MD: National Center for Health Statistics, Hospital Care Statistics Branch, 1991.

Vahdat LT, Papadopoulos K, Balmaceda C, et al. Phase I trial of sequential high-dose chemotherapy with escalating dose paclitaxel, melphalan, and cyclophosphamide, thiotepa, and carboplatin with peripheral blood progenitor support in women with responding metastatic breast cancer. *Clin Cancer Res* 1998; 4:1689–95.

West W. *The Deposition of William West, M.D., October 30, 1992, re: Denise Montes, Plaintiff, v. Blue Cross and Blue Shield of Florida, Defendant, Case No. 92–1865,* U.S. District Court, Southern District of Florida. 1992.

Chapter 6

Angell M. *Science on Trial: The Clash of Medical Evidence and the Law in the Breast Implant Case.* New York: Norton, 1996.

Brinkley J. Cost down, coverage up for federal employees; mental health, marrow transplants, inoculations among benefits some say should be available to all. *Rocky Mountain News* September 22, 1994:14A.

Cancer Letter. Duke physician, BMT patients lobby for reimbursement. *Cancer Lett* October 22, 1993; 19(41):4–5.

Caplan A. It might not be wise to require new cancer treatment coverage. *St. Paul Pioneer Press,* April 12, 1995.

Clinton WJ. Remarks to the National Breast Cancer Coalition, October 18, 1993. *Public Papers of the Presidents: William J. Clinton, 1993, Vol. 2* (pp. 1761–1763). Washington, D.C., Government Printing Office, 1994.

Darby M. FEHBP plans scramble to meet order to cover cancer treatment. *Managed Care Outlook* September 23, 1994; 7(18):1, 9–10.

DeMott K. OPM orders ABMT/HDC coverage before evidence is in. *Med Guidelines Outcomes Res* December 1, 1994; 5(23):1–2, 5.

Devoy A. Clinton health bill opens Hill debate. *Washington Post* October 28, 1993:A1.

Dickersin K. Interview by RA Rettig, July 19, 2004.

Dienst ER. High dose chemotherapy and autologous bone marrow transplant (HDC/ABMT) for breast cancer, part 1. *Breast Cancer Action Newsletter* June 1993a; 18: 1–3. Available at http://www.bcaction.org/Pages/SearchablePages/1993Newsletters/Newsletter018a. html. Accessed June 30, 2006.

Dienst ER. High dose chemotherapy and autologous bone marrow transplant (HDC/ABMT) for breast cancer, part 2. *Breast Cancer Action Newsletter* August 1993b; 19:1–3. Available at http://www.bcaction.org/Pages/SearchablePages/1993Newsletters/Newsletter019a. html. Accessed June 30, 2006.

Dienst ER. One woman's dying wish. *Breast Cancer Action Newsletter* October 1995; 32. Available at http://www.bcaction.org/Pages/SearchablePages/1993Newsletters/ Newsletter018a.html. Accessed June 30, 2006.

Flynn WE III, associate director for retirement and insurance, Office of Personnel Management. Letter to Alphonse O'Neil-White, Group Health Association of America, January 17, 1995.

Goldstein A. A growing chorus against breast cancer. *Washington Post* October 19, 1993:A1.

Groch AG. Political action to compel the federal government to mandate insurers of federal employees cease excluding bone marrow transplants for women with breast cancer while covering the same treatment for men with testicular cancer. Memorandum to Betsey Lambert, Esq., and Board of the NBCC, December 17, 1992.

Groch AG. High dose chemotherapy with bone marrow or autologous progenitor cell rescue [HDC/BMT/APCR] as a treatment option for women with breast cancer; the issue: access to HDC/BMT/APCR, an accepted medical treatment for advanced breast cancer, and women's right to choose among treatment options. Memorandum to individuals concerned about breast cancer. February 7, 1993. (Widely distributed to interested parties.)

Grow D. Breast cancer battle may not require fight for insurance. *Minneapolis Star Tribune* March 30, 1995:3B.

Harris SR. Chief, Health Benefits Contrast Division III, Office of Personnel Management. Letter to Dear FEHB Plan. Washington, DC: Office of Personnel Management, September 20, 1994.

Ignagni K. President and CEO, Group Health Association of America. Letter to the Hon. Eleanor Holmes Norton, September 27, 1994.

Jones R, Peters W, Williams S, Spitzer G, Champlin R, Davidson N. Letter to Hon. James King, Director, Office of Personnel Management, June 6, 1994. In U.S. House hearing, 1994:81–83.

Jordan MW. Letter to Mr. Ed Flynn, Associate Director for Retirement and Insurance, Office of Personnel Management: Kaiser Foundation Health Plan, Inc., October 19, 1994.

King JB. Letter to Hon. EH Norton, U.S. House of Representatives, September 28, 1994. In U.S. House hearing 1994:60–64.

Kroft S. The most promising treatment? Is bone marrow transplant really the answer to curing breast cancer? *60 Minutes* September 26, 1993.

Lambert B. Interview by RA Rettig, August 12, 2004.

Langer A. Interview by RA Rettig, April 2, 2004.

Love SM. Interview by RA Rettig, September 1, 2004.

Minnesota House of Representatives. 79th Session. House File No. 1742, March 29, 1995.

Minnesota 2004. Clifton Jacobson conducted interviews in March, April, and May 2004. Interviewees were granted anonymity.

Myers LF, Assistant Director for Insurance Programs, Office of Personnel Management. Letter to Clifton R. Gaus, Sc.D., Administrator, Agency for Health Care Policy and Research, July 26, 1995.

National Breast Cancer Coalition. Minutes of National Breast Cancer Coalition Meeting, Bel-Air, California, January 9, 1993.

Norton EH. Letter to Hon. James B. King, Director, Office of Personnel Management, August 16, 1994. In U.S. House hearing 1994:60.

Office of Personnel Management, Federal Employees Health Benefits Program. *Blue Cross and Blue Shield Service Benefit Plan.* Washington, DC: Office of Personnel Management, 1994a.

Office of Personnel Management, Federal Employees Health Benefits Program. *Government Employees Hospital Association, Inc. Benefit Plan, Washington, DC, 1994.* Washington, DC: Office of Personnel Management, 1994b.

Office of Personnel Management, Federal Employees Health Benefits Program. *Kaiser Foundation Health Plan of the Mid-Atlantic States, Inc.* Washington, DC: Office of Personnel Management, 1994c.

Office of Personnel Management. 1995 FEHB Program Open Season Highlights. Press release. September 20, 1994d. Available at http://www.opm.gov/pressrel/1994/PR940920.htm. Accessed January 7, 2005.

Office of Personnel Management, Federal Employees Health Benefits Program. *Blue Cross and Blue Shield Service Benefit Plan.* Washington, DC: Office of Personnel Management, 1995a.

Office of Personnel Management, Federal Employees Health Benefits Program. *Government Employees Hospital Association, Inc. Benefit Plan, Washington, DC, 1994.* Washington, DC: Office of Personnel Management, 1995b.

Office of Personnel Management, Federal Employees Health Benefits Program. *Kaiser Foundation Health Plan of the Mid-Atlantic States, Inc.* Washington, DC: Office of Personnel Management, 1995c.

O'Neill-White A, vice president and general counsel, Group Health Association of America. Letter to William E. Flynn, III, associate director for retirement and insurance, Office of Personnel Management, December 23, 1994.

Pearson C. Interview by RA Rettig, April 8, 2004.

Peters WP, Ross M, Vredenburgh JJ, et al. High-dose chemotherapy and autologous bone marrow support as consolidation after standard-dose adjuvant therapy for high-risk primary breast cancer. *J Clin Oncol* 1993; 11:1132–43.

Presidential panel calls breast cancer research underfunded. *Washington Post* October 28, 1993:A25.

Rich S, Brown D. Federal worker health program to add benefits; slightly lower premiums accompany improvements. *Washington Post* September 21, 1994:A1.

Sage WM. Lessons from breast implant litigation. *Health Aff* 1996; 15:206–10.

Schroeder P. Interview by Rachel Turow, October 29, 2002.

Schroeder P, Norton EH, et al. Letter by 53 Members of Congress to Hon. James B. King, Director, Office of Personnel Management, October 29, 1993. In U.S. House hearing, 1994:146.

Schroeder P, Norton EH. Letter to Hon. James B. King, Director, Office of Personnel Management, August 12, 1994. In U.S. House hearing, 1994:59.

Shayer B. Interview by RA Rettig, August 13, 2004.

Slatella M. Panel: Up the ante on breast cancer. *Newsday* October 28, 1993:17.

Smith CJ. Interview by RA Rettig, September 3, 2004.

U.S. House of Representatives, Committee on Post Office and Civil Service, Subcommittee on Compensation and Employee Benefits. *Oversight Hearing on the Federal Employee Health Benefits Plan (FEHBP) Coverage of HDC/ABMT Treatment for Breast Cancer.* Washington, DC: 103rd Congress, 2nd Session, August 11, 1994:1–149. (Abbreviated as U.S. House hearing 1994.)

Winslow R. Political pressure pushed a U.S. agency to back new therapy—health plans were ordered to pay for experimental, costly cancer regimen—many scientists doubt value. *Wall Street Journal* 1994:A1.

Chapter 7

American Medical Association Diagnostic and Therapeutic Technology Assessment. Autologous bone marrow transplantation: reassessment. *JAMA* 1990; 263:881–7.

Aubry WM. Summary presentation prepared for RA Rettig, CM Farquhar, and PD Jacobson, March 5, 2002.

Banta HD, Behney CJ, Willems JS. *Toward Rational Technology in Medicine: Considerations for Health Policy.* New York: Springer, 1981.

Bezwoda WR, Seymour L, Dansey RD. High-dose chemotherapy with hematopoietic rescue as primary treatment for metastatic breast cancer: a randomized trial. *J Clin Oncol* 1995; 13:2483–9.

Blue Cross Blue Shield Association. BCBSA TEC Program re-evaluates high-dose chemotherapy with ABMT for metastatic breast cancer. News release, with attachment. February 29, 1996.

Blue Cross Blue Shield Association. Site visit by RA Rettig, PD Jacobson, and WM Aubry and extended interview with N Aronson and others associated with the Technology Evaluation Center, Chicago, IL, March 14, 2002.

Brown EF, director, Department of Technology Assessment, American Medical Association. Letter to Gary Tisch of Shernoff, Bidart, Darras, Claremont, California. Copy in project files. February 27, 1990.

Bunker JP, Fowles J, Schaffarzick R. Evaluation of medical-technology strategies: effects of coverage and reimbursement (first of two parts). *N Engl J Med* 1982a; 306:620–4.

Bunker JP, Fowles J, Schaffarzick R. Evaluation of medical-technology strategies: proposal for an institute for health-care evaluation (second of two parts). *N Engl J Med* 1982b; 306:687–92.

CalPERS. Memorandum to CALPERS Health Benefits Committee, from Health Plan Administration Division, subject: Benefit policy on autologous bone marrow transplant (ABMT) for PERSCare and PERS Choice, February 21, California Public Employees Retirement System, 1996a.

CalPERS. Memorandum to CalPERS Health Benefits Committee, from Health Plan Administration Division, subject: Benefit policy on autologous bone marrow transplant (ABMT), California Public Employees Retirement System, March 19, 1996b.

CalPERS. Memorandum to CalPERS Health Benefits Committee, from Health Plan Administration Division, subject: Benefit policy on high dose chemotherapy/autologous bone marrow transplant (HDC/ABMT) for breast cancer, California Public Employees Retirement System, April 16, 1996c.

Cancer Letter. BMT appropriate for some breast cancer patients, Blues advisory panel says. *Cancer Lett* March 8, 1996:5.

Chuang KH, Aubry WM, Dudley RA. Independent medical review of health plan coverage denials: early trends. *Health Aff* 2004; 23:163–9.

Coates VH, Vice President, ECRI. Letter with analysis attached to Mary Horowitz, MD, MS, Scientific Director, North American Autologous Bone Marrow Transplant Registry, January 17, 1995.

Cova JL. A swift response to a modest proposal. *J Natl Cancer Inst* 1992; 84:744–5.

ECRI. Evidence lacking for efficacy of HDC/ASCR for metastatic breast cancer. *Health Technol Assess News* [ECRI newsletter] November–December 1994:3.

ECRI. *High-Dose Chemotherapy with Autologous Bone Marrow Transplantation and/or Blood Cell Transplantation for the Treatment of Metastatic Breast Cancer.* Plymouth Meeting, PA: ECRI, February 1995a.

ECRI. *High-dose Chemotherapy with Bone Marrow Transplant for Metastatic Breast Cancer: Patient Reference Guide.* Plymouth Meeting, PA: ECRI, 1995b.

ECRI. *Should I Enter a Clinical Trial: A Patient Reference Guide for Adults with a Serious or Life-Threatening Illness. A Report by ECRI Commissioned by AAHP.* Plymouth Meeting, PA: ECRI, 2002.

Eddy DM. *Common screening tests.* Philadelphia: American College of Physicians, 1991.

Eddy DM. High-dose chemotherapy with autologous bone marrow transplantation for the treatment of metastatic breast cancer. *J Clin Oncol* 1992; 10:657–70.

Friedman MA, McCabe MS. Assigning care costs associated with therapeutic oncology research: a modest proposal. *J Natl Cancer Inst* 1992; 84:760–3.

Gleeson S. Paying for innovations in surgery. *Bull Am College Surg* 1996; 81:10–13.

Gleeson S. Interview by RA Rettig, October 19, 2002.

Grow D. Breast cancer battle may not require fight for insurance. *Minneapolis Star Tribune* March 30, 1995:3B.

Handelsman H. Reassessment of autologous bone marrow transplantation (SuDoc HE 20.6512/7:988/3). Health Technology Assessment Reports, 1988. Rockville, MD: National Center for Health Services Research and Health Care Technology Assessment, U.S. Dept. of Health and Human Services, Public Health Service, 1988.

Henderson C. Interview by RA Rettig, May 17, 2002.

Institute for Clinical Systems Integration. *Technology Assessment Report.* Cover sheet. Bloomington, MN: Institute for Clinical Systems Integration, n.d.

Institute for Clinical Systems Integration. *Technology Assessment Report #2: High-Dose Chemotherapy with Autologous Stem Cell Support for the Treatment of Breast Cancer* (Prepared July 1993). Bloomington, MN: Institute for Clinical Systems Integration, January 11, 1994.

Institute for Clinical Systems Integration. *Technology Assessment Report #2 Update: High-Dose Chemotherapy with Autologous Stem Cell Support for the Treatment of Breast Cancer.* Bloomington, MN: Institute for Clinical Systems Integration, July 1996.

Institute for Clinical Systems Integration. *Technology Assessment Report #2 Second Update: High-Dose Chemotherapy with Autologous Stem Cell Support for the Treatment of Breast Cancer.* Bloomington, MN: Institute for Clinical Systems Integration, April 2002.

Institute of Medicine. *Assessing Medical Technologies.* Washington, DC: National Academy Press, 1985.

Kennedy MJ. High-dose chemotherapy of breast cancer: is the question answered? *J Clin Oncol* 1995; 13:2477–9.

Francine Klopert v. Los Angeles Unified School District and California Physicians' Service dba Blue Shield of California, No. BC 033741, Superior Court, State of California for the County of Los Angeles, 1992.

Lerner J, Turkelson C, Robertson D. Interview by RA Rettig, March 25, 2002.

McGivney WT. ABMT (autologous bone marrow transplantation): a microcosm of the U.S. health care system. *Physician Exec* 1992a; 18:45–7.

McGivney WT. Proposal for assuring technology competency and leadership in medicine. *J Natl Cancer Inst* 1992b; 84:742–4.

McGivney WT. Ensuring technological competence and leadership in medicine. *Physician Exec* 1993; 19:50–1.

McGivney WT. Autologous bone marrow transplantation: a microcosm of the U.S. health care system. In: Gelijns A, Dawkins HV, eds. *Medical Innovation at the Crossroads: Adopting New Medical Technology,* Vol. 4. Washington, DC: National Academy Press, 1994a:109–16.

McGivney WT. Technology assessment and coverage decision making. *AAPPO J.* 1994b; 4:11–17.

McGivney WT. Interview by RA Rettig, March 26, 2002.

Monaco G. Interview by RA Rettig, June 23, 2003.

National Comprehensive Cancer Network. NCCN breast cancer practice guidelines. *Oncology* 1996; 10(11):Suppl.47–75.

National Comprehensive Cancer Network. Update of the NCCN guidelines for treatment of breast cancer. *Oncology* 1997; 11(11a):199–220.

Nugent M, Information Specialist, North American Autologous Bone Marrow Transplant Registry. Letter to Vivian Coates, ECRI, August 19, 1994.

Peters WP. High-dose chemotherapy with autologous bone marrow transplantation for the treatment of breast cancer: yes. In: Rosenberg SA, ed. *Important Advances in Oncology 1995.* Philadelphia: Lippincott, 1995:215–230.

Peters WP, Berry DA, Vredenburgh JJ, et al. Five year follow-up of high-dose combination alkylating agents with ABMT as consolidation after standard-dose CAF for primary breast cancer involving greater than or equal to 10 axillary lymph nodes (DUKE/CALGB 8782). Abstract, American Society of Clinical Oncology 1995 annual meeting, Los Angeles, May 21–23, 1995. Available at http://www.asco.org/asco/publications/abstract_print_view/ 0,1144,_12–002324–00_29–00. Accessed October 14, 2002.

Peters WP, Ross M, Vredenburgh JJ, et al. High-dose chemotherapy and autologous bone marrow support as consolidation after standard-dose adjuvant therapy for high-risk primary breast cancer. *J Clin Oncol* 1993; 11:1132–43.

Rettig RA. Technology assessment—an update. *Invest Radiol* 1991; 26:165–73.

Rettig RA. *Health Care in Transition: Technology Assessment in the Private Sector.* Santa Monica, CA: RAND, 1997.

Ruzek S. Envisioning women's health from social and biomedical perspectives. Presentation, Reframing Women's Health conference, University of Illinois, Chicago Circle, July 19–24, 1994.

Ruzek S. Interview by RA Rettig, July 26, 2004, 2004.

Smith GA, Henderson IC. High-dose chemotherapy (HDC) with autologous bone marrow transplantation (ABMT) for the treatment of breast cancer: the jury is still out. In: DeVita VT, Hellman S, Rosenberg SA, eds. *Important Advances in Oncology 1995.* Philadelphia: Lippincott, 1995:201–14.

Smith TJ, Somerfield MR. The ASCO experience with evidence-based clinical practice guidelines. *Oncology* 1997; 11:223–7.

Sox HC. *Common Diagnostic Tests: Use and Interpretation.* Philadelphia: American College of Physicians, 1987.

Sox HC. *Common Diagnostic Tests: Use and Interpretation.* Philadelphia: American College of Physicians, 1990.

Triozzi PL. Autologous bone marrow and peripheral blood progenitor transplant for breast cancer. *Lancet,* August 13, 1994; 344:418–419.

Visco F. Interview by RA Rettig, June 11, 2004.

Vredenburgh J, Silva O, de Sombre K, et al. The significance of bone marrow micrometastases for patients (pts) with breast cancer and greater than or equal to 10+ lymph nodes treated with high-dose chemotherapy and hematopoietic support... Abstract, American Society of Clinical Oncology 1995 annual meeting, Los Angeles, May 21–23,1995. Available at http://www.asco.org/asco/publications/abstract_print_view/ 0,1144,_ 12–002324–00_29–00. Accessed October 14, 2002.

Weiss RB. Interview by RA Rettig, May 14, 2002.

Winslow R. Political pressure pushed a U.S. agency to back new therapy—health plans were ordered to pay for experimental, costly cancer regimen—many scientists doubt value. *Wall Street Journal* November 17, 1994:A1.

Zones JS, PhD, Chair, Board of Directors, and Co-Chair, Breast Cancer Committee, National Women's Health Network. Letter to Kathleen Connell, Controller of the State of California, March 13, 1996.

Zones JS. Interview by RA Rettig, June 23, 2004.

Chapter 8

Abrams J. Interview by RA Rettig September 17, 2003.

American Society of Clinical Oncology. American Society of Clinical Oncology commends Administration's cancer initiative. Press release. January 29, 1998a. Available at: http://www.asco.org/asco/shared/asco_print_view/1,1168,_12–002112–00_15–002104–00_18–0010833–00_19–0010834–00_20–001,00.html. Accessed January 25, 2005.

American Society of Clinical Oncology. ASCO urges swift passage of bill to guarantee Medicare coverage of cancer clinical trials. Press release. May 5, 1998b. Available at: http://www.asco.org/asco/shared/asco_print_view/1,1168,_12–002227–00_18–0010829–00_19–0010832–00_20–001,00.html. Accessed January 25, 2005.

American Society of Clinical Oncology. Momentum in cancer treatment threatened by crisis in clinical research. Press release. July 17, 1998c. Available at: http://www.asco.org/asco/shared/asco_print_view/1,1168,_12–002112–00_15–002417–00_18–0010827–00_19–0010828–00_20–001,00.html. Accessed January 25, 2005.

American Society of Clinical Oncology Online:1999 Plenary Session Abstracts Plus: the role of high-dose chemotherapy and bone marrow transplant or peripheral stem-cell support in the treatment of breast cancer: background and preliminary results of five studies to be presented at ASCO's annual meeting, May 15–18, in Atlanta, GA, 1999. Available at: http://www.asco.org; http://www.ucsfbreastcarecenter.org/forum/1999/newsApr.html. Accessed March 2, 2000.

Antman KH. Randomized trials of high dose chemotherapy for breast cancer. *Biochim Biophys Acta* 2001; 1471:M89–98.

Aubry WM. Summary presentation prepared for RA Rettig, CM Farquhar, and PD Jacobson, March 5, 2002.

Basser R, O'Neil A, Martinelli G, et al., Randomized trial comparing up-front, multi-cycle dose-intensive chemotherapy (CT) versus standard dose CT in women with high-risk stage 2 or 3 breast cancer (BC): first results from IBCSG Trial 15–95, 2003. Available at http://www.asco.org/asco/publications/abstract_print_view/1,1148,_12–002643–00_18–0023–00_19–00102679,00.html. Accessed June 5, 2003.

Bergh J, Wiklund T, Erikstein B, et al. Tailored fluorouracil, epirubicin, and cyclophosphamide compared with marrow-supported high-dose chemotherapy as adjuvant treatment for high-risk breast cancer: a randomised trial. Scandinavian Breast Group 9401 study. *Lancet* 2000; 356:1384–91.

Berry D. Interview by RA Rettig, October 31, 2003.

Bezwoda WR. 1999 ASCO Annual Meeting abstract no. 4, p. 21d: Randomized, controlled trial of high dose chemotherapy (HD-CNVp) versus standard dose (CAF) chemotherapy for high risk, surgically treated, primary breast cancer. 1999. Available at: http://www.asco.org/asco/publications/abstract_print_view/1,1148,_12–002643–00_18–0017–00_19–0014261,00.html. Accessed January 25, 2005.

Bezwoda WR, Seymour L, Dansey RD. High-dose chemotherapy with hematopoietic rescue as primary treatment for metastatic breast cancer: a randomized trial. *J Clin Oncol* 1995; 13:2483–9.

Bliss JM, Vigushin D, Kanfer E, et al. 2003 ASCO Annual Meeting abstract: randomized trial of high dose therapy using cyclophosphamide, thiotepa and carboplatin in primary breast cancer patients with 4 or more historically involved positive nodes. ISRCTN: 52623943.

2003. Available at http://www.asco.org/asco/publications/abstract_print_view/ 1,1148,_12–002643–00_18–0023–00_19–00102675,00.html. Accessed June 11, 2003.

Blue Cross Blue Shield Association. Site visit by RA Rettig, PD Jacobson, and WM Aubry and extended interview with Naomi Aronson and others associated with the Technology Evaluation Center, Chicago, IL, March 14, 2002.

Cancer Letter. Trial of bone marrow transplantation for breast cancer to begin in Philly. *Cancer Lett* April 5, 1991:7.

Cancer Letter. ABMT trials unlikely to show clear benefit for breast cancer; data release debated. *Cancer Lett* March 12, 1999:1–5.

Cheson BD, Lacerna L, Leyland-Jones B, Sarosy G, Wittes RE. Autologous bone marrow transplantation. Current status and future directions. *Ann Intern Med* 1989; 110:51–65.

Clinical Cancer Letter. NCI plans ABMT trials for breast cancer; survival, cost, QoL are endpoints. *Clin Cancer Lett* January 1991a; 14:5.

Clinical Cancer Letter. Clinical trials testing bone marrow transplants as breast adjuvant are underway; researchers, patients, insurers discuss trials in forum. *Clin Cancer Lett* September 1991b; 14:1.

Clinical Cancer Letter. Trials show no advantage for high-dose chemotherapy plus ABMT in breast cancer. *Clin Cancer Lett* April 1999:3.

Coffier B, Philip T, Burnett AK, Symann ML. Consensus Conference on Intensive Chemotherapy Plus Hematopoietic Stem-Cell Transplantation in Malignancies. Lyon, France, June 4–6, 1993. *J Clin Oncol* 1994; 12:226–31.

Comis RL, Miller JD, Aldige CR, Krebs L, Stoval E. Public attitudes toward participation in cancer clinical trials. *J Clin Oncol* 2003; 21:830–5.

Corrie P, Shaw J, Harris R. Rate limiting factors in recruitment of patients to clinical trials in cancer research: descriptive study. *BMJ* 2003; 327:320–1.

Crown JP, Lind M, Gould A, et al. 2002 ASCO Annual Meeting abstract: high-dose chemotherapy (HDC) with autograft (PBP) support is not superior to cyclophosphamide (CPA), methotrexate and 5-FU (CMF) following doxorubicin (D) induction in patients with breast cancer (BC) and 4 or more involved axillary lymph nodes (4+LN): the Anglo-Celtic I study. 2002. Available at http://www.asco.org/asco/publications/abstract_print_view/ 1,1148,_12–002643–00_18–0016–00_19–00166,00.html. Accessed June 28, 2002.

Crown J, Perey L, Lind M, et al. 2003 ASCO Annual Meeting abstract: superiority of tandem high-dose chemotherapy (HDC) versus optimized conventionally-dosed chemotherapy (CDC) in patients (pts) with metastatic breast cancer (MBC): The International Randomized Breast Cancer Dose Intensity Study (IBDIS 1). 2003. Available at http://www.asco.org/asco/publications/abstract_print_view/1,1148,_12–002643–00_18– 0023–00_19–00103811,00.html. Accessed June 11, 2003.

Eastern Cooperative Oncology Group. ECOG protocol for EST 2190, revised 7/94, revised 1/95. Philadelphia: Eastern Cooperative Oncology Group, 1995:i–vii.

Eddy DM. High-dose chemotherapy with autologous bone marrow transplantation for the treatment of metastatic breast cancer. *J Clin Oncol* 1992; 10:657–70.

Eddy DM. and Henderson C. A cancer treatment under a cloud. New York Times, April 17, 1999:A17.

Ellis PM, Butow PN, Tattersall MH, Dunn SM, Houssami N. Randomized clinical trials in oncology: understanding and attitudes predict willingness to participate. *J Clin Oncol* 2001; 19:3554–61.

Fallowfield L, Ratcliffe D, Souhami R. Clinicians' attitudes to clinical trials of cancer therapy. *Eur J Cancer* 1997; 33:2221–9.

Forum on Emerging Treatments for Breast Cancer. Proceedings: presenting clinical trials sponsored by the National Cancer Institute, Bethesda, Maryland, June 11, 1991. National Cancer Institute; Health Improvement Institute; Candlelighters Childhood Cancer Foundation.

Fox RC, Swazey JP. *The Courage to Fail : A Social View of Organ Transplants and Dialysis*. Chicago: University of Chicago Press, 1978.

Gianni A, Bonadonna G. 2001 ASCO Annual Meeting abstract: five-year results of the randomized clinical trial comparing standard versus high-dose myeloablative chemotherapy in the adjuvant treatment of breast cancer with > 3 positive nodes (LN+). 2001. Available at http://www.asco.org/asco/publications/abstract_print_view/1,1148,_12–002643–00_18–0010–00_19–0080,00.html. Accessed June 27, 2002.

Glick J. Interview by RA Rettig, March 25, 2002.

Glück S, Crump M, Stewart D, et al. Summary of current studies in breast cancer using high-dose chemotherapy in autologous blood and marrow transplantation, including NCI-C CTG MA.16, X. In: Proceedings of the 10th International Symposium. The National Cancer Institute of Canada Clinical Trials Group. 2001. Available at http://mmserver.cjp.com/gems/blood/ABMT.10.Glück.pdf. Accessed May 2001.

Grady D. Doubts raised on a breast cancer procedure. *New York Times* April 16, 1999a:A1.

Grady D. Conference divided over high-dose breast cancer treatment. *New York Times* May 18, 1999b:A19.

Henderson IC, Canellos GP. Cancer of the breast: the past decade (first of two parts). *N Engl J Med* 1980a; 302:17–30.

Henderson IC, Canellos GP. Cancer of the breast: the past decade (second of two parts). *N Engl J Med* 1980b; 302:78–90.

Henderson C. Interview by RA Rettig, May 17, 2002.

Hortobagyi GN. Interview by RA Rettig, July 10, 2002.

Hurd DD, Peters WP. Randomized, comparative study of high-dose (with autologous bone marrow support) versus low-dose cyclophosphamide, cisplatin, and carmustine as consolidation to adjuvant cyclophosphamide, doxorubicin, and fluorouracil for patients with operable stage II or III breast cancer involving 10 or more axillary lymph nodes (CALGB Protocol 9082). Cancer and Leukemia Group B. *J Natl Cancer Inst Monogr* 1995;19:41–4.

Jeffrey NA, Waldholz M. Oncologists will speed release of results of breast-cancer studies. *Wall Street Journal* March 11, 1999:B2. Available at http://online.wsj.com/search/full.html. Accessed on June 30, 2006.

Kahn HR. Interview by RA Rettig, December 1, 2003.

Kelahan AF. Interview by RA Rettig, March 26, 2002.

Klabunde CN, Springer BC, Butler B, White MS, Atkins J. Factors influencing enrollment in clinical trials for cancer treatment. *South Med J* 1999; 92:1189–93.

Kolata G. Women resist trials to test marrow transplants. *New York Times* February 15, 1995:C8.

Kroger N, Kruger W, Zander AR. High-dose chemotherapy in breast cancer: current status of ongoing German trials. In: Dicke KA, Keating A, eds. *Autologous Blood and Marrow Transplantation X: Proceedings of the 10th International Symposium*. Charlottesville, VA: Carden Jennings, 2001. Available at: http://www.bloodline.net. Accessed July 2003.

Lerner BH. *The Breast Cancer Wars: Hope, Fear, and the Pursuit of a Cure in 20th-Century America.* New York: Oxford University Press, 2001.

Lotz J, Cure H, Janvier M, et al. 1999 ASCO Annual Meeting abstract no. 161: high-dose chemotherapy (HD-CT) with hematopoietic stem cell transplantation (HSCT) for metastatic breast cancer (MBC): results of the French protocol PEGASE 04. 1999. Available at http://www.asco.org/asco/publications/abstract_print_view/1,1148,_12–002643–00_18–0017–00_19–0014417,00.html.

National Breast Cancer Coalition. Statement on bone marrow and stem-cell transplants. For immediate release. National Breast Cancer Coaltion, Washington, D.C. April 15, 1999.

National Cancer Institute. Strategy meeting minutes, high-dose chemotherapy with stem cell support for the treatment of breast cancer, Bethesda, MD, March 30, 1995a.

National Cancer Institute. *Patient Referral to the National Cancer Institute's Autologous Bone Marrow Transplantation Clinical Trials: The Physician's Perspective.* Bethesda, MD: National Cancer Institute, August 1995b.

National Cancer Institute. *The Road to an Autologous Bone Marrow Transplant Trial: Breast Cancer Patients' Decision-Making Process: Qualitative Research with Breast Cancer Patients.* Bethesda, MD: National Cancer Institute, 1996.

National Cancer Institute. NCI high priority clinical trial—phase iii randomized study of adjuvant CAF (cyclophosphamide/doxorubicin/fluorouracil) vs adjuvant CAF followed by intensification with high-dose cyclophosphamide/thiotepa plus autologous stem cell rescue in women with stage II/III breast cancer at high risk of recurrence (summary last modified 12/98). Bethesda, MD. National Cancer Institute, 1998.

National Cancer Institute. High-dose chemotherapy/bone marrow transplant studies for breast cancer. Press release. March 10, 1999a. Available at http://www.cancer.gov/newscenter/chemo. Accessed January 25, 2005.

National Cancer Institute. Interim results of large trials of high-dose chemotherapy with bone marrow or stem cell transplants for breast cancer. Press release. 1999b. Available at http://www.cancer.gov/newscenter/interim1. Accessed April 15, 1999.

National Cancer Institute. Questions and answers: high-dose chemotherapy with bone marrow or stem cell transplants for breast cancer. Press Release. April 15, 1999c. Available at http://www.cancer.gov/newscenter/interimqa. Accessed January 25, 2005.

National Cancer Institute. High-dose chemotherapy for breast cancer: history. April 26, 2001. Available at http://www.cancer.gov/clinicaltrials/developments/high-dose-chemo-history0501. Accessed October 1, 2002.

Neymark N, Rosti G. Patient management strategies and transplantation techniques in European stem cell transplantation centers offering breast cancer patients high-dose chemotherapy with peripheral blood stem cell support: a joint report from the EORTC and EBMT. *Haematologica* 2000; 85:733–44.

Nitz UA, Frick M, Mohrmann S, et al. 2003 ASCO Annual Meeting abstract: tandem high-dose chemotherapy versus dose-dense conventional chemotherapy for patients with high risk breast cancer: interim results from a multicenter phase III trial. 2003. Available at http://www.asco.org/asco/publications/abstract_print_view/1,1148,_12–002643–00_18–0023–00_19–00102903,00.html. Accessed July 31, 2003.

Pedrazzoli P, Da Prada GA, Robustelli della Cuna G. High-dose chemotherapy and stem-cell support in breast cancer. *Lancet* 1998; 352:1220.

Peters W, Rosner G, Vredenburgh J, et al. 1999 ASCO Annual Meeting abstract no. 2, p. 21b:

A prospective, randomized comparison of two doses of combination alkyating agents (AA) as consolidation after CAF in high-risk primary breast cancer involving 10 or more axillary lymph nodes (LN): preliminary results of CALGB 9082/SWOG 9114/NCIC MA-13. 1999. Available at http://www.asco.org/asco/publications/abstract_print_view/ 1,1148,_12–002643–00_18–0017–00_19–0014259,00.html. Accessed January 25, 2005.

Peters WP, Shpall EJ, Jones RB, et al. High-dose combination alkylating agents with bone marrow support as initial treatment for metastatic breast cancer. *J Clin Oncol* 1988; 6:1368–76.

Peters WP, Rosner G, Vredenburgh J, et al. Updated results of a prospective, randomized comparison of two doses of combination alkylating agents (AA) as consolidation after CAF in high-rsik primary breast cancer involving ten or more axillary lymph nodes (LN): CALGB 9082/SWOG9114/NCIC. March 13, 2001. Available at http://www.asco.org. Accessed June 28, 2002.

Price LA. High-dose chemotherapy in high-risk breast cancer. *Lancet* 1998; 352:1551–2.

Pusztai L, Hortobagyi GN. Discouraging news for high-dose chemotherapy in high-risk breast cancer. *Lancet* 1998a; 352:501–2.

Pusztai L, Hortobagyi GN. High-dose chemotherapy in high-risk breast cancer. *Lancet* 1998b; 352:1552.

Roche H, Viens P, Biron P, Lotz JP, Asselain B. High-dose chemotherapy for breast cancer: the French PEGASE experience. *Cancer Control* 2003; 10:42–7.

Rodenhuis S, Bontenbal M, Beex LV, et al. 2000 ASCO Annual Meeting abstract: randomized phase III study of high-dose chemotherapy with cyclophosphamide, thiotepa and carboplatin in operable breast cancer with 4 or more axillary lymph nodes. 2000. Available at http://www.asco.org/asco/publications/abstract_print_view/ 1,1148,_12–002640–00_ 18–002–00_19–00201199,00.html. Accessed January 25, 2005.

Rodenhuis S, Bontenbal M, Beex LV, et al. High-dose chemotherapy with hematopoietic stem-cell rescue for high-risk breast cancer. *N Engl J Med* 2003; 349:7–16.

Rodenhuis S, Richel DJ, van der Wall E, et al. Randomised trial of high-dose chemotherapy and haemopoietic progenitor-cell support in operable breast cancer with extensive axillary lymph-node involvement. *Lancet* 1998; 352:515–21.

Scandinavian Breast Cancer Study Group. 1999 ASCO Annual Meeting abstract no. 3, p. 21c: results from a randomized adjuvant breast cancer study with high dose chemotherapy with CTCb supported by autologous bone marrow cells versus dose escalated and tailored FEC therapy. 1999. Available at http://www.asco.org/asco/publications/abstract_print_view/ 1,1148,_12–002643–00_18–0017–00_19–007631,00.html. Accessed June 2002.

Schrama JG, Faneyte IF, Schornagel JH, et al. Randomized trial of high-dose chemotherapy and hematopoietic progenitor-cell support in operable breast cancer with extensive lymph node involvement: final analysis with 7 years of follow-up. *Ann Oncol* 2002; 13:689–98.

Siminoff LA, Zhang A, Colabianchi N, Sturm CM, Shen Q. Factors that predict the referral of breast cancer patients onto clinical trials by their surgeons and medical oncologists. *J Clin Oncol* 2000; 18:1203–11.

Stadtmauer E. Interview by RA Rettig, May 20, 2002.

Stadtmauer E, O'Neill A, Goldstein L, et al. 1999 ASCO Annual Meeting abstract no. 1, p. 21a: phase III randomized trial of high-dose chemotherapy (HDC) and stem cell support (SCT) shows no difference in overall survival or severe toxicity compared to maintenance chemotherapy with cyclophosphamide, methotrexate and 5-fluorouracil (CMF) for women with metastatic breast cancer who are responding to conventional induction chemotherapy: the "Philadelphia" Intergroup Study (PBT-1). 1999. Available at: http://www.asco.org/asco/publications/abstract_print_view/1,1148,_12–002636–00_18–0017–00_19–0014258, 00.html. Accessed January 25, 2005.

Tokuda Y, Tajima T, Narabayashi M, et al. ASCO Annual Meeting 2001 poster presentation: randomized phase III study of high-dose chemotherapy (hdc) with autologous stem cell support as consolidation in high-risk postoperative breast cancer: Japan Clinical Oncology Group (jcog9208). 2001. Available at http://www.asco.org/ac/1,1003,_12–002511–00_18–0010–00_19–002252–00_28–002,00.asp. Accessed January 25, 2005.

Zander AR, Krüger W, Kröger N, et al. 2002 ASCO Annual Meeting abstract: high-dose chemotherapy with autologous hematopoietic stem-cell support (HSCS) vs. standard-dose chemotherapy in breast cancer patients with 10 or more positive lymph nodes: first results of a randomized trial. 2002. Available at http://www.asco.org/. Accessed April 16, 2002.

Zujewski J, Nelson A, Abrams J. Much ado about not . . . enough data: high-dose chemotherapy with autologous stem cell rescue for breast cancer. *J Natl Cancer Inst* 1998; 90:200–9.

Chapter 9

Antman KH. Overview of the six available randomized trials of high-dose chemotherapy with blood or marrow transplant in breast cancer. *J Natl Cancer Inst Monogr* 2001a; 30:114–6.

Antman KH. Randomized trials of high dose chemotherapy for breast cancer. *Biochim Biophys Acta* 2001b; 1471:M89–98.

ASCO Online. Statement of the American Society of Clinical Oncology on potential misconduct in south african trial—improprieties in breast cancer study of high-dose chemotherapy reported to ASCO. February 4, 2000. Available at http://www.asco.org/people/nr/html/genpr/m_0200trialpr.htm. Accessed March 13, 2000.

Bearman SI, Green S. Gralow J, Barlow W, Hudis C, Wolff A, Ingle J, Hortobagyi G, Livingston R, Martin S. SWOG/Intergroup 9623: A phase III comparison of intensive sequential chemotherapy to high dose chemotherapy and autologous hematopoietic progenitor cell support (AHPCS) for primary breast cancer in women with ≥4 involved axillary lymph nodes. *J Clin Oncol,* 2005 Annual Meeting Proceedings, Vol. 23, No. 16S, Part I of II (June 1 Supplement), 2005:572.

Bergh J. Where next with stem-cell-supported high-dose therapy for breast cancer? *Lancet* 2000; 355:944–5.

Bezwoda WR. 1999 ASCO Annual Meeting abstract: randomised, controlled trial of high dose chemotherapy (HD-CNVp) versus standard dose (CAF) chemotherapy for high risk, surgically treated, primary breast cancer. 1999. Available at http://www.asco.org/asco/publications/abstract_print_view/1,1148,_12–002643–00_18–0017–00_19–0014261,00.html. Accessed January 25, 2005.

Bezwoda WR, Seymour L, Dansey RD. High-dose chemotherapy with hematopoietic rescue as primary treatment for metastatic breast cancer: a randomized trial. *J Clin Oncol* 1995; 13:2483–9.

Cleaton-Jones P. Scientific misconduct in a breast-cancer chemotherapy trial: response of University of the Witwatersrand. *Lancet* 2000; 355:1011–12.

Crown J. Smart bombs versus blunderbusses: high-dose chemotherapy for breast cancer. *Lancet* 2004; 364:1299–300.

Grant A. Horrorific high dose: quality of life concerns ignored. *MAMM* September/October 1999:30–2.

Grant G. Letter in reply to Groopman. *The New Yorker* October 1998:20.

Groopman J. A healing hell: why bone-marrow transplantation is the cancer cure of last resort. *The New Yorker* October 19, 1998:34–9.

Hetrick V. Interview by RA Rettig, April 6, 2004a.

Hetrick V. Interview by RA Rettig, December 17, 2004b.

Hortobagyi GN. What is the role of high-dose chemotherapy in the era of targeted therapies? *J Clin Oncology* 2004; 22:2263–66.

Horton R. After Bezwoda. *Lancet* 2000; 355:942–3.

Journal of Clinical Oncology. Retraction. *J Clin Oncol* 2001; 19:2973.

Kennedy MJ. High-dose chemotherapy of breast cancer: is the question answered? *J Clin Oncol* 1995; 13:2477–9.

Kolata G, Eichenwald K. Business thrives on unproven care, leaving science behind. *New York Times* October 3, 1999:A1.

Kolata G, Eichenwald K. Insurer drops a therapy for breast cancer. *New York Times* February 16, 2000:A24.

Lippman ME. High-dose chemotherapy plus autologous bone marrow transplantation for metastatic breast cancer. *N Engl J Med* 2000; 342:1119–20.

Love SM. Interview by RA Rettig, September 1, 2004.

Medical Care Management Corporation Consultants. Express Medical Technology Assessment: High dose chemotherapy with blood stem-cell transplantation for breast cancer. Bethesda, Maryland, September 1999.

Medical Care Ombudsman Program (MCOP) Consultants. Dose-intensive chemotherapy and progenitor cell transplant for breast cancer. Unpublished document prepared by Raymond B. Weiss. June 1999.

National Cancer Institute. Misconduct suspected in South African study. February 4, 2000. Available at http://www.cancer.gov/templates/page_print.aspx?viewid=125CFB5D-3D8F-413B-B49. Accessed October 1, 2002.

National Cancer Institute. Journal retracts fraudulent South African breast cancer study. April 26, 2001. Available at http://www.cancer.gov/templates/page_print.aspx?viewid=38BB4AF9-D97F-4F85-A18A. Accessed October 1, 2002.

National Comprehensive Cancer Network. Update of the NCCN guidelines for treatment of breast cancer. *Oncology* 1997; 11:199–220.

Nieto Y. The verdict is not in yet. Analysis of the randomized trials of high-dose chemotherapy for breast cancer. *Haematologica* 2003; 88:201–11.

Nieto Y, Champlin RE, Wingard JR, et al. Status of high-dose chemotherapy for breast cancer: a review. *Biol Blood Marrow Transplant* 2000; 6:476–95.

Norton L. High-dose chemotherapy for breast cancer: "how do you know?" *J Clin Oncol* 2001; 19:2769–70.

Peters WP, Rosner GL, Vredenburgh JJ, et al. A prospective, randomized comparison of high-dose chemotherapy with stem-cell support versus intermediate-dose chemotherapy after surgery and adjuvant chemotherapy in women with high-risk primary breast cancer: a report of CALGB 9082, SWOG 9114, and NCIC MA-13. *J Clin Oncol.* 2005; 23:2191–2200.

Philipson A. Interview by S Brownlee, November 2000.

Rahman ZU, Frye DK, Buzdar AU, et al. Impact of selection process on response rate and long-term survival of potential high-dose chemotherapy candidates treated with standard-dose doxorubicin-containing chemotherapy in patients with metastatic breast cancer. *J Clin Oncol* 1997; 15:3171–7.

Rahman ZU, Hortobagyi GN, Buzdar AU, Champlin R. High-dose chemotherapy with autologous stem cell support in patients with breast cancer. *Cancer Treat Rev* 1998; 24:249–63.

Rodenhuis S, Bontenbal M, Beex LV, et al. High-dose chemotherapy with hematopoietic stem-cell rescue for high-risk breast cancer. *N Engl J Med* 2003; 349:7–16.

Spector C. Jane Sprague Zones tapped to lead BCA. Breast Cancer Action Newsletter, no. 59. May/June 2000. Available at http://www.bcaction.org/Pages/SearchablePages/2000Newsletters/Newsletter059F.html. Accessed January 25, 2005.

Stadtmauer EA, O'Neill A, Goldstein LJ, et al. Conventional-dose chemotherapy compared with high-dose chemotherapy plus autologous hematopoietic stem-cell transplantation for metastatic breast cancer. Philadelphia Bone Marrow Transplant Group. *N Engl J Med* 2000; 342:1069–76.

Tallman M, Gray R, Robert N, et al. 2003 ASCO Annual Meeting abstract: phase III study of conventional adjuvant chemotherapy with or without high-dose chemotherapy and autologous stem cell transplantation in patients with stage II and III breast cancer at high risk of recurrence (INT 0121). 2003a. Available at http://www.asco.org/asco/publications/abstract_print_view/1,1148,_12–002640–00_18–0023–00_19–00104205,00.html. Accessed January 25, 2005.

Tallman MS, Gray R, Robert NJ, et al. Conventional adjuvant chemotherapy with or without high-dose chemotherapy and autologous stem-cell transplantation in high-risk breast cancer. *N Engl J Med* 2003b; 349:17–26.

Weiss RB. Systems of protocol review, quality assurance, and data audit. *Cancer Chemother Pharmacol* 1998; 42 Suppl:S88–92.

Weiss RB. The randomized trials of dose-intensive therapy for breast cancer: what do they mean for patient care and where do we go from here? *Oncologist* 1999; 4:450–8.

Weiss RB. Interview by RA Rettig, May 14, 2002a.

Weiss RB. Interview by RA Rettig, May 18, 2002b.

Weiss RB. Interview by RA Rettig, October 10, 2002c.

Weiss RB. E-mail to RA Rettig, forwarding e-mail to RB Weiss from Mphengoa Phooko, September 1, 2003.

Weiss RB, Gill GG, Hudis CA. An on-site audit of the South African trial of high-dose chemotherapy for metastatic breast cancer and associated publications. *J Clin Oncol* 2001; 19:2771–7.

Weiss RB, Rifkin RM, Stewart FM, et al. High-dose chemotherapy for high-risk primary breast cancer: an on-site review of the Bezwoda study. *Lancet* 2000; 355:999–1003.

Weiss RB, Vogelzang NJ, Peterson BA, et al. A successful system of scientific data audits for clinical trials. A report from the Cancer and Leukemia Group B. *JAMA* 1993; 270:459–64.

Wright-Browne V, Hortobagyi GN. High-dose chemotherapy for breast cancer: twenty years later. Whom should we treat? And when? *Tumori* 1996; 82:187–92.

Zones JS. What is the price of hope? Breast Cancer Action Newsletter, no. 33, 1995. Available at http://www.bcaction.org/Pages/SearchablePages/1995Newsletters/Newsletter033A.html. Accessed January 25, 2005.

Zones JS. Despite growing use of HDC, many questions remain. Breast Cancer Action Newsletter, No. 50, October/November 1998. Available at http://www.bcaction.org/Pages/SearchablePages/1998Newsletters/Newsletter050A.html. Accessed January 25, 2005.

Zones JS. Preliminary results from NCI show HDC offers little benefit. Breast Cancer Action Newsletter, no. 54, June/July 1999. Available at http://www.bcaction.org/Pages/SearchablePages/1999Newsletters/Newsletter054A.html. Accessed January 25, 2005.

Zones JS. Disappointment and deceit in high-dose chemotherapy trials, Breast Cancer Action Newsletter, no. 59, May/June 2000. Available at http://www.bcaction.org/Pages/SearchablePages/2000Newsletters/Newsletter059A.html. Accessed January 25, 2005.

Chapter 10

Aaron HJ, Gelband H, Institute of Medicine, Committee on Routine Patient Care Costs in Clinical Trials for Medicare Beneficiaries. *Extending Medicare Reimbursement in Clinical Trials.* Washington, DC: National Academy Press, 2000.

Abrams JS. Interview by RA Rettig, May 10, 2002.

American Society of Clinical Oncology. Reimbursement and coverage implications of clinical trials in treatment of cancer: prepared on November 30, 1992, and adopted at the May 16–18, 1993 ASCO meeting, Orlando, Florida. Alexandria, VA: American Society of Clinical Oncology, 1992.

Brownlee S. Health, hope and hype: why the media oversells medical breakthroughs. *Washington Post* August 3, 2003:B1.

Chirikos TN, Ruckdeschel JC, Krischer JP. Impact of clinical trials on the cost of cancer care. *Med Care* 2001; 39:373–83.

Department of Defense/National Cancer Institute. *Interagency Agreement between the Department of Defense and National Cancer Institute for Partnership in Clinical Trials for Cancer.* Washington, DC, March 5, 1996. [Memorandum from Stephen C. Joseph, MD, MPH, Assistant Secretary of Defense (Health Affairs) to Assistant Secretary of the Army (M&RA), Assistant Secretary of the Navy (M&RA), Assistant Secretary of the Air Force (MRAI&E). Subject: DoD participation in clinical cancer trials.]

Department of Veterans Affairs/National Cancer Institute. *Interagency Agreement between the Department of Veterans Affairs and National Cancer Institute for Partnership in Clinical Trials for Cancer.* Washington, DC, Department of Veterans Affairs,1997.

Didion J. *The Year of Magical Thinking.* New York. Alfred A, Knopf. 2005.

Eddy DM. The individual versus society: is there a conflict? In: Eddy DM, ed. *Clinical Decision-Making: From Theory to Practice: A Collection of Essays from JAMA.* Boston: Jones and Bartlett, 1996:102–9.

Fireman BH, Fehrenbacher L, Gruskin EP, Ray GT. Cost of care for patients in cancer clinical trials. *J Natl Cancer Inst* 2000; 92:136–42.

Friedman M. Interview by RA Rettig, May 9, 2002.

Glasziou P. Non-randomized trials that changed medical practice. November 2003. Available at http://www.hsc.usf.edu/~bdjulbeg/oncology/NON-RCT-practice-change.htm. Accessed May 13, 2005.

Gleeson, Susan, memorandum, to plan medical directors, HMO medical directors, re Research-Urgent Treatments, September 28, 1998.

Glick JH. Interview by RA Rettig, March 25, 2002.

Goldberg KB. Medicare to seek coverage advice from NCI, oncologists. *Cancer Lett* June 11, 2004:1–4.

Goldman B. Combinations of targeted therapies take aim at multiple pathways. *J Natl Cancer Inst* 2003a; 95:1656–7.

Goldman B. For investigational targeted drugs, combination trials pose challenges. *J Natl Cancer Inst* 2003b; 95:1744–6.

Goldman DP, Berry SH, McCabe MS, et al. Incremental treatment costs in national cancer institute-sponsored clinical trials. *JAMA* 2003; 289:2970–7.

Grann A, Grann VR. The case for randomized trials in cancer treatment: new is not always better. *JAMA* 2005; 293:1001–3.

Groopman J. *The Anatomy of Hope: How People Prevail in the Face of Illness.* New York: Random House, 2004.

Guyatt G, Rennie D. Evidence-Based Medicine Working Group, American Medical Association. *Users' Guides to the Medical Literature: A Manual for Evidence-Based Clinical Practice.* Chicago: AMA Press, 2002.

Hortobagyi GN. Interview by RA Rettig, July 10, 2002.

Hortobagyi GN. What is the role of high-dose chemotherapy in the era of targeted therapies? *J Clin Oncol* 2004; 22:2263–6.

Horton R. A manifesto for reading medicine. *Lancet* 1997;349:872–74.

International Committee of Medical Journal Editors (ICMJE). Uniform requirements for manuscripts submitted to biomedical journals: writing and editing for biomedical publication. Updated February 2006. Available at http://www.icmje.org/. Accessed July 14, 2006.

Kolata G, Eichenwald K. Group of insurers to pay for experimental cancer therapy. *New York Times* December 16, 1999:C1.

Kroft S. The most promising treatment? Is bone marrow transplant really the answer to curing breast cancer? *60 Minutes* September 26, 1993.

Krueger G. The formation of the American Society of Clinical Oncology and the development of a medical specialty, 1964–1973. *Perspect Biol Med* 2004; 47:537–51.

Morreim EH. From the clinics to the courts: the role evidence should play in litigating medical care. *J Health Polit Policy Law* 2001; 26:409–27.

National Breast Cancer Coalition. Clinical Trials Initiative. 2004a. Available at http://www.stopbreastcancer.org.org/bin/index.asp?strid=98&depid=7. Accessed September 18, 2004.

National Breast Cancer Coalition. Project LEAD. 2004b. Available at http://www.stopbreastcancer.org/bin/index.asp?Strid=483&btnid=4&depid=7. Accessed September 17, 2004.

New Jersey Association of Health Plans. NJAHP says clinical cancer trials agreement establishes precedent for cooperation. January 2000. Available at: http://www.njahp.org/Newsletter/winter2000.html. Accessed December 8, 2004.

Physician Payment Review Commission. Coverage decisions and technology assessment. In Report to Congress, 1994. Washington, DC, Government Printing Office, March 1994:219–36.

Rothman DJ. *Beginnings Count: The Technological Imperative in American Health Care.* New York: Oxford University Press, 1997.

Soares HP, Kumar A, Daniels S, Swann S, Cantor A, Hozo I, Clark M, Serdarevic F, Gwede C, Trotti A, Djulbegovic B. Evaluation of new treatments in radiation oncology: are they better than standard treatments? *JAMA* 2005; 293:970–8.

Strasberg SM, Ludbrook PA. Who oversees innovative practice? Is there a structure that meets the monitoring needs of new techniques? *J Am Coll Surg* 2003; 196:938–48.

Temple R. Commentary on "The Architecture of Government Regulation of Medical Products." *Virginia Law Rev* 1996; 82:1901–2.

Wagner JL, Alberts SR, Sloan JA, et al. Incremental costs of enrolling cancer patients in clinical trials: a population-based study. *J Natl Cancer Inst* 1999; 91:847–53.

Williams M. *The Woman at the Washington Zoo: Writings on Politics, Family, and Fate.* Edited by Timothy Noah. New York, Public Affairs, 2005.

Index

ABMT. *See* bone marrow transplantation; HDC/ABMT
Abrams, Jeffrey S., 223, 233, 241
access versus evaluation, 5, 17, 264, 271, 278
  ability of state governments to weigh, 175
acute leukemia, 22, 25
Adams, Alexandra, 89
Adams v. Blue Cross/Blue Shield of Maryland, Inc.,
  89–90, 105, 303, 309
adjuvant therapy, 18, 24, 25–6, 210
  evaluation of, 184
admissibility of evidence, 77
Adriamycin. *See* doxorubicin
advertising, effect on reporting, 270
Aetna, 11, 191, 274
  external review, 204
  technology assessments, 38, 187–90
  termination of HDC/ABMT coverage for
    breast cancer, 239
Agency for Health Care Policy and Research, 167,
  191, 311
Agency for Healthcare Research and Quality, 130, 287,
  311, 313
AIDS advocacy, 61
  effect on FDA rules, 43
Albert Einstein Cancer Center, 57
alkylating agents, 22
  dose-response relationships, 31
"allogeneic," 98
allogeneic bone marrow transplantation, 25
American Association of Health Plans, 195, 313
American Cancer Society, 59
  support of coverage mandates, 173
American College of Physicians, 182
American Joint Committee on Cancer, 18
American Medical Association, 182, 272
  statements about ABMT, 55
  survey of physician views of HDC/ABMT, 115
  technology assessments, 186–7
American Medical Writers Association, 195
American Oncology Resources, Inc., 140, 148
American Society for Clinical Oncology
  (ASCO), 192
  annual meetings, 236
  influence on HDC/ABMT use, 231–8
  influence on patient enrollment, 219
  position on preliminary data, 235

press release on HDC/ABMT, 58
response to FDA recommendations, 44–5
role in clinical research, 272–3
statement on insurance coverage, 281
statement on South African trial audit, 246
Americans with Disabilities Act of 1993, litigation under
  alleged violation of, 96–7
Amgen, 27, 301, 312
Anderson, Phyllis, 170
anecdotal testimony, role in legislative debates, 171
Anglo Celtic Oncology Group, 229
  results of clinical trial, 250
antibiotics, antitumor, 22
antimetabolites, 22
Antman, Karen, 29–31, 49, 222
  clinical trials conducted, 210
  continued support of HDC/ABMT, 248
  court testimony, 87
  legal impact of studies by, 100, 115–6, 127
  views on funding clinical trials, 40, 48
apheresis, 35
arbitrary and capricious standard, 78, 92–3, 101, 309
  in FEHBP and CHAMPUS cases, 94–5
Aronson, Naomi, 49
ASCO. *See* American Society for Clinical Oncology
Associated Press, article on HDC/ABMT, 64
Atlanta Journal Constitution, article on HDC/ABMT, 65
attorneys. *See also* litigation; litigation strategies
  reactions to outcomes of HDC/ABMT, 252–4
  role of personal experience, 116
  view of HDC/ABMT litigation, 126
Aubry, Wade, 38, 47, 184, 200, 232–4, 302
audits
  importance of, 250–1
  of South African trials, 242–8
Autologous Blood and Marrow Transplant Registry, 7,
  130, 239
  refusal to allow use of data, 194–5
autologous bone marrow transplantation (ABMT).
    See bone marrow transplantation; HDC/ABMT
Aventis Oncology, 278
Avon Foundation, 60

Baber, Pam, 255
bad faith claims, 80–1, 119, 125
  role in litigation, 111–2, 127

343

Bailes, Joseph, 243
Barbara Ann Karmanos Cancer Institute, 312
    press release on CALGB trial results, 237
Bast v. Prudential Insurance Co., 96
Bazell, Robert, article on high-dose
        chemotherapy, 67
BCBSA. *See* Blue Cross Blue Shield Association
*Bechtold v. Physician's Health Plan of Northern
        Indiana, Inc.*, 91
Benefit Trust Life Insurance Company, 91
Berlex Laboratories, 27, 301
Betzner, Arline, 11
Beveridge, Roy, role in South African trial audit, 242
Bezwoda, Werner, 198, 237, 240
    attempt of Peters to recruit, 312
    conduct during audit, 242–4
    firing and hearing, 245
    suspension of medical license, 246
biologic outcomes, versus health outcomes, 50–1
Biotherapeutics, 141
Bishop v. CHAMPUS, 94
Bitran, J. D., 32
Black, Shirley Temple, 59
bladder inflammation, after high-dose chemotherapy, 21
blood cell production, 26
Blue Cross and Blue Shield of Minnesota, 191
Blue Cross and Blue Shield of Missouri, 12
Blue Cross and Blue Shield of Virginia, 11
Blue Cross and Blue Shield Service Benefit Plan,
        response to coverage mandate, 168
Blue Cross Blue Shield Association (BCBSA), 282, 302.
        See also Technology Evaluation Center
    assessments of HDC/ABMT, 182–6, 199–202
    Groch criticism of, 156
    meetings on HDC/ABMT, 49–52
    organization of, 311
    support of clinical trials, 48–9, 204, 208, 274
    technology assessments, 37
Blue Cross of New Jersey, litigation against, 155
Blue Shield of California, 47, 202
Blum, Diane, 62
Blume, Karl, 32
board certification, 272
bone marrow, 25
bone marrow transplantation, 20–1. *See also*
        HDC/ABMT
    allogeneic versus autologous, 25
    contamination, 198
    costs, 34
    development of, 28
    versus peripheral blood stem cell rescue, 147, 149
    requests for coverage, 47
    revenues from, 14
    training, 149–50
    trends for breast cancer patients, 138
bone marrow transplanters, as distinct subspecialty, 261
*Bossemeyer. See Healthcare America Plans, Inc. v.
        Bossemeyer*
Boston Globe, 67
Boston Women's Health Book Collective, 58
Bradley, Bill, 155

Braun, Susan, 234
breach of contract, 80
breach of duty, 76
breast cancer. *See also* metastatic breast cancer; patient
        advocacy groups
    evidence-based reviews of clinical trials, 287–8
    lay guides to, 59
    overview of, 17–20
    perceptions of, 269–70
    probability of developing, 18
    recurrent, 19, 25
    research, 152, 154
    staging, 119, 313
    statistics, 17–8
Breast Cancer Action, 60, 153, 256
    position on release of preliminary data, 234
Breast Cancer International Research Group, 278
breast-conserving surgery, 26
Breast Evaluation Center, 29
Brenner, Barbara, 234
Brinker, Nancy, 60
Broder, Samuel, 45
Brown, Elizabeth, 55, 308
    letter effectively endorsing HDC/ABMT, 186
Brownlee, Shannon, 65, 66
Bucci v. Blue Cross/Blue Shield of Connecticut, 93
Bush, H., 23

Calder, Kim, congressional testimony, 165–6
CALGB, 208, 213
    audit committee, 240
    clinical trial, 209–10, 214, 249
    patient enrollment in trials, 219, 223
    presentation of trial at ASCO meeting, 237
    release of preliminary data, 233
California
    coverage of HDC/ABMT, 202–4
    support of external review, 190
California Public Employees' Retirement System,
        202–4
California Women's Health Council, 203
CanAct, 60
Cancer and Leukemia Group B. *See* CALGB
Cancer Care, Inc., 62
    congressional testimony, 165
cancer deaths. *See* mortality
Cancer Letter, coverage of preliminary trial data, 233
cancer treatment and care
    capitating, 139
    financial incentives, 28
cancer treatment centers
    marketing, 141
    role in development of clinical oncology, 28
Candlelighters, 189
Canellos, G. P., 22, 25
Caplan, Arthur, 311
cardiac events, after high-dose chemotherapy, 21
case studies, value of, 4
Case Western Reserve University, 57
Caudill v. Blue Cross & Blue Shield of North Carolina,
        94

Center for International Blood and Marrow Transplant
    Research, 130, 310
Centers for Medicare and Medicaid Services, 39, 282.
    See also Health Care Financing Administration
Chamberlin, Thomas C., 4
Champlin, Richard, congressional testimony, 163
CHAMPUS
    arbitrary and capricious standards, 94–5
    judgment against, 305
chemotherapy. *See also* high-dose chemotherapy
    adjuvant, 25–6
    combination, 21–2
    costs of, 48, 136
    drugs and regimens, 23
    evaluation of drugs, 42
    physiological effects, 21
Cheson, Bruce, 149
    congressional testimony, 159–61, 164
    response to OPM coverage mandate, 167
    review of HDC/ABMT studies, 207–8
cisplatin, 29
City of Hope, phase 2 studies at, 32
Civilian Health and Medical Program for the Uniformed
    Services. *See* CHAMPUS
Civil Rights Act of 1964, litigation under alleged
    violation of, 96
Cleaton-Jones, Peter, 246, 247
Clinical Efficacy Assessment Project, 182
clinical practice guidelines, 191–2
clinical trials. *See also* randomized clinical trials
    costs, 302
    definition of, 167
    drop out, 219
    effect of litigation on, 206–7, 222
    funding. *See* funding
    gender inequities in, 61
    insurers' reliance on, 106
    lack of randomization, 147
    outcome bias, 215
    problems of, 51, 256
    relation to treatment, 39
Clinical Trials Initiative, 277–8
Clinton health plan, 152
Coates, Vivian, 195
Cochrane Collaboration, 287
cognitive impairment
    from high-dose chemotherapy, 255, 256
    statistics, 288
Coiffier, Bertrand, 226
Coleman, Sharon, 32
colony stimulating factors. *See* human growth factors
Common Diagnostic Tests: Use and Interpretation,
    182
Common Screening Tests, 182
communication
    improving, 225
    insurer-patient, 105
    physician-patient, 110, 215–6
Community Cooperative Oncology Program, 147
complete response, 302
computed tomography, 37

conflict management, institutionalized, 266, 270–1,
    278–83
conflict of interest, 307
congestive heart failure, 291
Connell, Kathleen, 202
consensus conferences. *See* NIH consensus conferences
contract language, 157, 309
    ambiguity in, 80, 89–92, 98–9, 106–7, 110–1, 126, 307
    interpretation, 79–80
    marketing and, 307
    understanding of, 81, 110
contract law, 79
contra proferentem, 80
cooperative cancer groups, formation and list of, 213
Cooper regimen, 22, 23
cost containment, 38–9, 125–6, 172
costs, 17, 117, 149, 188
    considered in clinical trials, 214
    of coverage mandates, 166
    role in court decisions, 81
Council on Health Care Technology, 181
courts. *See also* litigation
    authority of federal, 305
    deference to medical professionals, 76–7
    handling of scientific evidence, 87–9, 100, 115–6, 127,
        303
    inadequacy as evaluators, 266–7
    role in social policy, 73
Cova, John, 190
coverage mandates, 16, 66, 94, 107, 152, 268
    comparisons, 176–7
    costs of, 166
    effect on clinical trials, 164, 194, 207
    ERISA, 77
cross-examination, difficulties for defense, 113, 116
cross-subsidies, 48
Crown, John, 229, 250
Culp, Guterson, and Grader, 56
Current Procedural Terminology, 20
customary practice, 76
cyclophosphamide, 22, 29

Dahl-Eimers v. Mutual of Omaha Life of Insurance Co.,
    95
damages
    bad faith judgments and level of, 111
    limitations on, 96, 303
    punitive, 80, 106, 111, 222
Dana-Farber Cancer Institute, 28
    phase 2 studies at, 32
Dansey, Roger, 199, 312
    role in South African trial audit, 247
data safety monitoring committees, 233
Davidson, Nancy, 52
Davis, Angela, 12
demand for treatment. *See* patient demand
deMeurs, Christine, 12–3
de novo standard, 78, 92–3, 101
Department of Defense
    agreements to conduct clinical trials, 280
    breast cancer research, 62

Department of Veterans Affairs, agreements to conduct clinical trials, 280
depression, 21
desperation, patient, role in litigation, 105, 313
DeVita, Vincent, 24
    legitimation of HDC/ABMT, 55
Diagnostic and Therapeutic Technology Assessment program, 55, 186–7
dialysis, 37
Dickersin, Kay, 152–3
Didion, Joan, 285
Dienst, Ricki, 153
disease-free survival, 210, 214, 296
    data from CALGB trial, 237
    data from European trials, 227–8
    ECRI conclusions, 193
    statistics for breast cancer, 288, 291
distant-stage tumors, definition of, 18
diversity jurisdiction, 305
Doctor's Group, 58
Dodd v. Blue Cross & Blue Shield Association, 96
Dorr, Andrew, 208
dose-response relationship, 31, 185
    debates about, 22–4
doxorubicin, 22, 301
"Dream Team" document, 55–6, 249
    impact on use of HDC/ABMT, 251
drugs
    approval of chemotherapy, 147
    development and clinical trials, 42
    investigational new, 43, 44, 262
    off-label use, 20
    recognition of new, 46
    tests of combinations, 276
Duckwitz v. General American Life Insurance Co., 101
Duke University
    Bone Marrow Transplant Program, 26
    CALGB trial, 209
    phase 2 studies at, 32
Dutch Health Insurance Council, 227

ECOG (Eastern Cooperative Oncology Group), 208, 213
    randomized clinical trial, 209–10, 249
ECRI, 38, 204, 273, 311
    assessment of HDC/ABMT, 136, 174, 223, 239, 256
    meeting to share HDC/ABMT assessment, 195
    patient information brochure, 195, 275
    technology assessments, 192–5
Eddy, David, 50, 208, 214
    development of criteria for technology assessments, 183
    paper in *Journal of Clinical Oncology* (1992), 82
    op-ed in *New York Times*, 238
education. *See also* public information
    physician, 272
    to promote clinical trials, 225
effectiveness. *See* treatment effectiveness
Eichenwald, Kurt, 250
Elias, Anthony, 312
Emergency Care Research Institute. *See* ECRI

emerging technologies. *See also* experimental procedures
    cost-effectiveness, 181
    coverage exclusion, 123
    payment for, 284
Emory University, 56
emotion, 260
    role in legislative debates, 173, 175
    role in litigation strategies, 117–8
Empire Blue Cross and Blue Shield, 150
Employee Retirement Income Security Act. *See* ERISA
endpoints
    debate about appropriate, 52
    of randomized clinical trials, 208
    surrogate, 44, 45, 46
equipoise, 215–6, 312
    determining, 278
ERISA, 303, 309
    damages under, 112
    preemption provisions, 77–9, 95–6
    standards of review, 92–3
ethical issues, in randomized clinical trials, 212
Europe, randomized clinical trials of HDC/ABMT, 226–30
evaluation, 259–60. *See also* technology assessments
    consideration of need for, 177
    inadequacy of courts in, 266
evidence, admissibility of, 77
Evidence-based Discussion Group, 262
evidence-based medicine, 283–5
Evidence-based Practice Centers, 192, 287, 313
evidence of harm, ECRI conclusions, 193
exclusionary provisions, 36, 38, 40, 110–1, 157
    difficulties in, 123
    effect of mandates, 166
    litigation and, 90–2, 98–9, 106–7
"experimental"
    definitions of, 107, 157
    use in insurance contracts, 98, 99
experimental procedures, 12–3
    evaluating, 42–6
    motivations for pursuing, 14
    recognition of, 46–8
    subjects of, 27
    as treatment, 39
expert testimony, 87–9, 100, 112–3, 120, 303
    qualifications of witness, 99
    reliance on, 280
    reluctance of witnesses, 116
    researchers versus clinicians, 90, 171
external grievance processes, 112
    as response to *Fox* verdict, 120
external review, 125, 204, 274, 280, 309
    at Aetna, 188–9

false hope, 285–6
fatigue, 21, 291
federal deficit, 38–9
Federal Employees Health Benefits Program. *See* FEHBP
Federal Food and Drug Cosmetic Act, 181

federal government
  budgetary constraints, 281
  role in HDC/ABMT saga, 16, 268
fee-for-service, 36, 82
  relation to patient enrollment, 231
FEHBP, 268
  arbitrary and capricious standards, 94–5
  coverage mandates, 152, 155–9, 166–7, 311
feminism, 59
  role in coverage mandates, 166, 171, 173–6, 311
  role in HDC/ABMT saga, 4, 17, 268, 270
Filgrastin, 301
financial incentives
  conflict of interest and, 307
  to perform medical procedures, 14
  role in use of HDC/ABMT, 117, 138, 150–2, 263, 267, 281
5-fluorouracil, 22
Flatley, Sherry, 155
Flynn, Ed, 167
Food and Drug Administration, 261
  accelerated approval regulations, 45
  approval of human growth factors, 27
  authority to regulate medical devices, 181
  avoidance of regulation by, 141, 147
  investigational new drug regulations, 43–4
  possible role in evaluation of medical procedures, 276
  purview of, 5, 20
Ford, Betty, 59
Forum on Emerging Treatments for Breast Cancer, 208–9
Fox, Nelene, 74, 78
Fox Chase Cancer Center, 214
Fox v. HealthNet, 74, 103, 196, 307, 308
  claim of coverage inconsistency, 111
  effect on subsequent litigation, 83, 119–21, 239
  impact on settlements, 114
  role of sympathy, 118
France, randomized clinical trials, 238
Francine Klopert v. Los Angeles Unified School District, 185
Fred Hutchinson Cancer Center, 28
Freeman, Walter, 269
Frei, Emil (Tom) III, 22, 28–9, 31
  views on funding clinical trials, 40
Frendreis v. Blue Cross Blue Shield of Michigan, 95
Friedman, Michael, 50, 208
  comments on randomized clinical trials, 265
  proposal for patient care costs, 190
Friedman-Knowles Act, 190
Frye v. United States, 303
Fuja, Grace, 91
Fuja v. Benefit Trust Life Insurance Co., 304
funding
  breast cancer research, 61–2, 154
  clinical trials, 40–1, 48, 123, 211, 213, 273, 275
  public, 280–1
  research, 28
  in U.S. vs. Europe, 231

Gale, Robert, 139
Gaus, Clifton R., 167

Gelman, Rebecca, 24, 210
Genentech, 278
general reporters, coverage of medical stories, 67
Gentry, Carol, 66, 67
Germany, patient enrollment in clinical trials, 230
Gill, Geraldine, role in South African trial audit, 247
Glaspy, John, 13, 32
Gleeson, Sue, 48, 183
Glick, John, 216, 237, 265
Grady, Denise, 236
Grant, Anne, 254, 255
granulocyte colony-stimulating factor (G-CSF), 26, 301
granulocyte-macrophage colony-stimulating factor
      (GM-CSF), 26, 301
Green, Sharon, 152–3
Groch, Arlene Gilbert, 155–6
  congressional testimony, 166
Groopman, Jerome, 254, 285
Group Health, Inc., 191
Group Health Association of America, 167
Group Health Cooperative of Puget Sound, 38
Grow, Doug, 195
growth factors. *See* human growth factors
Gulf Health, Inc., 86

H. Lee Moffit Cancer Center and Research Institute, 56
Hackensack Medical Center, 217
Hahnemann University, 214
Halsted radical mastectomy, 16, 54, 224
Haney, Daniel, 64
Harkin, Tom, 62, 154
harm, evidence of, 193
Harris v. Mutual of Omaha Co., 94, 102, 302
Hatch, Mike, 169, 195
Hawkins v. Mail Handlers Benefit Plan, 305
Hayes, Daniel, 24
HDC/ABMT
  application by cancer stage, 27, 311
  assessments of. *See* technology assessments
  availability, 128, 206, 216–7, 226, 250, 263
  BCBSA meetings on, 49–52
  clinical trials. *See* clinical trials; randomized clinical
      trials
  conditions typically treated with, 310
  costs, 34, 48, 117, 136–7, 188, 191
  coverage of. *See* coverage mandates; insurance
      coverage
  decline in use, 237, 239
  description and overview, 5, 20
  drivers of use, 16, 58–69, 251, 256
  effectiveness. *See* treatment effectiveness
  financial incentives for providing. *See* financial
      incentives
  history of, 256
  legitimation by oncologists, 55–8
  means of discrediting, 106
  number of stories published about, 68
  pain and suffering associated with, 254–5
  patient knowledge of, 110
  payer data, 136–7
  pioneering work on, 33–4

HDC/ABMT (*continued*)
  portrayal of, 114, 171
  providers of, 139–51
  response of advocacy groups to, 62–4
  scientific debates, 197–9
  statistics, 3, 131–6, 207
  stories of individual outcomes, 251–5
  in terminally ill patients, 16
  use, 3, 35, 109, 111–2, 127, 129–30, 137–8, 222
HDCAMS (high-dose chemotherapy with autologous
      marrow support), 29
health care
  costs, 36, 38–9, 284
  effect of new medical technologies on, 37
  public perception of, 106
Healthcare America Plans, Inc. v. Bossemeyer, 90, 128
  role of contract language in outcome, 98–9
Healthcare Cost and Utilization Project, 130
Health Care Financing Administration, 39
Health Care Utilization Project database, 7
Health Insurance Association of America, 190
health maintenance organizations. *See also* managed care
      coverage of HDC/ABMT, 191
HealthNet, 12–4, 74. *See also Fox v. HealthNet*
health outcomes
  judgment of effectiveness and, 50–1
  lack of data on, 51–2, 188
  measurement in clinical trials, 214
Health Technology Advisory Committee, 174
Hellman, Samuel, 45
hematologists, role in cancer treatment, 28
Henderson, I. Craig, 37, 50, 150, 199, 209, 222, 224
  article in *Important Advances in Oncology*, 197
  congressional testimony, 158, 162
  criticism of dose-response claims, 24
  op-ed in *New York Times*, 238
  organization of Breast Evaluation Center, 29
Henderson, Karen, 97
Henderson v. Bodine Aluminum, Inc., 97
Herberman, Ronald B., 90
Herceptin trials, 278
Herman, Alan, role in South African trial audit, 242, 244
Hetrick, Virginia, 251–2
Hiepler, Mark, 13
high-dose chemotherapy. *See also* HDC/ABMT
  development and use of, 22–4
  long-term side effects, 255
  maximum tolerable dose, 31
  national market for, 146
  statistics, 132–4
  toxicity of, 21, 32, 291
high-dose chemotherapy with autologous bone marrow
      transplantation. *See* HDC/AMBT
HMO Group, 311
Hodgkin's disease, 22
Holder v. Prudential Insurance Co., 88–9
Holland, James, 29, 55
hormonal therapy, 19
Horowitz, Mary, 194–5, 199
Hortobagyi, Gabriel, 216, 223, 263
  comments on randomized clinical trials, 265
  suggestion of patient selection bias, 240
  views on HDC/ABMT, 248
Horton, Richard, 269
hospital charges, for HDC/ABMT, 34, 136
Hryniuk, W., 23, 24
Hudis, Clifford, role in South African trial audit, 247
Hughes, Bill, 155
human growth factors, 26–8, 214, 301
hypotheses, multiple working, 4

Ignagni, Karen, 167
Immunex, 27, 301, 312
IMPACT centers. *See* Response Oncology
induction chemotherapy, 209
industry custom, 302
infertility, after high-dose chemotherapy, 21
informed consent, 92, 215–6, 224, 283, 307
  role in litigation, 88–9, 100, 106, 110–1, 120, 127
initial conditions, importance of, 260, 261
injunctions, 13, 78, 83
  against Blue Shield of California, 185
  role of sympathy in hearings for, 117
inpatient treatment, 136
Institute for Clinical Systems Integration, 38
  HDC/ABMT assessments, 190–1
  response to Blue Cross policy changes, 202
Institute of Medicine, 181
insurance coverage. *See also* coverage mandates;
      exclusionary provisions .
  of bone marrow transplantation, 47
  congressional hearings, 158–68
  denials, 11–2, 89, 184
  challenges to, 36, 47–8. *See also* litigation
    effect of, 188
    interpretation of, 17
    under OPM, 94
    response to, 206
  external review. *See* external review
  factors in determinations, 75
  inconsistencies, 111, 115, 118, 120, 127, 307
  of investigational drugs, 44
  of patient care costs, 40, 185, 279
  withdrawal of, 239
insurance industry
  advocacy groups and, 66–7
  arrogance of, 105
  effect of mandates on premiums, 166
  lack of voice in media, 311
  legal defense of. *See* litigation strategies
  medical directors, 120, 308
  medicine and, 36–8, 45, 57
  perception of, 66, 171, 173, 175
  plan administrators, 93
  protection from liability, 77, 279
  response to new treatments, 36, 47
  response to randomized clinical trials, 48–9
  role in clinical trials, 41, 114
  role in institutionalized conflict management, 273–5
  technology assessments by. *See* technology
      assessments
  view of HDC/ABMT, 119, 172

intergroup trials, 209–10
  patient enrollment, 219, 223
  publication of final results, 249
International Bone Marrow Transplant Registry, 310
international trials, 226–31
  results of, 250
interstitial pneumonitis, 21
interviews, 6, 104
invasive breast cancer, 18
"investigational," definition, 107, 157, 186, 308
Investigational New Drug
  applications, 42, 262
  approval and coverage of, 44
  oncology protocols registered as, 147, 148
  treatment rule, 43
investigational treatments. *See* experimental procedures

James Graham Brown Cancer Center, 57
Japan, results of HDC/ABMT clinical trial, 229
Jenkins v. Blue Cross Blue Shield of Michigan, 88
Johns Hopkins University, phase 2 studies at, 32
Jones, Roy, 49, 150, 156, 157, 159, 194, 223, 310
  congressional testimony, 162–3
  involvement in deMeurs case, 13
Jordan, Mark, 167
journalism. *See also* medical reporting
  education, 270
  effect of women in, 66
Journal of Clinical Oncology, 52, 198
  Eddy review of literature, 82
  Henderson critique of Hryniuk study, 24
  publication of findings of first South African trial
    audit, 247–8
  reaction to Bezwoda fraud, 272
Journal of the National Cancer Institute, review of
    HDC/ABMT literature, 231–2
judicial bias, 123

Kahn, Hyman, 53, 210–1
Kaiser Permanente, 38, 167
Kelahan, Andrew, 49
Kennedy, M. John, 32, 198
kidney transplants, 37
Kiernan, Laura, 67
Killian v. Healthsource Provident Administrators, 93
King, James B., 163, 164
Klausner, Richard, 232
Kolata, Gina, 65, 66, 222, 250
Kulakowski v. Rochester Hospital Service Corp., 88, 93
Kushner, Rose, 59

Lambert, Betsy, 153
The Lancet, publication of South African trial audit, 245
Langer, Amy, 60, 61, 62, 63, 166
Larson, Erik, 12
Lasagna, Louis, 43
Lautenberg, Frank, 155
law, versus science, 124–5
Lazarus, Hillard, 32
Leff, Lisa, 65
legislators, response to science, 173

Lerner, Jeff, 193, 195, 223
letters of support, use in court, 115
letter-writing campaigns, 61
Leukine, 27
Levine, M. N., 24
liability, establishing, 75–7
Lichter, Allen S., 231, 233
life-threatening illnesses, use of investigational drugs
    against, 43
Lippman, Marc, 55, 249
litigation. *See also* courts; *specific cases*
  under alleged statute violations, 96–7
  avoiding, 125
  effect of managed care on, 77
  effect on clinical trials, 206–7, 222
  effect on legislative mandates, 170
  effect on use of HDC/ABMT, 16
  factors in health care, 81–2
  individualism of, 266
  outcomes, 84–5, 267
    factors affecting, 100–2, 126–8
  protection of insurers from, 77, 279
  role of contract language, 98–9
  role of expert testimony, 99–100
  role of standard of care, 121–2
  under state laws, 95–6
  trends in, 83–4
litigation strategies, 103
  analysis of, 119–21
  arousing sympathy, 117–8, 308
  bad faith focus, 111–2
  contract focus, 106–7
  defense, 103, 105–6, 122–3
  difficulties faced, 113, 116
  expert witness focus, 112–3
  informed consent focus, 110–1
  plaintiff, 103, 105
  presentation of science, 114
  role of quality of life, 118–9
  standard of care focus, 107–10
  treatment costs focus, 117
Livingston, Robert, 210
locality rule, 76
local recurrence, 19
local-stage tumors, definition of, 18
Long, Dee, 169
Loupe, Diane, 65
Love, Susan, 59, 60, 61, 150, 152–3

magnetic resonance imaging, 37
male bias, in medicine, 17, 59, 96, 155
MAMM, 255
managed care, 4, 75
  effect on health care litigation, 77
  in late 1980s, 82
  in Minnesota, 170
  perception of, 17, 105, 118, 120, 307, 309
  relation to patient enrollment, 231
mandatory reporting, 129
marketing, contract language and, 107, 307
Mashburn v. Mail Handlers Benefit Plan, 94

mastectomy. *See* radical mastectomy
maximum tolerable dose, 31
Mayo Clinic, 170, 171, 214
    involvement in clinical trials, 213
McCabe, Mary, 49
    proposal for patient care costs, 190
McClellan, Mark, 282
McGivney, William, 38, 187–90, 282
McGrory, Brian, 67
MCOP. *See* Medical Care Ombudsman Program
M. D. Anderson Cancer Center, 28, 32
MedCenters Health Plans, 191
media
    effect on legislative mandates, 170
    portrayal of insurers, 12, 311
    role in HDC/ABMT saga, 64–9, 268–70
Medica, 191
medical billing, 47
Medical Care Management Corporation, review of
    randomized trials, 241
Medical Care Ombudsman Program, 188–90, 204,
    274, 311
    Weiss's role in, 241
medical directors
    reliance on, 120
    testimony of, 308
medical entrepreneurs, testimony of, 124
medical innovations. *See also* experimental procedures
    conflicts surrounding, 260
medical interventions, terms for, 20
medical necessity, 36, 38, 75, 304
    definition of, 91, 309
    determinations and scientific literature, 47
medical procedures
    evaluation of, 5–6, 264, 283
    exploitation of, 14, 16
    lack of oversight, 261
medical profession. *See also* oncology community
    deference to, 76–7, 269
    definition of subspecialties, 312
    role in HDC/ABMT saga, 256
    role in institutionalized conflict management, 271–3
    role in setting standard of care, 76
    scientific controversy in, 108
    weakness of self-regulation, 272, 273
medical reporting, 65–6, 269–70. *See also* journalism
    failures of, 67
Medicare, 36, 302
    coverage of patient care costs, 231, 281
    prospective payment under, 39
    relation to National Center for Health Care
        Technology, 181
medicine
    as a business, 270
    insurance and, 36–8, 45, 57
Memorial Sloan-Kettering, 28, 150
menopause, premature after high-dose chemotherapy, 21
meta-analysis, 301
metastatic breast cancer
    combination chemotherapy for, 22
    disease-free survival, 214

evidence-based reviews of clinical trials, 288–91
    treatment with HDC/ABMT, 27
methodology issues, of randomized clinical trials, 212
methotrexate, 22
micrometastases, 198
Minnesota
    coverage mandates, 195
        background, 169–70
        effort to repeal, 174–5, 311
        legislative debates, 171–4
    technology assessment in, 190
Minnesota Medical Association, 174
Monaco, Grace, 189, 311
mortality. *See also* overall survival; treatment-related
        mortality
    rates for breast cancer, 17
multiple working hypotheses, 4
Murray, Joseph E., 301
myelodysplastic syndrome, 228
Myers, Lucretia F., 167

National Academy of Sciences, 181
National Alliance of Breast Cancer Organizations, 60
    absence at congressional hearings, 166
    relation with media, 64
    stance toward HDC/ABMT, 62–3
National Breast Cancer Coalition, 60, 61, 277
    absence at congressional hearings, 166
    attendance at ECRI meeting, 195
    discussions of insurance coverage, 152–3
    meeting with President Clinton, 154
    response to Blue Cross policy changes, 202
    stance toward HDC/ABMT, 63
    statement on clinical trial preliminary data, 236
National Cancer Act of 1971, 28
National Cancer Institute
    appropriations, 39
    determination of "promising treatments," 188
    position on convening clinical trials of HDC/ABMT,
        50
    position on HDC/ABMT, 160
    proposal for patient care costs, 190
    public financing of clinical trials, 280–1
    "Questions and Answers" document, 234–5
    release of negative trial results, 232–4
    response to charges of gender inequities, 61
    response to OPM coverage mandate, 167
    role in institutionalized conflict management, 275–7
    sponsorship of randomized clinical trials, 208
    system of clinical trail support, 53
National Cancer Institute of Canada Clinical Trials
        Group, 214
National Center for Health Care Technology, 181
National Center for Health Services Research,
        181, 182
National Committee to Review Current Procedures for
        Approval of New Drugs for Cancer and AIDS,
        43–4
National Comprehensive Cancer Network, 192
    response to Blue Cross policy changes, 202
    statement on HDC/ABMT for breast cancer, 239

National Institutes of Health. *See* NIH consensus
    conferences; *see also* National Cancer Institute
National Mammography Day, 154
National Marrow Donor Program, 310
National Women's Health Network
    attendance at ECRI meeting, 195
    creation of, 59
    opposition to HDC/ABMT coverage in California, 203
    stance on HDC/ABMT, 158
Nationwide Inpatient Sample, 130
NBC Nightly News, report of preliminary trial data, 232
NCI. *See* National Cancer Institute
negligence, 76–7
neoadjuvant therapy, 19, 27, 301
Netherlands, randomized clinical trials, 240, 250
Neupogen, 27
Newcomer, Lee, 194
New Drug Application, 42
New Jersey Association of Health Plans, 282
The New Republic, article on high-dose chemotherapy,
    67
New York Medical College, 57
New York Times
    1990 article on HDC/ABMT, 64
    coverage of frontal lobotomy procedure, 269
    coverage of HDC/ABMT clinical trials, 222,
    236, 250
Nichols v. Trustmark Insurance Co., 95
Nieto, Yago, views on HDC/ABMT, 248–9
NIH consensus conferences, 26, 37, 181, 301
NIS data, limitations of, 137
no-fault liability, 302
non-doxorubicin regimens, 19
non-Hodgkin's lymphoma, 22
noninvasive breast cancer, 18
North Western National Life, 191
Northwestern University Medical School, 210
Norton, Eleanor Holmes, 158–64
Norton, Larry, 248, 250

occult cancers, 25
Office of Cancer Communication, 225
Office of Personnel Management (OPM), 155, 268
    authority over FEHBP and CHAMPUS health plans,
    94
    contracts with insurers, 156–7
    coverage mandates, 152, 163–8, 222
    ECRI report and, 195
    outcome of court cases involving, 99
Office of Technology Assessment, 181
Office on Women's Health Research, 59
off-label drug use, 20
off-protocol treatment, 216–7, 224, 230. *See also*
    HDC/ABMT, availability
Ohio State University, 56
Oldham, Robert, 141
oncology
    as a business, 267
    emergence of clinical, 28
    regulation of practice, 260
    rise of for-profit, 139–40

oncology community
    court testimony, 309
    hostility toward insurers, 45, 57
    legitimation of HDC/ABMT, 16, 55–8, 263, 272
    marketing of HDC/ABMT, 207
    relation with Food and Drug Administration, 276
    Response Oncology and, 148
OPM. *See* Office of Personnel Management
opportunistic infections, 21
organ transplantation, 301
O'Rourke v. Access Health, Inc., 95
Our Bodies Ourselves, 58
outpatient treatment, 136, 141, 147, 189
    development of, 139
overall survival, 51, 214
    data from CALGB trial, 237
    data from European trials, 227, 228, 229
    data from Philadelphia trial, 236
    ECRI conclusions, 193
    effect of approved drugs on, 44
    lack of data on, 34
    reported in South African study, 238
    statistics for breast cancer, 288, 291
Oxford Group, 287

Pacific Presbyterian, phase 2 studies at, 32
Park, Ed, 139
partial response, 31, 32, 302
patient advocacy groups, 59–61, 263
    effect on insurance coverage, 66–7
    relationship with media, 64
    response to HDC/ABMT, 62–4
    role in coverage mandates, 176
    role in institutionalized conflict management, 277–8
patient care costs, in clinical trials, 185, 278, 281
    Medicare coverage, 231
    NCI proposal, 190
patient choice, 153, 171
    role in litigation, 105, 120
patient demand
    advocacy groups and, 63
    for early access to drugs, 43
    role in HDC/ABMT saga, 17, 49, 260, 263–4
patient enrollment, in clinical trials, 216, 235
    challenges of, 54, 217–21
    considerations, 215–6
    effect of standard of care on, 263
    factors complicating, 206
    refusal rates, 230–1
    selection bias, 136, 224, 240, 262
    strategies to increase, 223–5
    in U.S. vs. European trials, 230–1
patient information, 195, 225. *See also* public
    information
"Patient Reference Guide to HDC/ABMT," 195
patients
    consideration of needs, 265
    protection of, 16–17
    as trial witnesses, 118
    understanding of treatments, 224
Pearson, Cynthia, 158

Pecora, Andrew, 217, 222
peer review, 309
peripheral blood stem cell rescue, 20
   costs, 147, 149
   at Response Oncology, 141
peripheral neuropathy, 291
personal experiences, role in legislative response, 268
Peters, William, 29–31, 157
   article in *Important Advances in Oncology*, 196–8
   attempted recruitment of Bezwoda, 312
   CALGB trials, 209, 214, 237, 249
   Capitol Hill luncheon, 154
   comment on Blue Cross Blue Shield coverage
      changes, 202
   court citation of research by, 100, 115–6, 127
   court testimony, 87
   deference to, 269, 272
   legitimation of HDC/ABMT, 55
   pioneering use of HDC/ABMT, 33
   role in South African trial audit, 242
   studies of human growth factors, 26–7
   views of clinical trials, 54
pharmaceutical industry
   effect of advertising on media, 270
   funding clinical research, 40
phase 1 studies, of drugs, 42
phase 2 studies, 30–4, 217
   of drugs, 42
   inconclusiveness of, 249
   relation to randomized clinical trials, 164, 224
   results of, 207
   transition to randomized clinical trials, 262, 274, 275
phase 3 studies. *See* randomized clinical trials
Philadelphia trial, 210–1, 214
   effect of results, 237
   funding, 274
   initiation of, 53
   patient enrollment, 217, 223
   presentation at ASCO meeting, 236
   publication of final results, 249
Philip, Thierry, 226
Philipson, Alice, 252
physical and functional measures, statistics, 288
physician fees, 34, 139
physician-patient relationship, 14
   communication, 110, 215–6
   damages based on interference, 13
   role in litigation strategy, 105
Physician Payment Review Commission, 282
Physician Reliance Network, Inc., 140
physicians. *See also* physician-patient relationship
   academic, 116
   court testimony, 112–3, 303
   demand for coverage of HDC/ABMT, 49
   education and training, 149–50, 272
   enthusiasm for treatments, 260, 263
   ethical conflicts, 215–6
   getting information to, 195
   influence of recommendations, 105, 111, 231, 263,
      271
   presentation by media, 65

reimbursement, 216, 231
   relationship with insurers, 48, 112, 261, 262, 308
   treating, bias in favor of, 123
   view of randomized clinical trials, 54
Physicians Reliance Network, 148
Pirozzi, Pamela, 11, 87
Pirozzi v. Blue Cross-Blue Shield of Virginia, 87, 88, 89,
      92, 128, 307
policy implications, weight in court decisions, 101
political activism, 58–9, 260
political reporters, coverage of HDC/ABMT saga, 67
politics
   overriding science, 177
   role in coverage mandates, 170, 172, 174
postmarketing evaluation studies, 42
precedent, role in court decisions, 100–1
prednisone, 22
preponderance of evidence standard, 302
President's Cancer Panel, 155
PRN Research, 140
procedure codes, 5, 47
products liability law, 302
Project LEAD, 277
"promising treatments," Aetna's handling of, 187–8
protocols, 312
   individually tailored, 147
   violation, 219
public information
   from clinical trials, 284
   importance of, 274–6
   providing, 280
public perception, of healthcare, 106
public relations, role in coverage mandates, 173
pulmonary fibrosis, 291
punitive damages, 80
   bad faith and, 111
   effect on clinical trials, 222
   strength of case and, 106

quality of life, 51
   after high-dose chemotherapy, 255
   assessments and approval of new drugs, 44
   insurers' consideration of, 106
   measurement in clinical trials, 214
   role in litigation, 118–9, 127
   statistics for metastatic breast cancer, 288, 291

Race for a Cure, 60
Radiation Therapy Oncology Group, 260
radiation treatments, review of, 260–1
radical mastectomy, 16, 18, 26
radiologists, role in cancer treatment, 28
randomization, 312
   importance of, 262
   time required, 216
randomized clinical trials, 3, 16, 27, 206
   audits of, 241–8
   barriers to support, 225
   BCBSA support of, 49–52, 185
   characteristics, 212
   comparison and interpretation, 210, 214–5

congressional testimony, 160–1
costs, 275
criteria for, 262
of drugs, 42
effect of coverage mandates on, 164, 194
effect of treatment availability on, 206, 216–7, 226,
    250, 263
endpoints, 214–5
funding, 123, 211, 213. *See also* funding
initiation of, 208
limited commitment to, 55
in Minnesota, 191
motivations to participate in, 54
need for, 51, 53–4, 207
organization of, 213–4
relation to phase 2 studies, 30, 224, 262, 274, 275
response of insurers to, 48–9, 114
standard of care and, 122
Reach to Recovery program, 59
realism, 285
reasonableness, 76–7
recurrent breast cancer, 19, 25
Reger v. Espy, 96
regional-stage tumors, definition of, 18
registry data, 273
Regramostim, 301
Rehabilitation Act of 1973, litigation under alleged
    violations of, 96
remission rates, with combination chemotherapy, 22
reporting systems, 130
research
    funding, 28, 39, 61–2
    gender inequities, 59
    role of advocacy groups, 61
    translation to clinical practice, 148
    value of, 39
researchers, testimony of, 171
residency programs, 272
resistance, to chemotherapy, 21
respectable minority rule, 76, 108
response duration, ECRI conclusions, 193–4
Response Oncology, 136, 160, 163, 267, 310
    clinical trials, 217
    effect on outpatient treatment, 189
    establishment and development, 140–1
    position with insurers, 148
    revenues, 141, 147–7, 239
    treatment centers, 143–6
Response Technologies, Inc. *See* Response Oncology
revenues
    of American Oncology Resources, 140
    from bone marrow transplantation, 14
    revenue-cost differential, 138
    at not-for-profit medical centers, 150
    of Physician Reliance Network, Inc., 140
    of Response Oncology, 141, 146–7
risk-benefit decisions, 264–5
Robert, Nicholas J., 209
Robertson, Diane, 195
Rockefeller, Happy, 59
Rodenhuis, Sjoerd, 227, 250

Rogers, Paul, 311
Rose Kushner Award, 195
Rosen, Peter, 32
Rosenthal, Elizabeth, 64–5, 66
Rosner, Gary, 55
Ruzek, Sheryl, 195–6

Salick, Bernard, 139
Salick Health Care, 139–40, 150
Saral, Rein, 58
Sargramostim, 301
Scalamandre v. Oxford Health Plans, Inc., 92
Scandinavia, clinical trials of HDC/ABMT, 227–8
Schnipper, Lowell, 40
Schroeder, Patricia, 157–9, 165
science
    versus law, 124–5
    relation to clinical practice, 283
    role in legislative debates, 173
    role in litigation, 114–7, 128, 303
science courts, 123–4, 309
scientific fraud, 309
scientific literature, 7
    approach of courts to, 88
    claim of reliance on outdated, 115
    reliance of insurers on, 47
scientific process, 124
scientists
    court testimony of, 171
    independent panels of, 124
Scripps Clinic and Research Foundation, 56
secondary acute myeloid leukemia, 228
secondary malignancies, 21, 228, 291
settlements, 114, 303
    reasons against, 105–6
severe immunodeficiency, treatment with bone marrow
    transplantation, 25
sexism, 17
SHARE, 60
Shayer, Belle, 153
Shea, Thomas, 32
"Should I Enter a Clinical Trial?," 195
Simkins v. NevadaCare, 92
60 Minutes, story on HDC/ABMT, 149–50, 269
Slamon, Dennis, 13
small cell carcinoma, 22
Smith, Curtis, 158
    congressional testimony, 159, 161
Smith, Garret, 197
Smith v. CHAMPUS, 88, 95
social legitimacy, of medicine, 271
social policy, role of courts, 73
South African trial, 16, 204–5, 232, 237–8, 240–242, 272
    audit of first, 247–8
    audit of second, 242–7
    impact on use of HDC/ABMT, 251
    questions about, 199
    responses to audit findings, 245–6
    results, 198
Southwest Oncology Group. *See* SWOG
Spitzer, Gary, 32, 49

St. Petersburg Times, article on HDC/ABMT, 66, 67
St. Vincent's Hospital, New York, 150
St. Vincent's University Hospital, Dublin, 229
Stadtmauer, Edward, 216, 233, 249
staging, breast cancer, 17–9
STAMP (Solid Tumor Autologous Marrow Program), 29, 209
standard of care, 81, 309
    effect on treatment utilization, 263
    establishing, 76
    resource constraints and, 302
    role in litigation, 100, 107–10, 116, 121–2
standards of review, 98
Stanford University, phase 2 studies at, 32
state governments
    ability to weigh access versus evaluation issues, 175
    coverage mandates, 168–9
    role in HDC/ABMT saga, 268
state laws, litigation involving, 95–6
statistical power, 302
stem cells, effect of chemotherapy on, 21
study size, 51
Subcommittee on Compensation and Employee Benefits, 158–64
subjectivity, in endpoint judgments, 210
surgeons, role in cancer treatment, 28
surrogate endpoints, 44, 45
    versus health outcomes, 46
Susan G. Komen Breast Cancer Foundation, 60, 234
Sweeney v. Gerber Products Co. Medical Benefits Plan, 86
SWOG, 208, 213
    clinical trial, 209, 222, 226, 250
sympathy, role in litigation, 81, 101–2, 105, 117–8, 128, 267, 313
synthesis of information, 283

Tallman, Martin, 210, 224, 249
tandem transplants, 312
Taylor v. Blue Cross/Blue Shield of Michigan, 95
technology assessments, 6, 125, 181, 182
    impetus for, 37
    by insurance industry, 37, 204, 273–4
    lack of effect on clinical practice, 274
    role in legislative debates, 174
    weaknesses of centralized, 182
Technology Evaluation and Coverage program, 37
Technology Evaluation Center, 38
    criteria, 183
    explanation of coverage changes, 200–2
    review of ABMT, 49
Temple University, 214
Tennenbaum, David, 45
Tepe v. Rocky Mountain Hospital and Medical Services, 95
terminal illness
    policy of Aetna, 188–9
    use of HDC/AMBT and, 16
terminology, lack of standard, 214
testicular cancer, 17
Texas Oncology, 140

Thomas, E. Donnal, 28, 301
Thomas, Janice, 86
Time magazine, managed care coverage, 12
time to relapse, 210
time to tumor progression, 291
tissue transplants, ruling of ambiguity concerning term, 98
tort law, 75
tort reform, 303
toxicity, 51
    auditory, 21, 291
    hair loss, 21
    of high-dose chemotherapy, 21, 32, 291
    liver, 21, 32
    lung, 21
    mood disturbance, 21, 291
    myeloablation, 21
    neutropenia, 27, 291
    organ, 21, 291
    tissue, 21
    types of, 291
treatment bias, 262
treatment billing, 146
treatment costs, 17, 149
    litigation strategies involving, 117
treatment effectiveness, 89, 97
    evidence for, 206
    proof of, 116, 123
    role in litigation, 108
treatment-induced tumors, 228
treatment, Investigational New Drug rule, 43
treatment outcomes, ECRI evaluation, 193
treatment-related mortality, 31–2, 51, 185, 214
    data from CALGB trial, 237
    insurers' consideration of, 106
    role in litigation, 115, 120
    statistics, 133, 135–6, 291
Tufts University, 214
tumors, resistant, 21
tumor volume, 302
Turner v. Fallon Community Health Plan, 96
two schools of thought doctrine. *See* respectable minority rule

United HealthCare, view of coverage mandate, 194
U.S. Congress
    hearings on coverage of HDC/ABMT, 158–68
    meeting with Peters, 154
US HealthCare
    financing of Philadelphia trial, 210, 274
    support of randomized clinical trials, 52–3
U.S. Oncology, 140, 148, 312
University Hospital, Cleveland, phase 2 studies at, 32
University of Michigan Medical Center, 56
University of Minnesota, 57, 170
University of Nebraska, 57
    phase 2 studies at, 32
University of Nevada, 56
University of Pennsylvania, 214
University of Southern California, phase 2 studies at, 32

University of Utah Medical Center, 57
University of Witwatersrand
   handling of Bezwoda fraud, 245
   response to audit of first HDC/ABMT trial, 247

values, managing conflicting, 264
Vaughan, William, 32, 49, 223
vincristine, 22, 29
   use in South African trial, 240
Visco, Fran, 60, 61, 166, 202, 224, 232
voluntary reporting, 129
Walks for Breast Cancer, 60

Wall Street Journal
   coverage of OPM coverage mandate, 165, 194
   coverage of preliminary trial data, 232
Washington Post, article on HDC/ABMT, 65
Weiss, Raymond, 189, 251
   audits of HDC/ABMT clinical trials, 240–2
West, William, 141, 147, 160
   interview by *60 Minutes*, 149
White v. Caterpillar, 87–8, 93
Whitehead v. Federal Express Corp., 100
Whittington, Kelly, 89

Williams, Marjorie, 286
Williams, S. F., 32
Winslow, Ron, 165, 194
Wittes, Robert, 39, 49, 234
   recommendations for funding of clinical trials, 39–40
   review of HDC/ABMT studies, 207–8
Wolfe v. Prudential Insurance Co., 95
Women and Their Bodies, 58
Women's Community Cancer Center of Oakland, 60
women's health, 4. *See also* feminism
   perceptions of, 269–70
   role of movement in use of HDC/ABMT, 58–64
women's health conference, 1994, Ruzek's address, 195
Women's Health Equity Act, 59
Women's Health Initiative, 59
Yankee, Ron, 29
Y-ME National Breast Cancer Organization, 60
You Are Not Alone, 60, 252

Zander, Axel, 32
Zeneca Group, PLC, 310
Zones, Jane Sprague, 203, 255
Zweber, Corrine, 169